Social Work

What are the key ideas that underpin social work practice?

This inspiring reader brings together some of the most significant ideas which have informed social work practice over the last 40 years. Exploring these fundamental ideas, the book includes commentaries that allow the reader to understand the texts on their own terms as well as to be aware of their relations to each other and to the wider social work context.

An accessible introduction contextualises the reader, summarising the main themes and highlighting key issues. The book is then divided into three main sections, each presenting key texts which have contributed to the development of:

- The profession of social work
- Social work knowledge and values
- Social work skills and practice.

There is no settled view or easy consensus about what social work is and should be, and the ideas reflected in this volume are themselves diverse and complex. The contributions are drawn from a wide range of perspectives: psychological, sociological, philosophical, educational and political, as well as perspectives which are grounded in the experiences of practitioners and those who use services.

This important resource is essential reading for all social work students.

Viviene E. Cree is Professor of Social Work Studies at the University of Edinburgh. She is the author of *Sociology for Social Workers and Probation Officers*, editor of *Becoming a Social Worker* and co-author of *Social Work: Voices from the Inside*, all published by Routledge. She is also co-author of *Social Work: Making a Difference* and co-editor of the series, Social Work in Practice, published jointly by BASW and the Policy Press.

Student Social Work

This exciting new textbook series is ideal for all students studying to be qualified social workers, whether at undergraduate or Masters level. Covering key elements of the social work curriculum, the books are accessible, interactive and thought-provoking.

New titles

Human Growth and Development
John Sudbery

Mental Health Social Work in Context
Nick Gould

Social Work
A reader
Viviene E. Cree

Social Work and Social Policy
An introduction
Jonathan Dickens

Social Work Placements
Mark Doel

Forthcoming titles

Integrating Social Work Theory and Practice
Pam Green Lister

Building Relationships and Communicating with Young Children
A practical guide
Karen Winter

Sociology for Social Workers and Probation Officers
Viviene E. Cree

Social Work Law and Ethics
Jonathan Dickens

Social Work
A reader

Edited by Viviene E. Cree

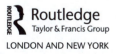

Routledge
Taylor & Francis Group

LONDON AND NEW YORK

First published 2011
by Routledge
2 Park Square, Milton Park, Abingdon, Oxon, OX14 4RN

Simultaneously published in the USA and Canada
by Routledge
270 Madison Avenue, New York, NY 10016

Routledge is an imprint of the Taylor & Francis Group, an informa business

Typeset in Times New Roman by
RefineCatch Ltd, Bungay, Suffolk
Printed and bound in Great Britain by
TJ International Ltd, Padstow, Cornwall

British Library Cataloguing in Publication Data
A catalogue record for this book is available
from the British Library

Library of Congress Cataloging in Publication Data
Social work : a reader / edited By Viviene E. Cree
   p. cm.
   1. Social service—Great Britain.   2. Social workers—Great Britain.   I. Cree, Viviene E., 1954–   .
   HV245.S62215 2011
   361.30941—dc22   2010016014

ISBN13: 978–0–415–49972–9 (hbk)
ISBN13: 978–0–415–49973–6 (pbk)

For Marianne

Contents

Acknowledgements

I would like to thank all the people who made this book possible: the team at Routledge (Grace McInnes, Commissioning Editor, who invited me to submit a proposal and Khanam Virjee who was responsible for arranging all permissions); my colleagues, Gary Clapton, Ruth Forbes, Susan Hunter, Richard Perry, Dina Sidhva and Mark Smith who chipped in with ideas for contributions and lent me books and articles for the reader; Comfort Jinadu, PhD student, who helped with photocopying and library visits; my friends, my partner, Alan, and sons, Calum and Iain, who all continued to believe that the manuscript would be ready before I set off on a sabbatical trip. I would also like to thank Marianne Hughes for her insight and inspiration.

The publishers would like to thank the following for permissions to reprint their material:

Chapter 1: Policy Press/BASW for permission to reprint M. Payne, *What is Professional Social Work?*, Revised 2nd edition, Bristol, (2006): 12–21

Chapter 2: Policy Press/BASW for permission to reprint V.E. Cree and S. Myers, *Social Work: Making a Difference*, Bristol (2008): 15–30

Chapter 3: SAGE Publications, London, Los Angeles, New Delhi and Singapore for permission to reprint James Midgley, 'Issues in international social work: Resolving critical debates in the profession', *Journal of Social Work*, 1 (1): 21–35 (2001)

Chapter 4: SAGE Publications, London, Los Angeles, New Delhi and Singapore for permission to reprint Jan Fook, 'Uncertainty: The defining characteristics of social work', in M. Lymbery and K. Postle (eds) *Social Work: A Companion to Learning* (2007): 31–9

Chapter 5: Taylor & Francis, UK for permission to reprint N. Parton (ed.) *Social Theory, Social Change and Social Work*, London: Routledge (1996): 98–113

Chapter 6: Palgrave Macmillan for permission to reprint Ian Butler and Mark Drakeford, *Social Policy, Social Welfare and Scandal: How British Public Policy is Made*, Basingstoke: Palgrave Macmillan, (2003): 207–25

Chapter 7: Ashgate Publications for permission to reprint Robin Lovelock, Karen Lyons and Jackie Powell, *Reflecting on Social Work – Discipline and Profession*, (2004): 145–162

Chapter 8: Oxford University Press for permission to reprint Jan Steyaert and Nick Gould, *British Journal of Social Work*, 39 (4): 740–53 (2009)

Chapter 9: Taylor & Francis Ltd (www.tandf.co.uk/journals) for permission to reprint Gina Tyler, *Social Work Education*, 25 (4): 385–92 (2006)

Chapter 10: Palgrave Macmillan for permission to reprint D. Howe, *Attachment Theory for Social Work Practice*, Basingstoke: Macmillan (1995): 45–57

Chapter 11: Acknowledgement is due to both of the following publishers who between them control the rights for this work:
Scribner, a Division of Simon & Schuster, Inc., for permission to reprint Elisabeth Kubler-Ross, *On Death and Dying*. Copyright © 1969 by Elisabeth Kubler-Ross; copyright renewed © 1997 by Elisabeth Kubler-Ross. All rights reserved
Taylor & Francis Books, UK for permission to reprint Elisabeth Kubler-Ross, *On Death and Dying*, (1970): 37–123. Copyright © 1969 by Elisabeth Kubler-Ross; copyright renewed © 1997 by Elisabeth Kubler-Ross.

Chapter 12: Acknowledgement is due to both of the following publishers who between them control the rights for this work:
HarperCollins Publishers for permission to reprint Thomas A. Harris, *I'm Okay – You're Okay* (1973): 16–34. Copyright © 1967, 1968, 1969, copyright renewed © 1995 by Amy Bjork Harris
The Random House Group Ltd for permission to reprint Thomas A. Harris, *I'm OK – You're OK* (1973): 16–34, published by Jonathan Cape

Chapter 13: Oxford University Press for permission to reprint C. Wright-Mills, *The Sociological Imagination*, Oxford: Oxford University Press (1959): 8–11

Chapter 14: Taylor & Francis Books UK for permission to reprint D.R. Tomlinson and W. Trew (eds) *Equalising Opportunities, Minimising Oppression: A Critical Review of Anti-discriminatory Policies in Health and Social Welfare*, London: Routledge: (2002): 41–54

Chapter 15: Taylor & Francis Books UK for permission to reprint P. Hill Collins, *Black Feminist Thought: Knowledge, Consciousness and the Politics of Empowerment*, 2nd edition, London: Routledge (2000): 251–90

Chapter 16: Acknowledgement is due to both of the following publishers who between them control the rights for this work:
Penguin Books Ltd for permission to reprint P. Freire, *Pedagogy of the Oppressed*, Harmondsworth: Penguin (1972): 45–58
The Continuum International Publishing Group for permission to reprint P. Freire, *Pedagogy of the Oppressed*, Harmondsworth: Penguin (1972): 45–58

Chapter 17: John Wiley and Sons for permission to reprint Braye Suzy, Preston-Shoot Michael, 'The role of law in welfare reform: critical perspectives on the relationship between law and social work practice', *International Journal of Social Welfare*, 15: 19–26 (2006)

Chapter 18: SAGE Publications, London, Los Angeles, New Delhi and Singapore for permission to reprint Chris Beckett and Andrew Maynard, *Values and Ethics in Social Work: An Introduction* (2005): 5–23

Chapter 19: Blackwell Publishing Ltd for permission to reprint M. Davies (ed.) *The Blackwell Companion to Social Work*, 3rd edition, Oxford: Blackwell, (2008): 442–8

Chapter 20: The British Association of Social Workers (www.basw.co.uk) for kind permission to reproduce Mekada Graham, *Social Work and African-centred Worldviews*, Birmingham: Venture Press (2001): 63–74

Chapter 21: Wadsworth, a part of Cengage Learning, Inc., Gerard Egan, for permission to reproduce *The Skilled Helper: A Problem-Management and Opportunity-Development Approach to Helping*, 9th edition, Belmont, CA: Brooks/Cole © 2010: 131–50

Chapter 22: Taylor & Francis Books UK for permission to reproduce Brian Sheldon and Geraldine MacDonald, *A Textbook of Social Work*, London: Routledge (2009): 95–111

Chapter 23: Jessica Kingsley Publishers for permission to reproduce M. Nash, R. Munford and K. O'Donogue (eds) *Social Work Theories in Action*, London: Jessica Kingsley (2005): 39–45

Chapter 24: Oxford University Press for permission to reproduce A.R. Roberts (ed.) *Crisis Intervention Handbook: Assessment, Treatment and Research*, Oxford: Oxford University Press (2005): 11–21

Chapter 25: Pearson Education, Inc. for permission to reproduce D. Saleebey, *The Strengths Perspective Social Work Practice*, 4th edition, Boston, MA: Pearson Education © 2006: 7–22

Chapter 26: Taylor & Francis Ltd (www.tandf.co.uk/journals) for permission to reproduce Simon Prideaux, Alan Roulstone, Jennifer Harris and Colin Barnes, 'Disabled People and Self-directed Support Schemes: Reconceptualising Work and Welfare in the 21stCentury', *Disability & Society*, 24 (5): 557–69 (2009)

Chapter 27: Taylor & Francis Books UK for permission to reprint A. Leathard (ed.) *Interprofessional Collaboration: From Policy to Practice in Health and Social Care*, London: Brunner-Routledge (2003): 94–113

Chapter 28: Palgrave Macmillan for permission to reprint Lena Dominelli, *Feminist Social Work Theory and Practice*, Basingstoke: Palgrave (2002): 17–40

Chapter 29: Edward Arnold for permission to reproduce M. Brake and R. Bailey (eds) *Radical Social Work and Practice*, London: Edward Arnold (1980): 7–24

Chapter 30: SAGE Publications, London, Los Angeles, New Delhi and Singapore for permission to reprint M. Gray and S. Webb (eds) *Social Work Theories and Methods*, Sage, London (2009): 119–28

Introduction

Reading social work

Viviene E. Cree

Social work as a profession has 'come of age' in recent years. It is now a registered profession in the UK with an Honours degree as its minimum qualification and statutory requirements in place for continuing professional development beyond qualification. Social work has also developed exponentially at both graduate and postgraduate levels throughout the world over the last 20 years, with increasing numbers of countries requiring (at least) degree-level entry and professional registration. The growth in accreditation, unsurprisingly, has been matched by a corresponding expansion in the social work literature. Social work students today are faced with a raft of reading lists, publications and web resources which they are expected to read and understand. In consequence, what they often do is turn to textbooks which provide an overview of the subject. These books may contain little original thinking, and instead summarise existing ideas and knowledge, some more successfully than others. What they cannot do, however, is allow students to read seminal texts first-hand. This reader, in contrast, invites students and practitioners to do just that: to read key source material (or, more accurately, extracts of this) for themselves, so that they can make up their own minds and draw their own conclusions about the usefulness or otherwise of these texts. A brief commentary will, I hope, enable readers to locate the texts in their wider contexts. But the primary objective of this reader is that key authors and texts should be able to speak for themselves.

Selecting the material for the reader

Selecting material for the reader has proved to be a considerable challenge. As an applied discipline, social work draws on a formidable and disparate body of knowledge, which includes psychology, sociology, social policy, politics, education, economics, health studies, philosophy, theology and law. As a professional activity, it makes use of a similarly wide range of practice skills, from one-to-one therapeutic interventions to family work, group work and community development. As an enterprise which seeks to engage with the human condition, all of art, history, literature and music have something to contribute to social work. So, what to include in and, more importantly, what to leave out of this collection?

I began by inviting academic and practice colleagues, service users, carers and students to make their own selections. The number of possible topics grew and grew, as visitors to my office added their ideas to the large and increasingly hectic list on the whiteboard on the wall. What this exercise reminded me was that the distinction social work often makes between knowledge, skills and values is an artificial one which breaks down as soon as we explore a given topic in more detail (more on this below).

My next tack was to think about the book 'show-casing' the writing and research which has changed social work practice most over the years: classic studies like *Social Diagnosis* (Richmond 1917), *The Client Speaks* (Mayer and Timms 1970) or *Children Who Wait* (Rowe 1973) all have something important to tell us about how social work has developed and why it is, as it is, today. But the problem with this approach was that students might receive a very partial view of social work; either that or the commentary would have to be lengthy in order to explain what went on before and after each study. The reader might also have seemed somewhat dated; a collection about what social work was in the past, rather than a helpful book for twenty-first century practice.

I then had a brainwave. Could the UK's National Occupational Standards for Social Work offer an effective way of structuring the source material? Anyone who has worked with students to make sense of the six standards, 22 learning foci and seemingly never-ending list of knowledge, skills and competences will agree that this road can only lead to disappointment, if not, despair. The standards, as I will outline below, contain a confusing and sometimes repetitive mix of themes, and could not be expected to give the enlightenment that I was searching for.

This brought me, finally, to consider what has inspired me most on my journey in and through social work. Some authors are my all-time favourites: the sociologists Michel Foucault, Zygmunt Bauman and Richard Sennett are at the top of my personal wish-list, but I have to acknowledge that they are not primarily resources for social work. Furthermore, if this reader is to be truly useful for social work students, it must reflect social work across the board, in all its differing positions and contexts.

What appears in this book, then, is a combination of the authors and books that are on most people's 'top ten' lists, alongside some of the texts which have influenced my ideas and practice most over my time in social work. Students and practitioners will find a deliberately broad range of ideas and practices included. They will also, it is hoped, find inspiration and, at times, courage to go on, faced with the usual ups and downs of life in what is always a contested, and at times, beleaguered profession.

Structure and contents of the reader

The reader is structured into three sections. The first section of the book introduces the reader to key texts which are important in understanding social work as a profession. The second section presents a range of source material which encompasses some of the central knowledge and ideas in social work. Some of these extracts are by social work authors. Others are by authors who, I believe, can make a significant contribution to social work's knowledge and value base. The final section of the book brings together excerpts related to skills and practice, acknowledging from the outset that the division between knowledge, values and skills is inevitably a false one, since each works together to make social work practice what it is today. Some texts are short extracts, others longer, depending on the nature of the subject being presented. A brief commentary will introduce each of the three sections, providing an overview so that readers may understand better the nature of the different texts in relation to one another and in relation to the wider social work context. In addition, each text is prefaced by a short introduction, and concludes with recommendations for further reading selected by me.

Before moving onto the extracts proper, it is essential that we take a step back to address some of the wider questions which will inform all the material which follows. Is social work a profession? What is social work knowledge? What do social workers do? I will then offer a few observations about social work in the future.

Is social work a profession?

When Abraham Flexner posed the question 'Is social work a profession?' at a conference of American charities in 1915, his conclusion was 'not yet'. Although he acknowledged that social work was intellectual in character and required analysis and judgement, he felt that the social worker was, in essence, a mediator; there was no defined scope to his or her actions and no clear end-product. He ended his speech by urging those present at the conference to go out and build a profession. The social work pioneer Mary Richmond was the first to take up the challenge in her book, *Social Diagnosis*, which was published in 1917. Here she laid down the process of investigation, analysis and treatment which, she argued, defined casework.

Since that time, social workers have struggled with the question of whether social work is, and should be, a profession. Some have continued to assert social work's professional aspirations while others have been resistant to the idea that social work should seek professional status, claiming that professional bodies are self-serving organisations which protect middle-class interests at the expense of the community (see Heraud 1979; Hugman 1991; Freidson 2001). Some have acknowledged that while social work may be professional in its activities and values, its work is defined not by the profession, but by the state: it is the state which produces its service users (see Johnson 1972, 1977). This gives social work a particular character, and inevitably contributes to this sense of it being caught in the middle, 'between the individual and the state, the powerful and the excluded, negotiating, and at times in conflict with both' (Cree 2008: 289). This is clearly demonstrated in the fact that registration in the UK is government, not professional led. Moreover, its future is never certain; on the contrary, there is always someone writing about the demise of social work as we know it! Maybe that is inevitable, given social work's location. And maybe this is where creativity and transformational change can come about, if those of us who are involved in social work are prepared to work together to make this happen (Cree 2008).

What is social work knowledge?

It was the Central Council for Education and Training in Social Work (CCETSW), which institutionalised the division in social work education between knowledge, skills and values. *Paper 30*, introduced in September 1989, brought together two existing social work awards, the Certificate in Social Service (CSS) and the Certificate of Qualification in Social Work (CQSW), to create the new Diploma in Social Work (DipSW). In doing so, CCETSW introduced a set of rules and requirements which had to be met for social work qualification, and, with them, the notion of competence, made up of knowledge, skills and values. The undergraduate social work degrees in the UK, launched in 2003 and 2004, moved away from what had been experienced as a 'tick box' approach to competences (see Barnett 1994; Ford 1996; Kemshall 2000), and replaced this with the National Occupational Standards for Social Work (NOS).

One of the problems with a framework built on discrete knowledge, skills and values is that they are not distinct entities. On the contrary, knowledge is much more than simply academic, theoretical knowledge. Skills are likewise built on theoretical ideas. Meanwhile, values underpin all theories and skills. Educational researchers have argued that it is better to think about 'knowledge' as a general term which incorporates theory and skills. So, for example, Cust (1995) proposes that knowledge which is involved in action or while undertaking a task includes conceptual knowledge (knowing *that*), procedural knowledge (knowing *how*), and strategic knowledge (knowing *what to do when*). Macaulay (2000) describes this more fully. She explains that conceptual knowledge (sometimes referred to as propositional or declarative knowledge) consists of concepts, facts, propositions and theories. These may be acquired through experience or through comprehension of written and verbal materials. Procedural knowledge, in contrast, specifies actions to be taken when the right conditions are present. Strategic knowledge (sometimes referred to as conditional knowledge) is an awareness of when to use conceptual and procedural knowledge and why (2000: 9–10). Conceptual, procedural and strategic knowledge are all underpinned by what Eraut (1994) calls 'personal' knowledge, based on the individual's own idiosyncratic apprehension of experience. I hope that this reader will increase students' ability to build their own ideas, by offering a way of thinking about knowledge which conceptualises it as a broad and ever-changing concept, to be engaged with and challenged, rather than regurgitated as theory with a capital 'T'.

What do social workers do?

Neil Thompson, writing in an introduction to social work, asserts that 'Social work is what social workers do' (2000: 13). But what, then, do social workers do? A simple way of answering this question is to turn to the UK's National Occupational Standards for Social Work for guidance. National Occupational Standards have been devised for a large number of occupations and professional groups. The National Occupational Standards for Social Work offer a set of descriptions of the functions of social workers, aiming to provide a benchmark of 'best practice' in social work competence across the UK. They form the basis for the new degree introduced in 2003 in England and in 2004 in the rest of the UK. The standards were developed from a detailed analysis of what social workers do through consultation with employers and practitioners and they include service users' own statements of their expectations of social workers. The statutory Codes of Practice for Social Care (Social Service) Employers and Employees have also been incorporated into the National Occupational Standards. The standards are for all kinds of social workers, statutory or independent sector-based, working for health, education or for social services (and from justice agencies in Scotland), regardless of whom their service users are (Cree and Myers 2008).

There are slight differences in the way that the standards are presented in different parts of the UK, but the substance remains the same. In England, Wales and Northern Ireland, the standards are described as key roles, with units and elements within each key role. The key roles are as follows:

1   prepare for, and work with individuals, families, carers, groups and communities to assess their needs and circumstances;

2   plan, carry out, review and evaluate social work practice, with individuals, families, carers, groups, communities and other professionals;
3   support individuals to represent their needs, views and circumstances;
4   manage risk to individuals, families, carers, groups, communities, self and colleagues;
5   manage and be accountable, with supervision and support, for your own social work practice within your organisation;
6   demonstrate professional competence in social work practice.

The problem with the standards is, of course, the same problem we have already come up against in relation to the earlier discussion of theory, skills and values, that is, different concepts are central to more than one standard, and it is extraordinarily difficult to separate out one key role from another. There has also been considerable debate within social work about why some parts of the social work task (for example, managing risk) have been given such prominence, whereas others (for example, community development) are barely visible (see Doel and Shardlow 2005; Slater 2004). At the end of the day, these are the standards we have to work with, and the pragmatist in me accepts that the reader needs to demonstrate some of this thinking if it is to be useful for student social workers. But we need to hold in check the idea that this is only or all that social workers do, or all that they will do in the future. Any exploration of social work in different countries of the world (especially in what is commonly called the 'developing world' or 'the South') shows just how parochial and culturally and context-specific the UK standards are. These should therefore be worked with using the same critical approach which has already been identified in our discussion about social work as a profession (see also Cree and Myers 2008 for a vignette-based approach to understanding and using the UK standards).

Looking ahead

It is not certain what the future will hold for the profession of social work, but given the course of social work's history and its recent experience (see Cree 2009), it seems likely that more organisational and institutional upheaval lies ahead, in the UK at least. Social work in England and Wales is currently working out the detailed implications of its Social Work Taskforce review which took place during 2009, a review which has called for, amongst other recommendations, a probationary year for newly qualified workers and the creation of a new College of Social Work. Scotland, meanwhile, is striving to consolidate on the basis of its own review of social work, *Changing Lives* (Scottish Executive 2006). We may find, in the future, that something has been lost in the scramble to reorganise social work and social services departments; increasing specialisation may not make for better services for those with whom we are working. In that case, we may find the pendulum shifting back again towards the principle of generic services. But it seems unlikely that we will be able to recover the heady days of the 1970s when it was genuinely believed that social work had a significant role to play in promoting social welfare for all. Social work in the UK has gone so far down the road of individualised, personalised services that it is difficult to imagine how this might be turned around (see Dominelli 2004). At the same time, the impact of the economic recession on the public and voluntary sectors is only just being felt and will, undoubtedly, get worse in the short term.

Nevertheless, I believe that there are spaces for optimism. On the one hand, there continue to be a great many voices of opposition within social work: practitioners who want to work alongside service users and carers to bring about change; managers who are willing to go the extra mile; academics who continue to ask critical questions of themselves and of social work. Many of these voices are represented in this reader, and are also to be found in Cree and Davis (2007) and in the various collectives and alliances which have emerged in recent years, including the Social Work and Health Inequalities Network, Shaping Our Lives, the National Service User Network and the Social Work Action Network (SWAN). See Ferguson and Woodward (2009) for a fuller discussion of these initiatives. There are also, significantly, alternative views of social work which continue to exist and to grow in the developing world, as Hugman (2009) indicates. In a polemic article, he argues that social work in the 'global North' has much to learn from social work in the 'global South'. The international definition of social work, adopted by the International Federation of Social Work at its general meeting in Montréal, Canada, in July 2000 and co-opted as the Key Purpose of Social Work within the National Occupational Standards in Social Work, gives a small clue as to what this re-imagining of social work might entail:

> Social work is a profession which promotes social change, problem solving in human relationships and the empowerment and liberation of people to enhance well-being. Utilising theories of human behaviour and social systems, social work intervenes at the points where people interact with their environments. Principles of human rights and social justice are fundamental to social work.
>
> (www.ifsw.org/f38000138.html/accessed 22 June 2010).

References

Barnett, R. (1994) *The Limits of Competence: Knowledge, Higher Education and Society*, Buckingham: SRHE and Open University Press.

CCETSW (1989) *Paper 30: Rules and Requirements for the Diploma in Social Work*, London: CCETSW.

Cree, V.E. (2008) 'Social work and society', in M. Davies (ed.) *Blackwell Companion to Social Work*, 3rd edition, Oxford, Blackwell, 289–302.

——(2009) 'The changing nature of social work', in R. Adams, L. Dominelli and M. Payne, (eds) *Social Work: Themes Issues and Critical Debates*, 3rd edition, Basingstoke, Palgrave Macmillan, 26–36.

Cree, V.E. and Davis, A. (2007) *Social Work: Voices from the Inside*, London, Routledge.

Cree, V.E. and Myers, S. (2008) *Social Work: Making a Difference*, Bristol: Policy Press/BASW.

Cust, J. (1995) 'Recent cognitive perspectives on learning-implications for nurse education', *Nurse Education Today*, 15: 280–90.

Doel, M. and Shardlow, S.M. (2005) *Modern Social Work Practice: Teaching and Learning in Practice Settings*, Aldershot: Ashgate.

Dominelli, L. (2004) *Social Work: Theory and Practice for a Changing Profession*, Cambridge: Polity Press.

Eraut, M. (1994) *Developing Professional Knowledge and Competence*, London: Falmer Press.

Ferguson, I. and Woodward, R. (2009) *Radical Social Work in Practice: Making a Difference*, Bristol: Policy Press/BASW.

Flexner, A. (1915) 'Is social work a profession?', Proceedings of the National Conference of Charities and Corrections, 42nd Annual Session, held in Baltimore, Maryland, 12–19 May 1915, reproduced in *Research on Social Work Practice*, 11(2) March (2001): 152–65.

Ford, P. (1996) 'Competences: their use and misuse', in P. Ford and P. Hayes (eds) *Educating for Social Work: Arguments for Optimism*, Aldershot: Avebury.

Freidson, E. (2001) *Professionalism: The Third Logic*, Cambridge: Polity Press.

Heraud. B. (1979). *Sociology of the Professions*, London: Open Books.

Hugman, R. (1991) *Power in Caring Professions*, Basingstoke: Macmillan.

—— (2009) 'But is it social work? Some reflections on mistaken identities', *British Journal of Social Work*, 39: 1138–53.

Johnson, T.J. (1972) *Professions and Power*, Basingstoke: Macmillan.

—— (1977) 'The professions in the class structure', in R. Scase (ed.) *Industrial Society, Class Cleavage and Control*, London: Allen & Unwin, 93–109.

Kemshall, H. (2000) 'Competence and risk assessment', in V.E. Cree and C. Macaulay (eds) *Transfer of Learning in Professional and Vocational Education*, London: Routledge, 53–76.

Macaulay, C. (2000) 'Transfer of learning', in V.E. Cree and C. Macaulay (eds) *Transfer of Learning in Professional and Vocational Education*, London: Routledge, 1–26.

Mayer, J.E. and Timms, N. (1970) *The Client Speaks: Working Class Impressions of Casework*, London: Routledge & Kegan Paul.

Richmond, M.E. (1917) *Social Diagnosis*, New York: Russell Sage Foundation.

Rowe, J. (1973) *Children Who Wait: A Study of Children Needing Substitute Families*, London: Association of British Adoption Agencies.

Scottish Executive (2006) *Changing Lives: Report of the 21st Century Social Work Review*, Edinburgh: Scottish Executive. Available at: www.scotland.gov.uk/Resource/Doc/91931/0021949.pdf (accessed on 14 June 2010).

Slater, P. (2004) 'Reforming professional training and protecting vulnerable adults from abuse: A thematic analysis of the new social work degree's prescribed curriculum', *British Journal of Social Work*, 34: 649–61.

Thompson, N. (2000) *Understanding Social Work, Preparing for Practice*, Basingstoke: Macmillan.

Part I

The profession of social work

Commentary 1

I have written extensively about the profession of social work in previous publications, most recently in Cree (2008 and 2009), Cree and Davis (2007) and Cree and Myers (2008). (See also Dominelli 2004; Fook *et al.* 2000; Lovelock *et al.* 2004.) I pointed out that social work is not an easy thing to sum up or describe. On the contrary, history shows that social work has always been 'up for grabs'; its task and its future direction by no means self-evident (Cree 1995: 153). The term 'social work' in the UK today encompasses a wide range of activities and functions which take place across the statutory, voluntary and private sectors, and, increasingly, within settings such as health and education where social work is not the dominant or only professional grouping. Social work in the developing world remains a much broader and more community oriented activity (see Hugman 2009; Midgley 1997). It is vital given this complex reality that social workers have a critical awareness of the nature of social work, and an understanding of some of the issues and dilemmas at the heart of social work's professional endeavours.

This section of the book provides the 'big picture' of social work, presenting the location within which it operates, historically and in the present day. The extracts highlight important themes which have emerged in the development of the profession of social work and introduce some of the central issues and debates within social work today. All the extracts are written by people working within social work practice and education.

Key questions:

1   Is social work a profession?
2   What sense does it make to talk about international social work?
3   Who defines the task of social work, nationally and internationally?

References

Cree, V.E. (1995) *From Public Streets to Private Lives: The Changing Task of Social Work*, Aldershot: Avebury.
——(2008) 'Social work and society', in M. Davies (ed.) *Blackwell Companion to Social Work*, 3rd edition, Oxford: Blackwell, 289–302.
——(2009) 'The changing nature of social work', in R. Adams, L. Dominelli and

M. Payne (eds) *Social Work: Themes Issues and Critical Debates*, 3rd edition, Basingstoke: Palgrave Macmillan, 26–36.

Cree, V.E. and Davis, A. (2007) *Social Work: Voices from the Inside*, London: Routledge.

Cree, V.E. and Myers, S. (2008) *Social Work: Making a Difference*, Bristol: Policy Press/BASW.

Dominelli, L. (2004) *Social Work: Theory and Practice for a Changing Profession*, Cambridge: Polity Press.

Fook, J., Ryan, M. and Hawkins, L. (2000) *Professional Expertise: Practice Theory and Education for Working in Uncertainty*, London: Whiting & Birch.

Hugman, R. (2009) 'But is it social work? Some reflections on mistaken identities', *British Journal of Social Work*, 39: 1138–53.

Lovelock, R., Lyons, K. and Powell, J. (eds) (2004) *Reflecting on Social Work: Discipline and Profession*, Aldershot: Ashgate.

Midgley, J. (1997) 'Social work and international social development: Promoting a developmental perspective in the profession', in M.C. Hokenstad and J. Midgley (eds) *Issues in International Social Work*, Washington, DC: NASW Press, 11–26.

1   What is professional social work?

Malcolm Payne

Malcolm Payne is one of the most prominent social work academics in the UK. He has been writing about social work for over 30 years, much of this work concerned with the history and profession of social work, as well as theory and practice skills, social work knowledge, organisations and structures, social work futures, and, in recent years, social work's role in palliative care. I have chosen an extract from his book on professional social work which was first published in 1996 by Venture Press, a publishing arm of BASW. The book was revised and republished in 2006.

From *What is Professional Social Work?*, Revised 2nd edition, Bristol: Policy Press/BASW (2006): 12–21.

Social work's three-way discourse

The argument in this book is that social work is a three-way discourse; every bit of practice, all practice ideas, all social work agency organisation and all welfare policy is a rubbing up of three views of social work against each other. I argue that this discourse plays out the struggle about the claim: these three views are different ways of dealing with the claim. Figure 1.1 shows them at the corners of a triangle; the triangle represents the discourse between them, a field of debate that covers all social work. When I first described these three views, in the first edition of this book, I used complex names for them, but more recently, people have used simpler terms, so in this edition, I concentrate on the simpler terms, and give the complex names in this figure for reference. The important differences between these views of social work connect with different political views about how welfare should be provided.

Therapeutic views.   These see social work as seeking the best possible well-being for individuals, groups and communities in society, by promoting and facilitating growth and self-fulfilment. A constant spiral of interaction between workers and clients modifies clients' ideas and allows workers to influence them; in the same way, clients affect workers' understandings of their world as they gain experience of it. This process of mutual influence is called reflexiveness. Because it is reflexive in this way, social work responds to the social concerns that workers find and gain understanding of as they practise, and feeds back into society knowledge about these problems and how society might tackle them. Through this process of mutual interaction with social workers,

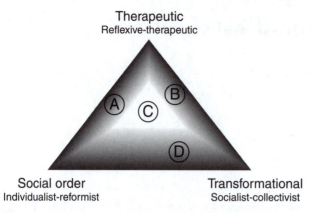

Figure 1.1 The three views of social work.

clients gain power over their own feelings and way of life. Such personal power enables them to overcome or rise above suffering and disadvantage, so they experience the work to help them gain this power as therapeutic. I originally called this kind of social work 'reflexive-therapeutic'. This view expresses in social work the social democratic political philosophy that economic and social development should go hand-in-hand to achieve individual and social improvement.

This view is basic to many ideas of the nature of social work, but two other views modify and dispute it.

Transformational views.   These views (for example, Pease and Fook, 1999) argue that we must transform societies for the benefit of the poorest and most oppressed. Social work aims to develop cooperation and mutual support in society so that the most oppressed and disadvantaged people can gain power over their own lives. It facilitates this by empowering people to take part in a process of learning and cooperation, which creates institutions that all can own and participate in. Elites accumulate and perpetuate power and resources in society for their own benefit. By doing so, they create the oppression and disadvantage that social work tries to supplant with more egalitarian relationships in society. Transformational views imply that disadvantaged and oppressed people will never gain personal or social empowerment unless society makes these transformations. Value statements about social work, such as codes of ethics, represent this objective by proposing social justice as an important value of all social work. This view expresses the socialist political philosophy that planned economies and social provision promotes equality and social justice, and I originally called it 'socialist-collectivist'.

Social order views.   These see social work as an aspect of welfare services to individuals in societies. It meets individuals' needs and improves services of which it is a part, so that social work and the services can operate more effectively. Dominelli (2002) calls these maintenance approaches, reflecting the term used by Davies (1994); I originally called them 'individualist-reformist'. They see social work as maintaining the social order and social fabric of society, and maintaining people during any period of difficulties that they may be experiencing, so that they can recover stability again.

This view expresses the liberal or rational economic political philosophy, that personal freedom in economic markets, supported by the rule of law, is the best way of organising societies.

Each view says something about the activities and purposes of social work in welfare provision in any society, and so they are each different implementations of social work's claim. Therapeutic social work says: 'Help everyone to self-fulfilment and society will be a better place'. Social order social work says: 'Solve people's problems in society, by providing help or services, and they will fit in with general social expectations better; promoting social change to stop the problems arising will produce all-round improvements'. Transformational social work says: 'Identify and work out how social relations cause people's problems, and make social changes so that the problems do not arise'.

Each view criticises or seeks to modify the others. For example, seeking personal and social fulfilment, as in therapeutic views, is impossible to transformers because the interests of elites obstruct many possibilities for oppressed peoples, unless we achieve significant social change. They argue that merely accepting the social order, as therapeutic and social order views do, supports and enhances the interests of elites. To the transformer, therefore, the alternative views involve practice that will obstruct the opportunities of oppressed people who should be the main beneficiaries of social work. To take another example, social order views say that trying to change societies to make them more equal or create personal and social fulfilment through individual and community growth are unrealistic in everyday practice, and inconsistent with the natural organisation of societies in competitive markets. This is because most practical objectives of social work activity refer to small-scale individual change, which cannot lead to major social and personal changes. Also, stakeholders in the social services that finance and give social approval to social work activities mainly want a better fit between society and individuals. They do not seek major changes. That is why social order views prefer their approach.

However, these different views also have affinities. For example, both therapeutic and transformational views are centrally about change and development. Also, therapeutic and social order views are about individual rather than social change. Generally, therefore, most conceptions of social work include elements of each of these views. Alternatively, they sometimes acknowledge the validity of elements of the others. For example, transformational views criticise unthinking acceptance of the present social order, which is often taken for granted in social order and therapeutic views. Nevertheless, most people who take this view of social work accept helping individuals to fulfil their potential within present social systems. They often see this as a stepping-stone to a changed society by promoting a series of small changes aiming towards bigger ones.

So these different views fit together or compete with each other in social work practice. Looking at Figure 1.1, if you or your agency were positioned at A (very common especially for beginning social workers), your main focus might be providing services in a therapeutic, helping relationship, as a care manager (in managed care) or in child protection. You might do very little in the way of seeking to change the world, and by being part of an official or service system, you are accepting the pattern of welfare services as it is. However, in your individual work, what you do may well be guided by eventual change objectives. For example, if you believe that relationships between men and women should be more equal, your work in families will probably reflect your views. Position B might represent someone working in a refuge for women suffering domestic violence. Much of their work is helping therapeutically, but the very basis of their agency is changing attitudes towards women in society, and you might do some campaigning work as part of your helping role. Position C is equally balanced; some change, some service provision; some therapeutic helping. My present job is like that: to promote community development so that communities become more resilient about and respond better to people who are dying or bereaved, but I also provide help for individuals and I am responsible for liaison with other services so that our service system becomes more effective. Position D is mainly transformational but partly maintenance. This reflects the reality that seeking social change is not, in the social services, completely revolutionary, but will also seek to make the service system more effective. Many community workers, for example, are seeking quite major change in the lives of the people they serve by achieving better cooperation and sharing, but they may act by helping local groups make their area safe from crime, by providing welfare rights advocacy or by organising self-help playgroups in the school holidays.

Conclusion: the claim and the perspectives

Social work's claim, unique among similar professions, is to combine in a professional role both social transformation and also individual improvement through interpersonal relationships. Because the social world is constantly in flux and individual humanity is infinitely variable, the only valid approach to understanding social work is to examine its social construction. However, a completely relative social construction, premised on constant variation in response to social and human contexts, does not reflect the world that most people experience. There are many continuities in social work, which is constructed in a shared language of concepts about its nature, contained in a discourse among three views of it: therapeutic, social order and transformational views. Social workers construct their own social work practice by following pathways towards, through, and sometimes away from, a nexus of ideas and debate that is the centre of social work. Thus, any particular social work act, any case, any social work role, any agency, any welfare system reflects a constantly changing balance among these three views about how to meet the claim. However, the three views are consistently present.

References

Davies, M. (1994) *The Essential Social Worker: A Guide to Positive Practice*, 3rd edition, Aldershot: Arena.

Dominelli, L. (2002) *Anti-oppressive Social Work Theory and Practice*, Basingstoke: Palgrave.

Pease, B. and Fook, J. (eds) (1999) *Transforming Social Work Practice: Postmodern Critical Perspectives*, London: Routledge.

Further reading

Cree, V.E. and Myers, S. (2008) *Social Work: Making a Difference*, Bristol: Policy Press/BASW.

Dominelli, L. (2004) *Social Work: Theory and Practice for a Changing Profession*, Cambridge: Polity Press.

Fook, J., Ryan, M. and Hawkins, L. (2000) *Professional Expertise: Practice, Theory and Education for Working in Uncertainty*, London: Whiting & Birch.

Higham, P. (2006) *Social Work: Introducing Professional Practice*, London: Sage.

Johnson, T.J. (1972) *Professions and Power*, Basingstoke: Macmillan.

—— (1977) 'The professions in the class structure', in R. Scase (ed.) *Industrial Society, Class Cleavage and Control*, London: Allen & Unwin, 93–109.

Lovelock, R., Lyons, K. and Powell, J. (eds) (2004) *Reflecting on Social Work: Discipline and Profession*, Aldershot: Ashgate.

Malin, N. (ed.) (2000) *Professionalism, Boundaries and the Workplace*, London: Routledge.

Parry, N. and Parry, J. (1976) *The Rise of the Medical Profession*, London: Croom Helm.

Witz, A. (1990) 'Patriarchy and the professions: The gendered politics of occupational closure', *Sociology*, 24(4): 675–90.

2 Making a difference

Lessons from history

Viviene E. Cree and Steve Myers

It may seem to the beginning social worker that social work history has little to offer in terms of understanding today's practice. However, in the following extracts we will see strong continuities between the past and the present: some of the core features at the heart of social work remain for good and ill, although the context in which social work is practised has changed greatly. We will also see that a historical analysis encourages us to be open to different points of view; to be not too quick to judge others from the standpoint of our own, inevitably partial, culture, society and personal biography. The extracts are drawn from a chapter by Viviene Cree and Steve Myers, both UK-based social work academics, which explores three case studies from history. There is not space here to include all three, so a selection has been made from two of the case studies.

From *Social Work: Making a Difference*, Bristol: Policy Press/BASW (2008): 15–30.

Newtown, 1820

Imagine a city on a cold winter's day in 1820. This could be any city in the UK – let's call it Newtown. What do you see, hear, and above all, smell?

You see a city which has undergone incredible expansion in the last 100 years. What was a small market town of 5,000 people has grown to be a sprawling city of over 80,000 men, women and children, all living on top of one another and competing for space in the narrow city centre streets. Buildings have been thrown up quickly, with little attention to planning or safety; evidence of industry is everywhere, from the breweries in the city centre to the mills and mines on the edge of town. You hear the din of the city streets: vendors yelling their wares, cattle being driven to market, music playing in the distance, children crying. You also hear the noise of industry: the clanking of machines, the blaring of factory sirens, the banging and shouts from the docks. You smell the overpowering stench of sewage flowing down the city streets, the rivers and streams polluted with waste, unwashed bodies, perfumes and spices from distant lands, smoke belching from chimneys. This is a city which has none of the social welfare systems which we take for granted in the twenty-first century. There is no health service free at the point of delivery for citizens, no universal education for children and no legislation regarding building control and sanitation. There is no system of social security and no public housing.

Stories from social work history

Social work emerged as a response to the social problems created by industrialisation and urbanisation. The late eighteenth and nineteenth centuries saw the creation of a vast number of statutory (public) schemes for sanitation, education, hospitals and clinics, policing and prisons, juvenile correction, workhouses and mental asylums. New laws governing working conditions and the treatment of children were introduced, at the same time as new mechanisms for recording population change (Cree 2002). On the voluntary front, there was an explosion in philanthropic activity, from visiting societies to charities dedicated to treating every conceivable social ill.

Workhouses

To understand where workhouses came from, we need to look much further back in history to the breakdown of mediaeval systems of care and patronage. In mediaeval times, care for those who were unable to look after themselves (that is, people who were too old to work, disabled people, orphans, the sick etc.) was seen as largely a problem for the individual and their families. Beyond this, landlords gave some support (financial and practical) to their tenants in times of short-term need. Voluntary collections were distributed by churches to those in need, whilst monasteries provided residential and hospital care (almshouses) for some sick and elderly people.

In 1601, the Elizabethan Poor Law Act (England & Wales) restated the principle of the paramountcy of family duty in welfare:

> It should be the duty of the father, grandfather, mother, grandmother, husband or child of a poor, old, blind, lame or impotent person, or other poor person, not able to work, if possessed of sufficient means, to relieve and maintain that person.

The 1601 Act authorised parishes to raise income through a tax on property to pay for help for those who had no family support. It also determined what help should be provided:

- the 'impotent poor' (the aged, chronic sick, blind and mentally ill who needed residential care) were to be accommodated in voluntary almshouses;
- the 'able-bodied poor' were to be set to work in a workhouse (they were felt to be able to work but were lazy);
- the 'able-bodied poor' who absconded or 'persistent idlers' who refused work were to be punished in a 'house of correction' (Fraser 2003).

An essential distinction is being made here, between those who were poor through no fault of their own (they were to receive care from voluntary agencies), and those who were to blame for their poverty (they were to receive statutory care). On a parallel track, Scottish parishes were permitted by a Poor Law Act of 1579 to raise taxes through rates to pay for poor relief. However, few did so, and in most areas, assistance remained in the hands of the church (through the Kirk Session) or the estate. Scotland differed from the rest of the UK in another key respect. Whilst England, Wales and Ireland built workhouses to set the able-bodied poor to work, Scotland preferred to build poor-houses for those who were unable to work, believing that there should be no statutory relief for the unemployed; the workhouses which were built (usually in the larger towns and cities) were run, not by parish authorities, but by charitable trusts (Levitt 1988). In the years which followed, workhouses and poorhouses sprang up in an uneven way across the UK. At the same time, localised income maintenance schemes (like the Speenhamland system) emerged from time to time to 'top up' low wages and so relieve extreme hardship.

The Poor Law Amendment Act of 1834 (England and Wales) (also known as 'the new poor law') demonstrates that by the nineteenth century, poverty and unemployment were still major problems for society. Not only this, industrialisation and urbanisation were actually increasing demands for poor relief, as more people left the countryside in search of work, and those left behind had no-one to turn to for help. The Poor Law Amendment Act stated that there should be no poor relief for the able-bodied unemployed outside the workhouse. It divided the poor into two groups:

- the 'deserving poor' (e.g. elderly, sick or disabled people, orphans and widows) who were to receive financial and practical support (often home-based) from charitable or voluntary organisations;
- the 'undeserving poor' (e.g. able-bodied unemployed men, single mothers, prostitutes) who were forced to turn to the state, and thus to the workhouse (Mooney 1998).

This legislation, for the first time, created a new administration process to oversee its implementation, organised around poor law unions with a central board. Following this, a major building programme turned rhetoric into reality, as workhouses were built in towns and cities across England, Wales and, after an 1838 Act, in Ireland. Scotland passed its own Poor Law Act in 1845, in large part because after the Disruption in the Church of Scotland in 1843 (when 40 per cent of ministers left to form the new Free Church of Scotland), there were simply not enough Kirk Session members to manage poor relief across Scotland. Poor relief gradually became passed to parish authorities, but still with the proviso that the able-bodied poor should not be given assistance.

Legacy

The legacy of workhouses, and of the Poor Law, can be seen throughout social work and social policy in the UK today. Three key principles remain:

- that the family should be the main provider of care;
- that poor people should be deterred from seeking help;
- that public assistance should be set at a level below that of a minimum wage.

But there are other, perhaps less explicit, messages which are just as influential in social work practice today, though we might wish to distance ourselves from them. For example, there is a fundamental notion that there are 'deserving' and 'undeserving' people, and that it is social work's task, on behalf of society, to make these distinctions (we call them 'assessments'). There is also the idea that help should only be available to those who are local. Refugees and asylum seekers today experience the same kind of discrimination and oppression as those who travelled much shorter distances in search of work in the past. There is also, finally, the belief that voluntary and statutory measures of care should function side by side, with statutory authorities carrying the major responsibility for containing and controlling – punishing? – those who are not deemed to be worthy of voluntary care.

Friendly visiting societies

The story of friendly visiting societies seems to offer a much more positive slant on social work history than that of workhouses; the very name 'friendly visiting' suggests something which we are likely to find more comfortable, more acceptable to our view of ourselves as a good, caring profession. In considering this in more detail, we will examine the story of one friendly visiting society, the Edinburgh based Indigent Old Women's Society, placing it in its wider context.

In 1797, a small group of middle-class ladies met in an Edinburgh drawing room to discuss what to do about the problem of their older domestic servants who were too old and too infirm to work. The ladies decided to form a visiting society, the 'Senior Female Society for Indigent Old Women' (later changed to the simpler Indigent Old Women's Society). In establishing the society, they each contributed a sum of money which would then be distributed in the form of a monthly pension to older women in need; they also held fundraising events (such as door-to-door collections and public sermons) to set the society on a firm financial footing.

The Indigent Old Women's Society provides a fairly typical example of a friendly visiting society; societies like this flourished throughout the eighteenth and nineteenth centuries in towns and cities across the UK. There would probably have been up to 50 visiting societies operating in Newtown by 1820, some connected with the many different branches of churches, and others not.

The growth in societies was not, however, without its critics. From the late 1860s onwards, branches of the new Charity Organisation Society (COS) became established in major cities, with the primary aim of coordinating (and controlling) voluntary effort. The system which the COS attempted to put in place was that any person in need should apply first to the COS. Their case would be assessed by a trained caseworker, who would recommend either help from a specified local voluntary society (if they were deemed to be 'deserving' of help, such as an older or sick person without family support) or referral to the poor law (if they were seen to be an 'undeserving' case, that is long-term unemployed, alcoholic or a prostitute). It was intended that no-one would receive help except by going through this formal procedure.

In practice, the COS never managed to exert the control it needed or wished over the voluntary societies or their service users. Needy people continued to apply direct to societies for help, and the COS was never able to attract enough visitors to carry out the necessary home visits and checks on claimants. Most crucially, the COS was never able to sustain the distinction between 'deserving' and 'undeserving' poor; there were simply too many people in need, and too many overlaps between the two groups (Mooney 1998). As a national organisation, the COS collapsed within 20 years, although local societies did continue to act as clearing houses for voluntary initiatives.

Legacy

The legacy of friendly visiting societies, like the legacy of workhouses, is complex and contradictory. It is clear that at their core, the two systems depended on one another:

just as the workhouse was there to control and punish the 'undeserving' poor, so the friendly visiting society (in common with housing associations and the settlement movement) existed to support the 'deserving' poor. They were, in the end, two sides of one coin.

But there is another important consideration here. The two systems were not, as might at first be thought, separable into systems of 'control' (the workhouses) and systems of 'care' (the friendly visiting societies). Instead, care and control operated together in both settings. While the workhouse provided food, shelter and medical care to those with nothing, so the friendly visiting society operated strict rules about behaviour which was, and was not, permitted by the older people in receipt of its care. So, for example, if an older woman was found with alcohol (or to have a man living with her) she would be removed from the society's list. This suggests that any categorisation of a voluntary agency as 'care' (and so, implicitly, 'good') and a statutory agency as 'control (hence 'bad') is not sustainable. Social work is always about care *and* control; we care for others through control, and an analysis of social work history shows that this has been the case at all times.

Conclusion

This chapter began with the picture of Newtown: a growing industrial city in the early stages of the development of industrial capitalism. Newtown is a very different place today. The industries on which it flourished have all but gone; the dockyards have been transformed into single person flats for the young and upwardly mobile; the city centre is a place for shopping and entertainment, not for living. Children are now at school until 18 years of age, and a welfare state guarantees a minimum level of care and protection for most citizens. But what has remained?

Newtown, in common with poor law times, is still a society which seeks to exclude and discriminate against those who do not belong – refugees and asylum seekers. They are no longer locked up in workhouses, but are held in detention centres and sometimes in prisons. Children are still separated from their parents; families are still forcibly evicted and transported to lands from which they have fled. Furthermore, there is evidence of changing patterns of poverty over the last 40 years or so, with increasing polarisation between rich and poor.

The family remains the main provider of care: whether in the community, or in residential institutions, there is still a fundamental acceptance that care should be provided by family members. Successive research studies have shown that this 'burden of caring' often falls on women – on wives, daughters and mothers, in spite of changes in women's employment. Yet studies have also shown that caring operates in the space of a relationship; it is usually reciprocal, and those who give and receive care do so willingly. They just wish that the state could provide more back-up, more respite, so that they could continue to care for longer.

Social work is still characterised by care and control. As all three examples have shown, social work continues to seek to mould the behaviour and standards of the poor and disenfranchised while helping and supporting them; social work, along with all the other 'psy' professions (Foucault 1977), is fundamentally in the business of managing populations and policing families. We do so, hopefully, in a respectful, empowering way, but this is nevertheless what we are paid to do on behalf of society. Whether we are working in the statutory or the voluntary sector, the reality is the same.

References

Cree, V.E. (2002) 'Social work and society', in M. Davies (ed.) *Blackwell Companion to Social Work*, 2nd edition, Oxford: Blackwell, 275–87.

Foucault, M. (1977) *Discipline and Punish*, London: Allen Lane.

Fraser, D. (2003) *The Evolution of the British Welfare State: A History of Social Policy since the Industrial Revolution*, 3rd edition, Basingstoke: Palgrave Macmillan.

Levitt, I. (1988) *Poverty and Welfare in Scotland 1890–1948*, Edinburgh: Edinburgh University Press.

Mooney, G. (1998) '"Remoralizing" the poor?: Gender, class and philanthropy in Victorian Britain', in G. Lewis (ed.) *Forming Nation, Framing Welfare*, London: Routledge, 55–104.

Further reading

Cree, V.E. (1995) *From Public Streets to Private Lives: The Changing Task of Social Work*, Aldershot: Avebury.

Jones, C. (2002) 'Social work and society', in R. Adams, L. Dominelli and M. Payne (eds) *Social Work: Themes, Issues and Critical Debates*, 2nd edition, London: Palgrave Macmillan.

Payne, M. (2005) *The Origins of Social Work: Continuity and Change*, Basingstoke: Palgrave Macmillan.

Sheldon, B. and Macdonald, G. (2009) 'A brief history of social work', in B. Sheldon and G. Macdonald, *A Textbook of Social Work*, London: Routledge, 3–34.

3   Issues in international social work

James Midgley

James Midgley, who is based at the University of California, Berkeley, has published widely on issues of international social work, social policy and social development. This extract is drawn from the first issue of the publication, *Journal of Social Work,* and explores some of the central themes which Midgley and others have been engaged in writing about for the last 20 years.

From *Journal of Social Work*, 1 (1): 21–35 (2001).

Terms such as 'shrinking world', 'global village' and 'international interdependence' are now used with monotonous regularity. Although commonplace, they signify the dramatic changes which are taking place in the way people experience the social world. For centuries, the immediate locality shaped and bounded reality. With the rise of nationalism in the nineteenth century, the nation state emerged to frame human experience and today people's identities are moulded by national affiliation. However, a global consciousness is also emerging and many more people now have a greater appreciation of their place within a complex, worldwide system of human activity. The emergence of a greater global awareness has, of course, been facilitated by objective changes in the way the social world impinges on human experience. The revolution in communications, the ability to travel readily to remote parts of the world, the increasing cultural diversity of national populations, enhanced global trade and economic activities as well as greater international political cooperation, have all fostered the globalization of the human experience.

While the profession of social work is also affected by the trend towards globalization, social workers have been engaged in international exchanges for many decades. Indeed, formative attempts to formulate a social work practice methodology involved extensive international contacts between the profession's founders in the United Kingdom, the United States and other industrializing countries in the late nineteenth century. Innovations such as charity visiting and settlement work in the United Kingdom diffused to the United States and, in turn, theoretical developments in American social work were adopted in Europe and elsewhere. Since then, as Hokenstad and Kendall (1995) report, international exchanges between social workers have increased significantly. Today, social workers are more interested in developments in other countries, they travel more often to international meetings and conferences, and they are more frequently engaged in international collaboration.

In spite of enhanced international engagement, social workers are sharply divided on a number of important international issues. There appears to be little agreement on what positions the profession should take on these issues. There is disagreement about the nature of international social work and the profession's commitment to internationalizing the curriculum and social work practice. The normative implications of globalization are also in dispute. Although many social workers stress the positive benefits that enhanced economic, political and cultural integration can bring, others are highly critical of these developments. There are differences of opinion on whether the profession should be primarily committed to remedial, activist or developmental forms of practice. This issue is particularly pertinent to the question of social work's proper role in the developing countries of the global South, but it is also relevant to the industrial nations. Finally, social workers are divided on the question of the universality of social work values and whether internationalism is a desirable normative position for the profession to adopt as it seeks to respond to the forces of globalization.

These and other issues pose a challenge to international social work. It is unlikely that they can be easily resolved, but this article seeks to clarify the debates attending each issue in the hope that clarification will result in a better appreciation of how differences of opinion might be reconciled or, at least, be better understood and respected. Although social work, like many other applied fields, has tended to polarize issues, it is possible to find ways to accommodate differences and propose resolutions that most social workers can accept.

The problem of definition

There is no standardized definition of the term 'international social work' or agreement about what international social work entails. Even the experts have different views about the meaning of the term. Healy (1995) reports that a plethora of definitions have emerged, and her own review of the terminologies employed by social workers shows that a large number of different terms are currently used.

Some writers define international social work as a field of practice, stressing the importance of specific skills and knowledge to enable social workers to work in international agencies. This definition is the oldest, having been formalized in the 1940s and 1950s. Friedlander (1955, 1975) uses the term to refer specifically to the social welfare activities of international agencies such as the Red Cross and the United Nations. Healy (1995) reports that this approach was widely accepted in the past and that it governed the first definition of international social work adopted by the Council on Social Work Education in the United States in 1957. A variation of this approach defines international social work as social work practice with immigrants or refugees. Sanders and Pedersen (1984) favour this definition, suggesting that social work education should include more international content to allow domestic social workers to properly comprehend the cultural backgrounds of immigrants and refugees and be more sensitive to their needs.

Yet another approach places less emphasis on practice and defines international social work as the contacts and exchanges that take place between social workers from different countries. Midgley (1990) questions the view that international social work is a distinctive field of practice and argues that it connotes instead a variety of international exchanges. Healy (1995: 422) agrees, suggesting that international social work is a 'broad umbrella term referring to any aspect of social work involving two or more nations'. Hokenstad *et al.* (1992: 4) develop this idea and say that international social work is concerned with 'the profession and practice in different parts of the world . . . the different roles social workers perform, the practice methods they use, the problems they deal with and the challenges they face'. This idea comes close to proposing the creation of an academic field of comparative social work that would systematically study social work in different countries (Nagy and Falk, 2000).

Yet others take an even broader view and define international social work as a global awareness that enhances the ability of social workers to transcend their preoccupation with the local and contextualize their role within a broad, global setting. This approach finds expression in the proposal by Asamoah *et al.* (1997) to end the international-domestic dichotomy in social work and to create a global mindset among social workers that transcends local concerns. This idea is similar to Robertson's (1992) belief that a global consciousness is gradually emerging among ordinary people today. Other writers have echoed this idea, with the notion that social work must enhance international linkages, provide a professional education that inculcates a greater global awareness among students, and address problems on a worldwide scale (Hokenstad and Midgley, 1997: 7).

Many writers believe that the issue of definition needs to be resolved. Unless the nature and scope of international social work can be defined in concrete terms, it is hardly likely that social workers will hasten to become more involved in the field. Similarly, if schools of social work are to increase international curriculum content, they need to know what this content should comprise. At present, as Healy (1995) points out, social work educators have a poorly defined conceptual and practical subject terrain on which to build an adequate curriculum. Nagy and Falk (2000) point out that the failure to resolve the issue of definition is a formidable barrier to internationalizing the curriculum.

One way to address this is to formulate a broad definition of international social work that incorporates different approaches. Instead of juxtaposing different definitions, it is possible to recognize that they all have merit. Beginning with a broad, encompassing perspective based on a global consciousness, it is possible to recognize different dimensions of internationalization that focus, in turn, on comparative enquiry, professional collaboration and specific forms of practice in international agencies that requires appropriate knowledge and skills. A comprehensive synthesis based on this hierarchy of interests can be constructed to accommodate and reconcile diverse approaches and create a viable understanding of what international social work entails. It remains to be seen whether social workers involved in international social work will accept a synthesis of this kind.

Remedial, activist or developmental social work?

Since its founding in the late nineteenth century, social work has used different practice methods to apply the skills, knowledge and values of its professional personnel to the task of enhancing human well-being. These methods include social casework (or clinical social work as it is now more widely known), group work and community work. Although there is general agreement that these different methods form an integral part of the profession's activities, preferences for these practice methods give rise to different conceptions of social work's wider commitments, roles and functions. While most social workers believe that the profession should be primarily concerned with treating the problems of needy people, others contend that it should be actively involved in social reform. Some stress the need for preventive forms of intervention, and others believe that social work should seek to promote development and progressive social change. Although these different views on the profession's proper role and function find expression in domestic debates, they are particularly marked in international circles, particularly with reference to the developing countries of the global South.

Most social workers today engage in direct practice, working with individuals and their families and treating the personal problems of their clients. This reflects the dominance of a remedial orientation within the profession and the widespread use of psychological behavioural and treatment theories. In the industrial countries, social work has become heavily involved in psychotherapy, resulting in criticisms that it has abandoned its formative mission to serve the poor and oppressed (Specht and Courtney, 1994; Lowe and Reid, 1999). In developing countries, social workers are also primarily engaged in remedial practice but their interventions often focus on the material needs of their clients. Although relatively few engage in psychotherapy, professional education in these countries often relies heavily on Western textbooks that emphasize the acquisition of psychotherapeutic skills. The result is a mismatch between the professional education these social workers receive and the tasks they are required to perform.

Criticisms of social work's concern with remediation have been expressed by many social work writers from the developing countries, who claim that the profession's individualized, therapeutic approach is unsuited to the pressing problems of poverty, unemployment, hunger, homelessness and ill-health that characterizes the global South. For example, Bose (1992) writes scathingly about the irrelevance of much social work in India to its pressing development needs. Professional social work in India has remained committed to remedial practice with individuals and families and has failed to contribute to wider efforts to address the problems of mass poverty and deprivation. Other social work writers from the developing world have previously made the same argument (Khinduka, 1971; Midgley 1981; Nagpaul, 1972; Shawkey, 1972).

These criticisms have enhanced awareness of the need for social work to play a more significant role in development, and in more recent years evidence of a greater commitment to developmental forms of social work practice has emerged both in the developing and the industrial countries. Community work principles have been applied not only to mobilize and organize local people but to promote their involvement in community projects that improve health, nutrition, literacy and infrastructure. Social workers have also become involved in productive activities through the creation of agricultural and manufacturing cooperatives and through the use of micro-credit and micro-enterprises (Else and Raheim, 1992; Gray, 1996; Livermore, 1996; Midgley, 1993; Midgley, 1997). These activities are compatible with international efforts by the United Nations to promote social development and they suggest that social work can make a useful contribution to addressing the pressing material needs of hundreds of millions of poor people around the world today.

But some writers believe that developmental forms of social work do not address underlying social inequalities and injustices, and that they fail to challenge the pervasive exploitation of the poor, women, gays and lesbians, people with disabilities and other oppressed groups. They argue for a more activist commitment that challenges oppression and promotes liberation. They point out that social work has in the past done little to contribute to this goal. Indeed, its commitment to remediation has deflected attention from these issues.

While it is true that social and political activism has not been a primary preoccupation in social work, the profession has since its early days advocated social reform and engaged in activist forms of practice. In the United States, many social workers associated with the settlements at the turn of the century campaigned for progressive social improvements, and in the 1930s the rank and file movement was inspired by socialist ideology. These social workers collaborated with the labour movement to advocate for progressive change. In the United Kingdom community work has long been identified with a vigorous form of local activism that challenges established political and social practices. In the 1970s many social workers in Latin American countries were inspired by the writings of Paulo Freire, and sought to apply his ideas in social work practice (Resnick, 1976). Activism also found expression in the efforts of some social workers to challenge oppressive dictatorship in countries such as Chile and South Africa (Jimenez and Alwyn, 1992; Mazibuko *et al.*, 1992; Patel, 1992).

However, it cannot be claimed that social activism has been popular in social work or that it has inspired many social workers. In fact, few social workers pay much attention to these activities and some even regard them as inappropriate. In turn, social workers who are committed to social action often regard therapeutic practice as little more than a tool for perpetuating entrenched inequalities and supporting the vested interests of elites.

It will be difficult to reconcile these different views about social work's proper role and function in society. Disagreements on this issue have been vigorously expressed for many decades and no real accommodation has yet been forged. Nevertheless, it is possible to conceive of a situation where the profession recognizes and institutionalizes its different commitments and places appropriate stress on their application in different situations. Obviously, the social needs of prosperous middle-class communities in the United States or other advanced industrial countries are not the same as those of impoverished slum-dwellers in Africa. Accordingly, social workers in these and other communities will emphasize different approaches when seeking to meet their needs. Also, remedial, preventive and developmental functions are not mutually exclusive and, as social workers in many developing countries are now demonstrating, it is possible to integrate these different functions within the same practice setting. For example, they have shown that the problems of child abuse and neglect can be managed more effectively within a wider developmental setting that promotes community involvement in pre-school education, child and maternal health, nutrition and greater economic independence for women. However, if these different functions are to be effectively integrated, social workers will need to recognize the value of the profession's diverse commitments and appreciate the extent to which they can all contribute to human welfare. This will, in turn, require a greater commitment from the profession's leadership to build consensus and end the internecine disagreements which have plagued social work since its formative years.

References

Asamoah, Y., Healy, L.M. and Mayadas, N. (1997) 'Ending the international–domestic dichotomy: New approaches to a global curriculum for the millennium', *Journal of Social Work Education*, 33 (2): 389–401.

Bose, A.B. (1992) 'Social work in India: Developmental roles for a helping profession', in M.C. Hokenstad, S.K. Khinduka and J. Midgley (eds) *Profiles in International Social Work*, Washington, DC: NASW Press, 71–84.

Else, J.F. and Raheim, S. (1992) 'AFDC clients as entrepreneurs: Self-employment offers an important option', *Public Welfare*, 50 (4): 36–41.

Friedlander, W. (1955) *Introduction to Social Welfare*, New York: Prentice Hall.

—— (1975) *International Social Welfare*, Englewood Cliffs, NJ: Prentice Hall.

Gray, M. (1996) 'Promoting social development through community social work', *Journal of Applied Social Sciences*, 21 (1): 45–52.

Healy, L.M. (1995) 'Comparative and international overview', in T.D. Watts, D. Elliott and N. Mayadas (eds) *International Handbook on Social Work Education*, Westport, CT: Greenwood Press, 421–40.

Hokenstad, M.C. and Kendall, K.A. (1995) 'International social work education', in National Association of Social Workers, *Encyclopedia of Social Work*, Washington, DC: NASW Press, 1511–20.

Hokenstad, M.C., Khinduka, S.K. and Midgley, J. (1992) 'The world of international social work', in M.C. Hokenstad, S.K. Khinduka and J. Midgley (eds) *Profiles in International Social Work*, Washington, DC: NASW Press, 1–10..

Hokenstad, M.C. and Midgley, J. (1997) 'Realities of global interdependence', in M.C. Hokenstad and J. Midgley (eds) *Issues in International Social Work*, Washington, DC: NASW Press, 1–11.

Jimenez, M. and Alwyn, N. (1992) 'Social work in Chile: Support for the struggle for justice in Latin America', in M.C. Hokenstad, S.K. Khinduka and J. Midgley (eds) *Profiles in International Social Work*, Washington, DC: NASW Press, 29–41.

Khinduka, S.K. (1971) 'Social work in the Third World', *Social Service Review*, 45 (1): 62–73.

Livermore, M. (1996) 'Social work, social development and microenterprises: Techniques and issues for implementation', *Journal of Applied Social Sciences*, 21 (1): 37–46.

Lowe, G.R. and Reid, N.P. (eds) (1999) *The Professionalization of Poverty: Social Work and the Poor in the Twentieth Century*, New York: Aldine de Gruyter.

Mazibuko, F., McKendrick, B. and Patel, L. (1992) 'Social work in South Africa: Coping with Apartheid and change', in M.C. Hokenstad, S.K. Khinduka and J. Midgley (eds) *Profiles in International Social Work*, Washington, DC: NASW Press, 115–28.

Midgley, J. (1981) *Professional Imperialism: Social Work in the Third World*, London: Heinemann.

—— (1990) 'International social work: Learning from the Third World', *Social Work*, 35 (4): 295–301.

—— (1993) 'Promoting a development focus in the community organization curriculum: Relevance of the African experience', *Journal of Social Work Education*, 29 (3): 269–78.

—— (1997) 'Social work and international social development: Promoting a developmental perspective in the profession', in M.C. Hokenstad and J. Midgley (eds) *Issues in International Social Work*, Washington, DC: NASW Press, 11–26.

Nagpaul, H. (1972) 'The diffusion of American social work education to India', *International Social Work*, 15 (1): 13–17.

Nagy, G. and Falk, D. (2000) 'Dilemmas in international and cross-cultural social work', *International Social Work*, 43 (1): 49–60.

Patel, L. (1992) *Restructuring Social Welfare: Options for South Africa*, Johannesburg: Raven Press.

Resnick, R.P. (1976) 'Conscientization: An indigenous approach to international social work', *International Social Work*, 19 (2): 21–9.

Robertson, R. (1992) *Globalization*, London: Sage Publications.

Sanders, D.S. and Pedersen, P. (eds) (1984) *Education for International Social Welfare*, Manoa, HI: University of Hawaii School of Social Work.

Shawkey, A. (1972) 'Social work education in Africa', *International Social Work*, 15 (1): 3–16.

Specht, H. and Courtney, M. (1994) *Unfaithful Angels: How Social Work Has Abandoned Its Mission*, New York: Free Press.

Further reading

Bywaters, P. and Napier, L. (2009) 'Revising social work's international policy statement on health: Process, outcomes and implications', *International Social Work* 52, 447–57.

Borrmann, S., Klassen, M. and Spatscheck, C. (eds) (2007) *International Social Work: Social Problems, Cultural Issues and Social Work Education*, Leverkusen Opladen: Verlag Barbara Budrich.

Cox, D. and Pawar, M. (2005) *International Social Work: Issues, Strategies, and Programs*, London: Sage.

Gray, M. (2010) 'Indigenization in a globalizing world: A response to Yunong and Xiong (2008)', *International Social Work*, 53, 115–27.

Healy, L.M. (2008) *International Social Work: Professional Action in an Interdependent World*, 2nd edition, Oxford: Oxford University Press.

Hugman, R. (2009) 'But is it social work? Some reflections on mistaken identities', *British Journal of Social Work*, 39: 1138–53.

—— (2010) *Understanding International Social Work: A Critical Analysis*, Basingstoke: Palgrave Macmillan.

Lyons, K., Manion, K. and Carlsen, M. (2006) *International Perspectives on Social Work: Global Conditions and Local Practice*, Basingstoke: Palgrave Macmillan.

4   Uncertainty

The defining characteristic of social work?

Jan Fook

Jan Fook's writing has been hugely influential in social work in the UK, in her native Australia, and across the world. She is probably best known for her writing on critical reflection. This extract, however, is broader than this, and picks up the vexing issue of uncertainty in social work. Fook argues that the idea of uncertainty is not a sufficient framework for defining the social work profession's contemporary mission. Instead, she suggests that 'contextuality' offers a more productive way forward. The extract is replete with many thought-provoking references which could be usefully followed up.

From M. Lymbery and K. Postle (eds) *Social Work: A Companion to Learning*, London: Sage (2007): 31–9.

Uncertainty

Thinking about uncertainty is aptly captured by Beck's (1992) description of contemporary times as 'reflexive modernity', which involves:

- a breakdown of predictable life stages, social rituals and norms because of uncertain social conditions;
- increased access to information, both through educational opportunities and technological advances;
- resulting shifts in social boundaries and categories and increased opportunity to remake them;
- emphasis on the importance of individual identity-making and life choices;
- contexts becoming more important;
- the breaking of traditional boundaries, people deriving their sense of community from a wide range of networks;
- different sources of power, less hierarchical and more mixed.

However, in this climate of greater choice and fluidity, there is also increased risk in charting a life course through uncertain conditions. Social institutions themselves cannot monitor and control these risks in personal lives, so there is a greater need for individuals to find their own sources of meaning and solidarity. Overall, the construction of the self within these fluid social contexts becomes the crucial task of living. Thus the self is a reflexive project (Giddens, 1991) in which 'critical reflection and incoming information are constantly used by people to constitute and (re)negotiate their identities' (Ferguson, 2001: 45). In reflexive modernity, this task of living, to create a meaningful sense of self in relation to changing social conditions, is what is uncertain.

Turner and Rojek (2001) add another dimension, 'vulnerability', to the idea of uncertainty: the vulnerability of our embodiment. Yet vulnerability also has positive aspects: it 'suggests an openness to the world and our capacity to respond to that openness in ways that are creative and transformative' (Turner and Rojek, 2001: xi). Furthermore, they argue that frailty implied in vulnerability is central to humanity, having the capacity to unite human beings. Uncertainty in this sense is borne out of our own physical vulnerability, carrying both positive and negative opportunities.

In broad terms, uncertainty experienced by individuals involves the interplay between breakdowns in taken-for-granted social institutions and people's need to make a meaningful sense of themselves in charting a successful life course in this context. This situation holds both positive and negative potential: positive in that opportunities may exist for creating new alliances and options and reaffirming universal bonds between people; negative in that increased competitiveness and fear of risk may lead to greater self-protection, narrowness, rigidity and social intolerance.

Uncertainty and implications for professional knowledge

There are specific implications of such uncertainty for the role of knowledge in society. Beck (1992) further theorises that within a 'risk society', *risk*, but also the *perception of risk*, becomes important. This perception fundamentally depends on external knowledge. Therefore, the nature of knowledge, its fallibility and control over its production become increasingly important in managing perception of risk. This has specific implications for professionals and their knowledge base, particularly for the expert knowledge base upon which professionals are presumed to practise.

Expert (scientific-technical) knowledge is coming under mounting public criticism, questioning its alleged value neutrality and, thus, emphasising the role of different political interests in determining knowledge, its interpretation and use. Pellizoni (2003: 328) terms this as 'radical uncertainty', characterised by problems whose very premises are indeterminate, in which knowledge may be interpreted in fundamentally different ways and about which there may not even be consensus on what is relevant. In this realm, 'facts and values overlap' (Pellizoni, 2003: 328).

How might some of this uncertainty play out in the daily dynamics of professional practice? 'Radical uncertainty' may provide a useful framework for understanding much indeterminacy that social workers experience. Banks (2001: 17–21) suggests that, for social workers, uncertainty may arise when 'technical rational' and 'moral' realms become confused – essentially technical-rational decisions gain moral overtones, and morality itself may become defined solely in terms of outcomes. This latter point refers to cases where the 'right' action may be determined by whether the 'right' outcome was achieved (only knowable in hindsight). To exemplify, she cites cases where a child protection worker may be deemed to have made the wrong decision (in not removing a child from parental care) only after the child is murdered. If the child appears to be subsequently unharmed, the decision is deemed right.

To summarise: uncertainty exhibits itself in several key ways. Broadly, there is uncertainty for individuals in both surviving and succeeding in life – this is the project of making selves and life courses when social structures are changing and no longer provide sufficient guidance. In this context arise particular uncertainties for professionals in trying to minimise risk and the perception of risk in situations and individuals' lives within uncertain environments. Professional knowledge is uncertain in several ways:

- There may be inadequacy in addressing new and changing situations.
- Outcomes may be unpredictable since contexts (and factors involved in those contexts) change.
- Meaning is indeterminate – since there may be multiple differing interpretations which may change according to context.
- Meaning systems may become confused so that moral and technical realms overlap.

Clearly, uncertainty of outcome is one of the major uncertainties facing professionals. Not only is it unclear which specific professional actions may lead to which specific outcomes (all other conditions remaining static), but having certain preconceived outcomes in mind may actually work against successful professional practice (Fook *et al.*, 2000: 134). Yet despite a wealth of research indicating the *certainty* of uncertainty, some practitioners still assume that uncertainty is something to be eliminated or controlled (Gibbs, 2002: 154–8).

Given clear acknowledgement of uncertainty in professional practice, how do we understand this persistent need for certainty? Perhaps professional status is somewhat dependent on management of risk or, at least, the perception of it – the conundrum for professionals is whether (and how) their knowledge can be made and applied in ways that effectively reduce these uncertainties, despite the fact that they are integral to current human and social experience. We might say that *the paradox of professional practice is the certainty of uncertainty, and the corresponding need to provide certainty within uncertainty*.

Recognising this sort of dilemma points to key ways to develop our characterisation of professionalism:

1   We need a better understanding of how we work and develop knowledge in relation to specific contexts, as opposed to how we develop more abstract and generalised knowledge. I term this *contextuality*.
2   As a result, we need to reconceptualise the nature of learning as contextual.
3   We need to develop openness and tolerance for difference in the light of vulnerability – this is not only a challenge but also a necessity.
4   We need to frame uncertainty and lack of control as positive opportunities.

New professionalism and the nature of professional knowledge and expertise

'New professionalism' (Leicht and Fennell, 2001) is a way of reconceptualising professionalism to incorporate some of these issues and challenges. It is presented as an alternative to 'old professionalism', in which it was assumed that professionals, as experts, could master the requisite knowledge in imposing order and reducing uncertainty (Gallagher, 2005). By contrast, 'new professionals' recognise there must also be openness to scrutiny. The 'new professionalism' therefore 'blends control through expertise with an openness to inspection and evaluation by peers and the public at large' (Leicht and Fennell, 2001: 14). We see calls for increased accountability in current trends in the UK towards service users (GSCC, 2002) and inclusion of their perspective in research, service design and delivery. This may entail recognition that scientific knowledge 'becomes more and more necessary but less sufficient' (Beck, 1992: 156), so that professionals must consider new ways of creating, using and reviewing knowledge. This has led to calls for a more reflective approach to practice (Sullivan, 1995: Chapter 6) valuing the role of intuition and the ability to develop expertise directly from experience itself (Gallagher, 2005).

The idea of working with uncertainty provides a useful conceptual framework to underpin our understanding of the expertise of the 'new professionalism'. How do professionals make certainty out of uncertainty, that is, act with relative confidence and commitment in situations where knowledge, outcomes and conditions are indeterminate?

Studies of social workers' actual practice indicate that they work in a large range of settings requiring diverse and multiple skills and knowledge. These situations often involve an array of competing interests, so it is not always clear who the client is, and workers' practice may be in part determined by context (Fook *et al.*, 2000: 111). These complexities lead to the need to develop the following features of expertise (summarised from Fook, 2004: 35–8):

- contextuality;
- knowledge and theory creation (transferability);
- processuality;
- critical reflexivity;
- a transcendant vision.

Contextuality refers to the ability to work in and with the whole context and in relation to it. This involves appreciation of how specific contexts may influence actions and interpretations of players in it, but it also involves ability to work with the whole context, rather than focusing solely on individual players (Fook *et al.*, 2000; Fook, 2002).

Transferability involves the ability to create knowledge/theory relevant to context and the ability to take learning from one situation and make it relevant to a new situation. In this sense, it differs from generalising knowledge across situations. The former's focus is on using prior knowledge to illuminate new meanings, whereas the latter's focus is more on imposing meaning from other contexts.

Critical reflexivity (Fook *et al.*, 2000; 189–92) and an ability to critically reflect is important in this theory-creation process. It involves not only creating theory directly from practice by exposing the assumptions embedded therein but also an ability to locate oneself and one's own influence in the situation, particularly in relation to existing power arrangements.

It is vital in social work to retain a value position, and there are increasing calls to maintain the integrity of professional work by doing this (Sullivan, 1995). 'New' professional expertise must therefore include ability to maintain a higher order of values, termed a 'grounded yet transcendent vision' (Fook *et al.*, 2000: 196). This involves the ability not only to respond to daily conflicts in particular situations but also to continue to work, at another level, in terms of broader goals (what might be termed a 'calling' (Gustafson, 1982)). This broader vision gives meaning and allows a sense of continuity despite uncertainty.

In summary, the expertise of the new professional requires not only a contextual ability to make and remake appropriate knowledge but also an ability to ground this knowledge in specific contexts and yet to transcend those contexts through maintaining broader values. Professionals use values to provide continuity and certainty and as a guide for remaking contextual knowledge and practice.

Conclusion

How well does the concept of uncertainty work as a framework for social work in contemporary times? Uncertainty is most clearly an integral part of the contexts of social work practice, providing a key way of formulating our understanding of the profession, especially in terms of the ways in which professional knowledge is created and used. However, there are also some clear and ongoing values, approaches and skills relevant in current contexts. In fact, I have argued that some key guiding principles become more certain. Our foregoing discussion has thrown some aspects into sharp relief according to their relative certainty or uncertainty. For instance, if we recognise knowledge and practice situations are uncertain, there is one certainty that follows: knowledge and practice must be flexible. Also, uncertain and changing situations do not undermine the relevance of more abstractly conceived values. These still provide necessary guidance in diverse situations; they remain a constant, but what may change are their specific expressions as they are co-created in different contexts.

It is possible, and necessary, to frame social work as a profession whose fundamental values are certain, but which uses flexible processes to co-create meaningful expressions of these in various contexts. In this sense, I would conclude that rather than *uncertainty* being the defining characteristic of social work, *contextuality*, or *the ability to respond meaningfully in relation to different and changing contexts*, is a more useful and relevant framework for understanding its contemporary mission.

References

Banks, S. (2001) *Ethics and Values in Social Work*, 2nd edition, Basingstoke: Palgrave.

Beck, U. (1992) *Risk Society: Towards a New Modernity*, London: Sage.

Ferguson, H. (2001) 'Social work, individualisation and life politics', *British Journal of Social Work*, 31 (1): 41–55.

Fook, J. (2002) *Social Work: Critical Theory and Practice*, London: Sage.

—— (2004) 'What professionals need from research: Beyond evidence-based practice', in D. Smith (ed.) *Social Work and Evidence Based Practice*, London: Jessica Kingsley, 29–46.

Fook, J., Ryan, M. and Hawkins, L. (2000) *Professional Expertise: Practice, Theory and Education for Working in Uncertainty*, London: Whiting & Birch.

Gallagher, A. (2005) 'Too clever to care? Nurses are not best served by being precious about professionalism', *Nursing Standard*, 12 (8): 14.

Gibbs, J. (2002) *Sink or Swim: Changing the Story in Child Protection. A Study of the Crisis in Recruitment and Retention of Staff in Rural Victoria*, Unpublished PhD thesis, Melbourne: La Trobe University.

Giddens, A. (1991) *Modernity and Self-identity*, Oxford: Polity Press.

GSCC (2002) *Codes of Practice for Social Care Workers and Employers*, London: GSCC.

Gustafson, J.M. (1982) 'Professions as "callings"', *Social Service Review*, 56 (4): 501–15.

Leicht, K. and Fennell, M. (2001) *Professional Work: A Sociological Approach*, Oxford: Blackwell.

Pellizoni, L. (2003) 'Knowledge, uncertainty and the transformation of the public sphere', *European Journal of Social Theory*, 6 (3): 227–55.

Sullivan, W. (1995) *Work and Integrity: The Crisis and Promise of Professionalism in America*, New York: Harper Business.

Turner, B. and Rojek, C. (2001) *Society and Culture: Principles of Scarcity and Solidarity*, London: Sage.

Further reading

Barnett, R. (2007) *A Will to Learn: Being a Student in an Age of Uncertainty*, Maidenhead: Open University Press.

Bauman, Z. (1997) *Postmodernity and Its Discontents*, Cambridge: Polity Press.

—— (2001) *Community. Seeking Safety in an Insecure World*, Cambridge: Polity Press.

—— (2003) *Liquid Love: On the Frailty of Human Bonds*, Cambridge: Polity Press.

—— (2006) *Liquid Times: Living in an Age of Uncertainty*, Cambridge: Polity Press.

—— (2008) *The Art of Life*, Cambridge: Polity Press.

Beck, U. (1992) *Risk Society: Towards a New Modernity*, London: Sage.

—— (1999) *World Risk Society*, Cambridge: Polity Press.

Cree, V.E. (2009) 'The changing nature of social work', in R. Adams, L. Dominelli and M. Payne (eds) *Social Work: Themes Issues and Critical Debates*, 3rd edition, Basingstoke: Palgrave Macmillan, 26–36.

Napier, L. and Fook, J. (eds) (2000) *Breakthroughs in Practice: Theorising Critical Moments in Social Work*, London: Whiting & Birch.

Parton, N. and O'Byrne, P. (2000) *Constructive Social Work: Towards and New Practice*, Basingstoke: Macmillan.

White, S., Fook, J. and Gardner, F. (2006) *Critical Reflection in Health and Social Care*, Maidenhead: Open University Press.

5   Social work, risk and 'the blaming system'

Nigel Parton

Nigel Parton has published extensively on child abuse, child protection and the state and social work. This extract, published in 1996, is one of the earliest examples of an analysis of risk and social work, and, as such, it demonstrates the emergence of a preoccupation which now dominates both academic literature and procedural guidelines alike. Parton locates the new risk agenda in social work in the context of changes which have taken and are taking place in 'modern' society.

From *Social Theory, Social Change and Social Work*, London: Routledge (1996): 98–113.

Increasingly, social workers and social-welfare agencies are concerned in their day-to-day policies and practices with the issue of risk. Risk assessment, risk management, the monitoring of risk and risk-taking itself have become common activities for both practitioners and managers. Similarly, estimations about risks have become key in identifying priorities and making judgements about the quality of performance and what should be the central focus of professional activities. The purpose of this chapter is to identify some of the areas of social work where notions of risk have taken on a particular significance and to begin the process of analysing what is meant by the term. More fundamentally, however, I want to address why it is the issue has become so important in recent years. My central argument is essentially that risk is not a thing or a set of realities waiting to be unearthed but a way of thinking. As a consequence, social work's increasing obsession(s) with risk(s) point to important changes in both the way social workers think about and constitute their practices and the way social work is itself thought about and thereby constituted more widely.

However, until recently most mainstream social-work texts have had little explicit discussion of risk. As Brearley, in the only book which has centrally addressed the issue for social work, has noted, while 'social work already has a great deal of knowledge and ideas about risk ... it may not always be expressed in those terms' (1982: 31). Similarly, Alaszewski and Manthorpe (1991: 277) have suggested that, while for commercial institutions such as stock markets, insurance companies and banks the concept of risk is well established and there are clear procedures for measuring and managing risks, there is no equivalent technology within welfare agencies. It seems that it is only recently that the issue has been addressed within mainstream social work in terms of risk. This suggests that an analysis of risk will provide important insights into the changing nature of social work and may encapsulate in important ways the contemporary experiences of what it is to do social work and to be a social worker.

The development of modern social work, particularly in the postwar period, was based on optimistic notions of improvement and rehabilitation and played a small but key element in the growth of 'welfarism'. 'Welfarism' was premised on the wish to encourage social responsibility, the mutuality of social risk and the encouragement of social solidarity and security. The principle of state intervention was made explicit via the institutional framework for maintaining minimum standards. This involved pooling society's resources and spreading the risks across the population and through the life-course. Social insurance summed up the approach and provided the basis for welfare developments in other areas. Persons and activities were to be governed through society, symbolised and coordinated by the state, and based on notions of social citizenship. Professional experts were invested with considerable discretion and trust.

The collapse of 'welfarism' and the growth of neo-liberal critiques have ushered in a quite new situation and one where notions of risk are not simply re-cast but given a much greater significance. No longer is the emphasis on governing through 'society' but through the calculating choices of individuals (Rose, 1993). For neoliberalism the political subject is less a social citizen with powers and obligations deriving from membership of a collective body than an individual whose citizenship is active. It is an individualised conception of citizenship where the emphasis is upon personal fulfilment and individual responsibility. At the same time, the impact of global market forces has hastened dislocation in most areas of economic and social life, reinforcing a whole variety of insecurities, uncertainties and fears. Not only can changes in social work be seen to reflect these wider and rapid social and economic transformations but also the nature of social work is such that it is intimately implicated and involved. The growing concerns about risk in social work can thus be understood as both reflecting these increased anxieties, uncertainties and insecurities and as providing a rationale for coping, understanding and responding to the new situation. For while there is growing concern that certain sections of the population are increasingly marginalised and vulnerable, there is also a greater emphasis on professional responsibility and accountability for the safety and well-being of those they come into contact with. Concerns about risk can be seen to articulate and represent these tensions and contradictions most clearly.

The nature of risk

The concept [of risk] originally emerged in the seventeenth century in the context of gambling. For this purpose a specialised mathematical analysis of chance was developed. Risk then meant the probability of an event occurring, combined with the magnitude of the losses or gains entailed (Hacking, 1975). Subsequently the analysis of probabilities became the basis of scientific knowledge, transforming the nature of evidence, of knowledge, of authority and logic. Any process or activity had its probabilities of success or failures. In the eighteenth century the analysis of risk had important uses in marine insurance. The chances of a ship coming safely home were set against the chances of it being lost at sea. The idea of risk was neutral and simply took account of the probability of gains and losses. The calculation of risk became deeply entrenched in science and manufacturing as a theoretical base for decision-making. In the process, notions of probability became embedded in modern ways of thinking.

However, as Mary Douglas (1986, 1992) has argued, as notions of risk have become more central to politics and public policy its connection with technical calculations of probability has weakened. While it continues to combine a probabilistic measure of the occurrence of the primary event(s) with a measure of the consequences of those events, the concept of risk is now only associated with negative outcomes. Definitions of risk are now only associated with notions of hazard, danger, exposure, harm and loss. For example, the Royal Society Study Group recently defined 'risk' 'as the probability that a particular adverse event occurs during a stated period of time, or results from a particular challenge' (1992: 2). The risk that is the central concept for policy debates has now not got much to do with neutral probability calculations. 'The original connection is only indicated by arm-waving in the direction of possible science: the word *risk* now means danger; *high risk* means a lot of danger' (Douglas, 1992: 24, original emphasis).

Whereas originally a high risk meant a game in which a throw of the die had a strong probability of bringing great pain or great loss, risk now only refers to negative outcomes. The word now only means bad risks. The language of risk is reserved for talk of undesirable outcomes. Whereas previously 'danger' would have been the right word, '*danger* does not have the aura of science or afford the pretension of a possible precise calculation' (Douglas, 1992: 25, original emphasis). The language of danger having turned into the language of risk thus gives the impression of being calculable and scientific. But this is not simply about linguistic style. The possibility of a scientifically objective decision about exposure to danger is part of the new complex of ideas. Not only is risk superficially scientific, it is also future-orientated and predictive. It looks forward to assess the dangers ahead.

However, Douglas argues that while this is an important shift it is not the major significance of the contemporary emphasis on risk. 'The big difference is not in the predictive uses of risk, but in its forensic functions' (1992: 27). The concept of risk emerges as a key idea for contemporary times because of its uses as a forensic resource. The more culturally individualised a society becomes, the more significant becomes the forensic potential of the idea of risk. Its forensic uses are particularly important in the development of different types of blaming system, and 'the one we are in now is almost ready to treat every death as chargeable to someone's account, every accident as caused by someone's criminal negligence, every sickness a threatened prosecution' (1992: 15–16).

Douglas sees the contemporary concerns with risk as fulfilling a similar role to that previously played by 'sin' in earlier times but the emphasis and implications are quite different. Previously, disasters were explained in terms of sins. However, whereas risks are future-orientated, sins are backward-looking: first the disaster, then the explanation of its cause in an earlier transgression. There is, however, another important difference. To be 'at risk' is equivalent to being sinned against, being vulnerable to the events caused by others, whereas being 'in sin' means being the cause of harm. The rhetoric of sin used to uphold the community, vulnerable to the misbehaviour of the individual, while the rhetoric of risk upholds the individual who is seen as *vulnerable* to the behaviour of the community, bureaucrats or powerful experts. While sin acts to protect the *community* from vulnerability risk acts to protect the *individual* from vulnerability. It has come to play a key role in the contemporary blaming system.

The risk society

Ulrich Beck (1992a, 1992b) characterises contemporary society as a 'risk society'. This does not simply refer to the fact that contemporary social life introduces new forms of danger for humanity but that living in the risk society means living with a calculative attitude to the open possibilities of action with which we are continually confronted. In circumstances of increasing uncertainty and apparent doubt the notion of risk has a particular purchase.

In the shift from the modern society to the risk society, the quality and nature of communal concerns and values shift. According to Beck, in the former the focal concerns are with substantive and positive goals of social change, attaining something good and trying to ensure that everyone has a stake and a fair share. However, in the risk society the normative basis is safety and the Utopia is peculiarly negative and defensive – preventing the worst and protection from harm. As a result statements on risk become the 'moral statements' of society (Beck, 1992a: 176). The axial principle is the distribution not of goods but of bads – the distribution of hazards, dangers and risks.

The concept of risk becomes fundamental to the way both lay actors and experts experience and organise the social world. Risk assessment and management are crucial to the colonisation, understanding and control of the future, but at the same time necessarily open up the unknown. Risk assessment suggests precision, and even quantification, but by its nature is imperfect. Given the mobile character of the social world and the mutable and controversial nature of abstract systems of knowledge, most forms of assessment contain numerous imponderables. This issue – the central yet uncertain nature of risk and risk assessment – is key to understanding the changing nature and role of science and knowledge and hence experts in contemporary society (Luhmann, 1993).

The risk society is thus also a self-critical, reflexive society. Risks come into being where traditions and assumed values have deteriorated. Determinations of risk straddle the distinction between objective and value dimensions. Moral standards are not asserted openly but in quantitative, theoretical and causal forms. But notions of risk are never settled and are continually moving. 'The concept of risk is like a probe which permits us over and over again to investigate the entire construction plan, as well as every individual speck of cement in the structure of civilization for potentials of self-endangerment' (Beck, 1992a: 176). Risk becomes central in a society which is taking leave of the past but which is also opening itself up to a problematic future. Risk becomes closely inter-related with reflexivity. For to assess risk in contemporary society requires the process of 'reflexive scientization' (Beck, 1992a) or 'reflexivity' (Giddens, 1990, 1991) in what we do and the way we do it, both individually and institutionally. The 'reflexive monitoring of risk is intrinsic to institutionalised risk systems' (Giddens, 1991: 119).

It is in this respect that it becomes evident that contemporary concerns with risk reflect ways of organising and thinking about the world rather than refer to some external or hidden reality. Thus while a significant part of expert thinking and public discourse is about risk profiling – analysing what, in the current state of knowledge and in current conditions, is the distribution of risks in the given milieu of action – such profiles are subject to continual critique and revision. No longer does expert knowledge create stable inductive arenas, for it is liable to produce unintended or unforeseen consequences or its findings may be open to diverse interpretations. The self and the wider institutional arrangements have to be continually assessed, monitored and reviewed and thereby reflexively made. Nothing can be taken for granted. So although science has become indispensable to this process, it is incapable of truth. 'Where science used to be convincing *qua* science, today, in view of the contradictory babble of scientific tongues, the *faith* in science or the *faith* in alternative science (or *this* method, *this* approach, *this* orientation) becomes decisive' (Beck, 1992a: 169, original emphasis). Under conditions of reflexive scientisation, the production or mobilisation of belief becomes a central source for the social enforcement of validity claims.

Thus the emergence of the risk society arises because of the undermining and loss of faith concerning science, knowledge and various hierarchies of truth and power. However, rather than replace these emerging doubts and uncertainties with new certainties, the process continues amidst growing complexities and scepticism such that reflexivity and calculative attitudes to the future become more pervasive. It is not by chance, then, that the increased focus on risk in social work has coincided with the decline in trust in social workers' expertise and decision-making, and the growing reliance on increasingly complex systems of audit, monitoring and quality controls. For audit has become central for responding to the pluralities of expertise and the inherent controversy and undecidability of their truth claims. As we have already noted, the key contemporary significance of risk is in its forensic functions and the importance this has for making experts accountable – justifying what they do and why they do it.

In recent years social-work practitioners and their managers have been subject to a range of new techniques for exercising critical scrutiny over their practice often formulated in budgetary and accountancy terms. What I am suggesting is that the emphasis on risk has also contributed to this increased role of auditing – in the widest sense – to which social work is both subject and in which it plays an active part. Whereas the trust in science, technology and experts – social workers – has been undermined, audit has increased, and this process is intimately related to our pervasive concerns about risk (Rose, 1993) which plays a key role in the 'blaming system' and new forms of accountability.

In short, the pervasiveness of risk in a context where the trust in science and experts is replaced by audit can lead to new forms of organisational defensiveness and authoritarianism. It is as if once concerns about risk become all-pervasive the requirement to develop and follow organisational procedures becomes dominant and the room for professional manoeuvre and creativity is severely limited. Ironically, once risk becomes institutionalised the ability and willingness of professionals to take risks – in the original sense of possible positive as well as negative outcomes – is curtailed.

References

Alaszewski, A. and Manthorpe, J. (1991) 'Literature review: measuring and managing risk in social welfare', *British Journal of Social Work*, 21 (3): 277–90.

Beck, U. (1992a) *Risk Society: Towards a New Modernity*, London: Sage.

—— (1992b) 'From industrial society to risk society: Questions of survival, social structure and ecological enlightenment', *Theory, Culture and Society*, 9 (1): 97–123.

Brearley, C.P. (1982) *Risk and Social Work*, London: Routledge & Kegan Paul.

Douglas, M. (1986) *Risk Acceptability according to the Social Sciences*, London: Routledge & Kegan Paul.

Douglas, M. (1992) *Risk and Blame: Essays in Cultural Theory*, London: Routledge.

Hacking, I. (1975) *The Emergence of Probability: A Philosophical Study of Early Ideas about Probability, Induction and Statistical Inferences*, Cambridge: Cambridge University Press.

Giddens, A. (1990) *The Consequences of Modernity*, Cambridge: Polity Press.

—— (1991) *Modernity and Self-identity: Self and Society in the Late Modern Age*, Cambridge: Polity Press.

Luhmann (1993) *Risk: A Sociological Theory*, Berlin: Walter de Gryter.

Rose, N. (1993) 'Government, authority and expertise in advanced liberalism', *Economy and Society*, 22 (3): 283–99.

Royal Society Study Group (1992) *Risk: Analysis, Perception and Management*, London: Royal Society.

Further reading

Alaszewski, A. (2001) 'Risk and dangerousness', in B. Bytheway, V. Bacigalupo, J. Bornat, J. Johnson and S. Spurr (eds) *Understanding Care, Welfare and Community: A Reader*, London: Routledge, 183–91.

Alaszewski, A.M. and Coxon, K. (2008) 'The everyday experience of living with risk and uncertainty', *Health, Risk & Society*, 10 (5): 413–20.

Beck, U. (1999) *World Risk Society*, Cambridge: Polity Press.

Beddoe, L. (2010) 'Surveillance or reflection: Professional supervision in "the Risk Society"', *British Journal of Social Work*, 40 (4): 1279–96.

Cree, V.E. and Wallace, S.J. (2009) 'Risk and protection', in R. Adams, M. Payne and L. Dominelli (eds) *Practising Social Work in a Complex World*, 2nd edition, Basingstoke: Palgrave Macmillan, 42–56.

Kemshall, H. (2002) *Risk, Social Policy and Welfare*, Buckingham: Open University Press.

Stanford, S. (2008) 'Taking a stand or playing it safe?: Resisting the moral conservatism of risk in social work practice', *European Journal of Social Work*, 11 (3): 209–20.

Tulloch, J. and Lupton, D. (2003) *Risk and Everyday Life*, London: Sage.

Warner, J. and Sharland, E. (2010) 'Editorial', *British Journal of Social Work Special Issue on Risk and Social Work: Critical Perspectives*, 40 (4): 1035–45.

Webb, S.A. (2006) *Social Work in a Risk Society: Social and Political Perspectives*, Basingstoke: Palgrave Macmillan.

6 Scandal, welfare and public policy

Ian Butler and Mark Drakeford

Ian Butler and Mark Drakeford are social work academics working in England and Wales respectively. In this extract, they review the main arguments in their book which explores landmark scandals in UK social work and health care from the post-Second World War to the early 2000s. They demonstrate not only how scandals are created, but also the ways in which they impact on policy and practice in social work thereafter. This is an important message for the social work profession, one which picks up a theme explored some years earlier by sociologists Stan Cohen (2002) in his work on 'Mods' and 'Rockers' in the 1970s, and by Stuart Hall and colleagues (1978) on their research into street theft ('mugging').

From *Social Policy, Social Welfare and Scandal: How British Public Policy is Made*, Basingstoke: Palgrave Macmillan (2003): 207–25.

Anatomising scandal

Characteristics of events themselves

At its most basic, scandal involves unanticipated exposure, followed by disapproval. Those involved in welfare scandals are almost always, in our assessment, taken unawares by the drama which engulfs their lives. Within institutions, as we have seen, the practices which become the focus of inquiry are usually of long-standing. Even afterwards, in many cases, such as at Farleigh Hospital, a significant body of internal opinion remained unconvinced that anything untoward, let alone scandalous, had ever taken place. It is only when institutional actors step outside the confines of internal routines that scandal becomes a conscious possibility. Nurses at Normansfield were alert to the scandalous possibilities of strike action. The authorities in Staffordshire were conscious that questions might be asked of Tony Latham's Fundwell activities. As to fieldwork scandals, the unanticipated element here refers to the events themselves. While Committees of Inquiry argue that the passage of affairs, in general, could have been altered by different decisions earlier in the chain of circumstances, few attempt to apply this rather banal conclusion to the particular event which form the focus of their investigation. The inherent unpredictability of acute mental illness and the stresses and volatility of circumstances in which child deaths occur are not amenable to anticipation. Scandal in social welfare, therefore, does not usually involve the sort of conscious risk-taking which is an integral part of scandals in other domains such as those involving politicians or big business (viz. Jeffrey Archer or Nick Lesson).[1] Rather, it involves processes whereby the private actions of individuals or the routine practices of institutions attract public censure in ways entirely unforeseen by those directly involved.

This lack of anticipation helps explain one of the paradoxes of social welfare scandal, which is the way in which, generally, Committees of Inquiry spend so little time in dealing with those individuals most directly responsible for what had taken place. The sense that staff within institutions and clients in the field were not consciously involved in deliberate wrongdoing (at least by the lights of their peers and the context within which they operated) means that culpability has to be sought in the wider, rather than the individual, sphere. The recent Inquiry into events at Bristol Royal Infirmary (Kennedy, 2001: 4), involving both an institution and the death of children, captures this feeling most directly in its claim that the Report provides:

> an account of people who cared greatly about human suffering, and were dedicated and well-motivated. Sadly, some lacked insight and their behaviour was flawed. Many failed to communicate with each other, and to work together effectively for the interests of their patients. There was a lack of leadership, and of teamwork.

Lack of anticipation is thus a crucial feature of social welfare scandals. It colours the nature of events, the reaction of those caught up in them and also the response of those appointed to inquire into them.

The second test identified earlier was that of exposure. Put simply, events and actions which remain undiscovered or unnoticed do not result in scandal, institutional scandals are particularly characterised by the exposure of practices which have been long embedded in the day-to-day culture of organisations. Nor, in these circumstances, is discovery usually an easy or unproblematic business. Institutions are especially capable of absorbing and minimising scandal. The Nolan Commission, reporting on that most venerable institution, the House of Commons, noted the 'culture of slackness' and 'the tolerance of corruption' which can characterise institutional responses to the behaviour of insiders. Even when the violations which lead to scandal concern the most basic human rights to life and liberty, institutions set up to provide care and promote welfare have proved remarkably resistant to investigation. In either case, however, scandals occur when a set of constituent elements engenders a particular response which transforms them into something beyond themselves. That response, is provided in scandal by energetic individuals, determined to bring attention to their discoveries. Sometimes this response is immediate in its transformative power, as in the case of the Ely Hospital Inquiry. At other times, such as in the case of Pindown, the process was long-drawn-out and was achieved only through considerable effort. Even fieldwork scandals, where the events themselves are more directly dramatic, can struggle for the sort of official exposure which Committees of Inquiry provide. Even Jayne Zito, involved in the most high-profile way in one of the landmark scandals of recent times, described the events which followed the murder of her husband in this way. 'We screamed from the rooftops' she told *Psychiatry in Practice* in 1996, 'to open the doors for the Ritchie Inquiry to take place publicly.' Moreover, the importance of exposure in social welfare scandals does not relate simply to the specific events themselves. Rather, as the series of Inquiries which followed Colwell and which continue to dominate newspaper headlines, discovery in one place, or one instance, produces further revelation in the same field. And in doing so, a further paradox emerges. Exposure, which is fundamental to scandal generation, becomes on repetition a barrier to that same generation. Scandal demands the unexpected, if not the unanticipated. Repeated uncovering of the same conditions means that this essential element is eroded to the point where its impact has ceased and scandal no longer arises.

Finally, comes the issue of disapproval. As noted earlier, Committees of Inquiry are often not centrally concerned with the most conspicuous targets of disapproval – those individuals at whose hands scandalous events have taken place. Rather, they focus primarily upon professional 'sin', and on the extent to which the particular events in question can be seen as characteristic or typical of such practices in general. In this way, scandal implies a ready audience of competing interests, within and beyond the organisations and individuals concerned, which makes the explication of the underlying actions and practices a matter of dispute and a struggle over meaning. Disapproval forms a crucial site of this struggle. Indeed, the transformation of particular occurrences into the raw material of scandal only takes place when it is possible to place a construction upon the underlying events which emphasises the extent to which they have departed from officially sanctioned, socially shared or emergent codes of conduct. The process of construction is often contentious and contested. The practices in Pindown, for example, were considered, by those held responsible, as simply administrative indiscretions, in which failure resided in violation of presentational rather than substantial rules. In the case of Normansfield, a direct struggle took place over public disapproval, with Dr Lawlor attempting to secure that disapproval for the nursing staff and the nursing staff attempting to secure it for him. All were involved in the disputed nature of events themselves. Where should disapproval rest in the Normansfield circumstances? Upon the strike action? Upon the reduced circumstances at the hospital? Upon the culpable neglect of those who had allowed this deterioration to take place? Even where the events at issue quite clearly represent an essential violation of shared moral norms – as in cases of murder – a struggle will take place to define the significance of contributory factors and to allocate responsibility between the individuals and organisations involved. Disapproval is thus a necessary condition for scandal, but the allocation of that disapproval is formed out of competing interpretations and the interests they represent.

Claims-making and counter-claims-making

Beyond the inherent characteristics of the raw material of scandal, a second element is required for their generation, that which social constructionists call claims-makers, individuals or interest groups which carry out Nichols' (1997) transformation of the raw material of routine events into landmark instances. For some writers, such as Fine (1997: 297), this element is the most important of all – 'a scandal suddenly appears, from the either – a chance occurrence that moral entrepreneurs seize for their own ends'. Best (1990) has suggested a classification of primary, secondary and tertiary claims-makers, in which the primary group are social problem activists – those who strive, for example, to bring the conditions of discharged mental health patients or young people in care to the attention of the public. Primary claims-makers in social welfare share one key characteristic. They are almost always outsiders, either in the sense of bringing a fresh eye to circumstances where general sensibilities have been blunted or in the sense of being part of a group who do not have a place on the dominant policy agenda.

The secondary group in Best's (1990) analysis are the representatives of the mass media who take up and publicise particular events or causes, conveying them to a wider public. The *Times* letter which led to the *Sans Everything* reports is an example at the simplest end of this process. Of course, as will have become clear from any of the individual scandals explored in this text, this 'conveyance' is a complex matter which involves direct and indirect interpretations of events, far more than any simple telling of the 'truth'. As Cavender *et al.* (1993: 153) make clear, 'the media do not simply report facts; instead, they convert events into news stories through frames of coverage – selection principles that determine what is reported as news, and how it is reported.' Katz (1987: 51–2) provides a useful insight into the frame most often adopted in the case of scandal when he suggests that virtually all such events 'deemed newsworthy are depicted as endangering one or another foundation of collective identity . . . Such stories have an unspoken melodramatic quality: they implicitly tap the folk ideas about vulnerability of collective identity'. The 'Cinderella' motif in press coverage of the Maria Colwell Inquiry is an excellent example of the direct connection between folk stories and scandal. More generally, the degree of force with which the danger to collective identity might be felt increases with the extent to which events occur in places which are themselves symbolic of such collectivism. Many of the social welfare scandals explored in this book have gained some of their momentum from the violation which thefts or neglect of duty represent in places ostensibly dedicated to the protection of the vulnerable and the provision of care. When patients can be killed by nurses in a hospital – as in the Whittingham scandal of the 1970s or the Allitt scandal of the 1990s – then a very direct assault has taken place also upon the collective sense of security. Secondary claims-makers develop this theme in social welfare to the point where they themselves become actors in the nexus between scandal and social policy.

What is it about social welfare which makes it so attractive to the news media? Clearly not all institutions are equally available for investigation or, more significantly in our context, representation as a source of scandal. Our suggestion would be that the organisations most vulnerable to such representation are those which already occupy an ambivalent or distrusted position within the public domain. Thus, politicians are always open to scandal because the involvement of any individual in moral or financial corruption strikes a chord with the public's view of politicians as a whole. So, too, with social welfare. Social workers, notoriously, have suffered a bad press at the hands of the powerful right-wing elements within the British media. 'Welfare' institutions, suspiciously regarded, provide a receptive context within which secondary claims-makers can operate relatively freely, knowing that individual mistakes or misdemeanours are unlikely to be sheltered within the protective shadow of a benignly-regarded institution or beneath the powerful legal policing of private corporations. Scandals, in this sense, occur when it is possible to present the unexpected and the exceptional as confirmation of a more hidden or submerged expectation. Thus, acts of cruelty in an institution, or the killing of someone by a discharged mental health patient are exceptional events – and newsworthy as such – but only become scandals, requiring a formal response at the level of a Committee of Inquiry, by tapping into a belief that they are emblematic of something far less unexpected. The folk-fear of the dangerous madman or the folk-memory of the workhouse lurk behind the social welfare scandals presented in this text. News values depend upon an initial appeal to novelty and moral distaste but rest, thereafter, on feeding rather than disrupting the prejudices, beliefs and mind sets of their audiences.

In the Best (1990) analysis, the audience for social welfare scandal represents the tertiary group of claims-makers, to whom the efforts of the first two groups are directed.

Public engagement is fundamental to the particular response to scandal. As Blom-Cooper (1996: 57) puts it, 'the most compelling reason' behind the decision to set up an independent Inquiry in social welfare, lies in 'the assuaging of public revulsion or repugnance that will not be satisfied by the traditional methods of remedial action'. Without a reaction of that sort from the public, the claim to scandal, particularly of any emblematic of symbolic significance, will have been lost.

Lastly, in this section it is important to discuss the crucial role played by counter-claims-makers in scandal generation, for as well as individuals and organisations who have an interest in attempting to mark out the general significance of a particular scandal, there are powerful players and institutional interests who will attempt the opposite: to suggest that the events under consideration, and their own part within them, have to be understood in quite different ways.

A number of such techniques have emerged in the accounts provided here, as well as those which are identified by Cavender *et al.* (1993: 153) as 'denials, mystification, and countercharges against those who demand accounts'.

Even where complete denial cannot be sustained, then counter-claims-making can attempt to mobilise denial by suggesting that code violations were either minor or understandable in the particular circumstances under investigation. Where complaints cannot be dismissed as simple misinterpretation of ordinary events, then organisations require other forms of denial. One which has been evident in a series of Inquiries investigated here is the 'bad-apple' denial. Sometimes this appears as a form of whole-class denial, usually when more powerful interest groups attempt to shift the blame for anything untoward down the chain of command, in a diffusion of responsibility which is characteristic of hierarchically-organised institutions.

Where whole classes of individuals could not be found wanting, then the 'bad-apple' denial often has recourse to a particular individual, or group of individuals. The 'bad-apple' approach reaches its height in the Normansfield Inquiry, where a whole barrelful are rounded on in the final sequence of the 800-page Report and expunged from the hospital and, in some cases, from the Health Service. Most importantly, however, the barrel itself is left intact. As Cavender *et al.* (1993: 163) suggest, 'the purging of problematic individuals confirms the system's legitimacy'.

In addition to denial, some counter-claims-makers can also follow a strategy of mystification. This occurs when individuals or organisations admit that something has gone wrong, but attempt to deny either the seriousness of such events, or their emblematic nature, by appealing to factors which either cannot be revealed, or which lie beyond the comprehension of outsiders or which, for reasons which cannot be fully explained, cannot be fully explained.

To denial and mystification can be added the counter-claims-making technique of counter-charging. Counter-charges in scandal exist, essentially, as means of attempting to discredit those claims-makers who attempt to offer a view of particular events which emphasies their emblematic nature, or which seeks to locate responsibility with more powerful actors within a policy context.

The point we seek to make is that scandal is not simply the product of those who seek to draw attention to its existence. It can also be formidably opposed by others, often in positions of relative power. The conditions in which scandal is generated involve disagreements not only about the explanations which lie behind events which all agree to be in need of explanation. More fundamental, first-principle disputes' can occur as to whether scandal has ever taken place.

Policy impact

If scandals are constructed, then, they are manufactured with a purpose.

Beyond the policies and practices of social welfare systems and workers there are a range of wider implications in the resolution of scandal through the mechanism of the Committee of Inquiry which need to be drawn together.

The conclusion to suggest that, beyond the detail of social welfare itself, the Inquiry is a process by which the immediate consequences of scandal can be managed, while leaving intact the wider institutional order. This finding is consistent with our earlier contention that, while scandal can accelerate a rising policy tide, it cannot, of itself, originate a change in policy direction, or alter the course of a policy which is already well established. The standard outcome of Inquiries is the identification of individual culpability or micro-systems failure. Larger questions of historical or structural significance are avoided, even where Inquiries deal with some of the most fundamental and contentious issues of contemporary society – the nature of parenting, children's rights, the treatment of mental illness, the operation of the criminal law and so on. In this way, as Cavender *et al.* (1993: 162) suggest, Inquiries contribute to a discourse in which scandals are treated as flaws in an essentially sound system, crises which will pass and where order and authority will be restored. Individual wrongdoing and minor policy adjustments attract the attention which might otherwise have been directed towards structural causes and thus minimise the need for extensive social change. Even when the corruption of care is as manifest as in some of the institutions which have appeared in the pages of this book, the weakness and cynicism which is characteristic of those organisations which are inherently incapable of making the image and the reality of care match each other only rarely emerges with any force from the pages of an Inquiry.

Notes

1 The possible exception to this is the Waterhouse Inquiry and the criminal activities of the paedophiles who preyed on children in their care. It should be noted that even here, there is some suggestion that abusers were able to persuade a great many others that their practices were not harmful or in any way exceptional.
2 *Psychiatry in Practice* is no longer available. The Zito Trust was closed in March 2009.

References

Best, J. (1990) *Threatened Children: Rhetoric and Concern about Child-victims*, Chicago: University of Chicago Press.
Blom-Cooper, L. (1996) 'Some reflections on Public Inquiries', in J. Peay (ed.) *Inquiries after Homicide*, London: Duckworth, 147–63.
Cavender, G., Jurik, N.C. and Cohen, A.K. (1993) 'The baffling case of the smoking gun: the social ecology of political accounts in the Iran-Contra Affair', *Social Problems*, 40 (2): 152–64.

Cohen, S. (2002) *Folk Devils and Moral Panics: Creation of Mods and Rockers*, 3rd edition, London: Routledge.

Fine, G.A. (1997) 'Scandal, social conditions and the creation of public attention: Fatty Arbuckle and the "problem of Hollywood" ', *Social Problems*, 44 (3): 297–323.

Hall, S., Critcher, C., Jefferson, T., Clarke, J.N., Roberts, B. (1978) *Policing the Crisis: Mugging, the State and Law and Order*, Basingstoke: Macmillan.

Katz, J. (1987) 'What makes crime "news"?', *Media, Culture and Society*, 9: 47–75.

Kennedy, I. (2001) *Inquiry into the Management and Care of Children Receiving Complex Heart Surgery at the Bristol Royal Infirmary*, Norwich: Stationery Office.

Nichols, L.T. (1997) 'Social problems as landmark narratives: Bank of Boston, mass media and "Money Laundering" ', *Social Problems*, 44: 324–41.

Further reading

Ayre, P. (2001) 'Child protection and the media: Lessons from the last three decades', *British Journal of Social Work*, 31: 887–901.

Burney, C. (2005) *Making People Behave: Anti-Social Behaviour, Politics and Policy*, Cullompton: Willan Publishing.

Galilee, J. (2005) *Literature Review on Media Representations of Social Work and Social Workers* (21st Century Social Work, Social Work Scotland), Edinburgh: Scottish Executive. Available at www.socialworkscotland.org.uk/ (accessed on 24 June 2010).

Gibelman, M. (2004) 'Television and the public image of social workers: Portrayal or betrayal?' *Social Work*, 49 (2): 331–5.

Hall, C. and Slembrouck, S. (2009) 'Professional categorization, risk management and inter-agency communication in public inquiries into disastrous outcomes', *British Journal of Social Work*, 39: 280–98.

Henderson, L. and Franklin, B. (2007) 'Sad not bad: Images of social care professionals in popular UK television drama', *Journal of Social Work*, 7 (2): 133–53.

LeCroy, C.W. and Stinson, E. (2004) 'The public's perception of social work: Is it what we think it is?', *Social Work*, 49 (2): 164–75.

Lester, H. and Glasby, J. (2006) *Mental Health Policy and Practice*, Basingstoke: Palgrave MacMillan.

Pearson, G. (1983) *Hooligan: A History of Respectable Fears*, Basingstoke: Macmillan.

Stevens, I. and Cox, P. (2008) 'Complexity theory: Developing new understandings of child protection in field settings and in residential child care', *British Journal of Social Work*, 38: 1320–36.

Zugazaga, C.B., Surette, R.B., Mendez, M. and Otto, C.W. (2006) 'Social worker perceptions of the portrayal of the profession in the news and entertainment media: An exploratory study', *Journal of Social Work Education*, 42 (3): 621–36.

7 Research as an element in social work's ongoing search for identity

Walter Lorenz

The relationship between social work and research is not straightforward. Some see it as politically neutral, a 'good thing' for social work and for service users, while others are highly critical of the connection between evidence-based practice (EBP) and managerialism. In this extract, Walter Lorenz, a social work professor based in Italy who co-founded the *European Journal of Social Work*, locates the controversies about research within the 'fundamental ambiguities' of social work. Lorenz draws on Habermas's (1987) distinction between 'the life-world' and 'the system' to present a wide-ranging argument about the nature of research and its contribution to the identity and profession of social work. Because this is such an important and contested topic, the list for further reading is inevitably lengthy.

From Robin Lovelock, Karen Lyons and Jackie Powell (eds) *Reflecting on Social Work: Discipline and Profession*, Aldershot: Ashgate (2004): 145–60.

Social work has always had an uneasy relationship with research. Undoubtedly, taking research findings and above all taking the debate about research methodology seriously contributes to the social status of the profession – an area of considerable uncertainty for British social work. Reviewing these developments in their wider social and political context reveals that the options being debated with regard to the research methodology most appropriate to social work do not just represent technical or instrumental possibilities for the achievement of given goals; rather, these controversies are closely linked to the issue of the identity of social work. Moreover, it is suggested here that these debates do not coincide accidentally but that there is in fact an intricate and historical connection between them. Thus an adequately comprehensive answer to the question of how to engage in social work research requires a clearer account and understanding of the formation of social work identities than has generally been evident.

The most striking feature of social work's current identity is the fragmentation of the profession and discipline, not just in an international context, where it presents a bewildering variety of professional titles and intellectual discourses, but also at national level, where in every country several professional profiles exist in parallel, sometimes contesting each other's territories. In the UK this relates not just to the still relatively recent split between social work and probation and to the older tensions in the relationship between social work and youth and community work, but above all to the dichotomy between social work and social care. The growing emphasis on care management in recent years has now begun to fragment the professional field further, and while the introduction of national Social Care Councils may formalise the relationship between the distinctive traditions concerned, it will do little to create a common sense of identity or to invigorate the intellectual dialogue amongst them. In fact, while creating a unified identity might be a justifiable interest for any profession in general terms, in the case of social work and social care this might run counter to the actual social mandate that this professional group has aquired and has striven to develop which involves setting the interests of service users above professional self-interests. Person-centred needs never correspond neatly to professional boundaries and the plurality of perspectives in the social professions can serve as a reminder of the creative, critical potential of inter-professional boundary disputes, as long as they are regarded as more than merely matters of power and group interests. It is precisely in order to unlock this potential that it is necessary to understand social work's inherent diversity and to identify common features across its different forms, which requires in turn a clear and careful historical and conceptual analysis.

Given the intermediary function of social work, the wider significance of discourses on research methodology cannot be elaborated adequately without reference to the intersection of these two sets of dynamics. They play a role on the one hand in the epistemological ambiguity between what has been described classically as the alternatives of social work as art and as science, and on the other hand in the ambivalence between striving for the status of a full, autonomous profession and retaining the empowering elements of 'voluntarism' and the solidarity with service users which they can convey.

Some elements of these complex interconnections have become visible in recent and current debates on social work research methods in the UK. While the pragmatism which prevails in the approach both to research and to practice methods in Britain (Powell, 2002) has hindered full recognition of the issues that are at stake, the political implications of the polarisation affecting professional practice as well as approaches to research nevertheless become apparent. Broadly speaking the debate divides into two camps, although in characterising it in this way we should not overlook the interlinking complexity of interests referred to above, which is present within each of the positions and which therefore gives rise to further differentiations in terms both of the pragmatics of organisational policies and of the impact of post-structuralist critiques (Kazi, 2000; Shaw, 1999).

On the one hand there is renewed interest in and advocacy for the relevance to social work of research methods which take up the traditions of positivism and empiricism, with the promise of providing accuracy of measurements, reliability of results, and transparency of actions, and hence of enhancing the public accountability of the profession (Dillenburger, 1998; MacDonald, 1994; Reid, 1994). Social work has always been suspected of lacking an empirical base for its methods of intervention, particularly an empirical base that was not borrowed from studies conducted by other disciplines, and there is certainly good reason to suggest that the profession has a need to confront data about the outcomes of its interventions (Shaw, 1999).

On the other hand this positivist stance is being contested from a perspective on research in social work which emphasises the elaboration and evaluation of subjective meanings as the key to understanding social phenomena. These meanings remain hidden to quantitative enquiry on account of the 'detachment' required by that method;

they can be captured best by qualitative approaches which aim at giving expression to the authentic voice of the 'research subject' (Ruckdeschel, 1985; Sherman and Reid, 1994; White, 1998). Among other things this approach inverts, or at least relativises, the relationship between 'experts' and 'people with mere experience', and thereby exposes and criticises the differentials in power involved (Beresford and Evans, 1999).

Categorising the parties to the ongoing debate about social work research in terms of such opposing methodological or philosophical positions is problematic, since the differences between the 'two sides' are far from simple and clear-cut. Crucially, the discussion is overlaid with a host of agendas which have a direct bearing on the gravitational pull of the various options and which can prompt curious 'border crossings' between theoretical perspectives. Chief among those is the renewed focus on assuring the quality of services, which itself has both a professional and a political side. The political agenda, noticeable particularly in the UK but spreading also to other parts of Europe, is about a restructuring of social work in terms of management criteria which emphasise cost-effectiveness and thereby outcome orientation. In research terms this is reflected in a shift from a focus on issues of principle and problem causation towards studies of policy implementation and effectiveness (Fisher, 1999; Gibbs, 2001). The professional agenda amounts to an attempt to reconstitute the status and to that extent the autonomy of the social work profession under these changed policy conditions by seeking to develop 'evidence-based practice', which of course feeds directly back into the same political agenda (see Webb (2001) for an incisive analysis consistent with the argument of the present chapter). This concern emphasises reliance on research findings rather than on established intervention methods as the constitutive part of professional social work (Taylor and White, 2001). It implies that once a secure knowledge base has been established with regard to a given situation, intervention becomes a matter of following given procedures (and thereby avoiding 'mistakes'). Achieving and maintaining service quality, in this version, seeks to combine a basically empiricist research framework with the underlying concern of 'quality assurance' for consumer views and participation. This approach purports to subvert the dichotomies of positivism and phenomenology, quantitative and qualitative methods, and adjustment (control) and emancipation which had beset the agenda, thereby seducing an insecure profession with the promise of bringing it intellectually into the fold of postmodernism while providing certain assurances against the angst of total relativism. In this line of development, not only is British pragmatism showing itself at its acrobatic best (Trinder, 1996), it also, by claiming to have resolved the various tensions referred to, marks a surrender to the logic (and the power) of the system, with action reduced to procedures.

It is not surprising, therefore, that intellectual discontent over such an alluring but flawed settlement is manifesting itself. The question is how to mobilise resistance and counter-arguments effectively against a development that takes colonisation to new heights. In the UK the concept of 'realism' (Kazi, 1998; Pawson and Tilley, 1997; Taylor and White, 2001) is being suggested as a reference point for a possible settlement of the at times strongly conflicting interests, and as a means of giving the social work profession a unifying profile and more secure social status while retaining the lifeworld link in the form of an action perspective. In 'realistic evaluation', 'Practitioners construct models of their practice, which include their theoretical orientation, practice wisdom, accepted knowledge amongst peers, tacit knowledge and previous experience of what works, for whom and in what contexts' (Kazi, 2000, p. 764). The process continues through the participative testing of the hypotheses thus derived to lead to a context-specific intervention programme that 'harnesses enabling mechanisms and steers clear of disabling mechanisms' (*ibid.*, pp. 764–5). The resultant models of 'scientific realism' (Kazi, 2000), 'sturdy relativism'/'realistic realism' (Taylor and White, 2001), or 'practice-focused reflexivity' (Sheppard, 1998), appear to satisfy the societal demands for greater accountability, the political interests in efficiency and effectiveness, and the professional concerns for autonomy based on scientific stringency.

However, there is a sense of premature settlement about these 'solutions', foreclosing on discussion, with a new emphasis on inclusiveness (empirical practice, interpretivist, and pragmatic approaches all under the roof of this type of 'realism') before the depth of the conflicts and the implications of social work's inherent diversity and plurality have been fully explored. Their concern with integration (of science and art, of rationality and emotions, of knowledge and values, of quantitative and qualitative models of research, of objectivity and subjectivity, of professional and consumer interests, of political agendas of control and of empowerment) paradoxically confirms their rootedness in and continued adherence to a dualistic epistemology disconnected from a theory of society. 'Realism' as the reliance on an objectivity which, though hidden and unreachable, serves as a given yardstick, surrenders the understanding of social processes to a scientific project which, by its very success in the area of science and technology, blocks the elaboration of values and meanings constitutive of societies and thereby the communicative potential constitutive of social work.

An alternative approach is explicitly to explore social work's intermediary role between lifeworld and system as this impacts in the area of research. This leads first of all to a sharper realisation of the conflicts and contradictions involved. But staying with this aspect of diversity, and acknowledging the apparent impossibility of uniting models of research and models of social work under one common approach, prompts the recognition that social work has its place in both lifeworld and system, and thereby releases its communicative potential. For Habermas the heuristic distinction between lifeworld and system marks two related realms of action in society, communicative and instrumental action, reflecting the sharp philosophical distinction he makes between communicative and instrumental reason (Habermas, 1987). The system is guided by principles and criteria of efficiency, necessary for the structural integration and material reproduction of society, by impersonal mechanisms best exemplified by the workings of the market. Communicative action, however, cannot come about on the basis of such 'given' reference points of meaning and understanding, but strives instead to constitute, out of the infinite diversity of subjective and conflicting meanings, the conditions for consensus. The openness of this process, its precarious ability to invoke reflection and critique, are for Habermas the very conditions – the only conditions – under which communication in its full sense can come about (Habermas, 1990).

Habermas emphasises the importance of the distinction between instrumental and communicative reason and action not only for the epistemological process of establishing different forms and regimes of knowing as such, but also for the creation of identities (Habermas, 1972). He elaborates on C.S. Peirce's observations that the (individual) human self which derives its identity solely from the success or failure of instrumental action can only develop in a negative way. It learns to become aware of itself only in moments where the discrepancy between its own position and the given, generalised consensus of 'common sense wisdom' becomes apparent. This observation could also be extended to the constitution of social work's professional identity, albeit that due care must be taken not to exaggerate the homogeneity of the latter. Once social work surrenders to the rationalistic requirements of the system and therefore adopts the dogma of positivism, it becomes set on an instrumental perspective on action and its identity becomes negatively constituted in terms of the 'remaining' discrepancy between claims (to efficiency and effectiveness) and resultant achievements. Since this discrepancy will always remain considerable, such negative constitution of the identity of social work is also likely to result in a negative public image.

These consequences cannot be avoided by means of the recourse to 'client participation' in research, at least not as long as such participation is conceived or employed purely as an instrumental device to give the results greater validity. Used in this way it simply preserves and transfers the basic underlying conception of research as instrumental action to an expanded 'community of researchers and practitioners'. Even though the results of such research can render themselves less vulnerable to criticism, seeming to satisfy both methodological and ideological criteria of 'representation' and 'representativeness' to a greater extent than does research conducted 'on them', the views of users, however representative they might be in statistical terms, are always going to be partial and in many ways 'parochial'. From an instrumental perspective on research the greater 'fit' of needs and outcomes achieved through client participation might represent a quantitative gain, but already in the application of such results the negative effects become tangible in as much as the approach renders those users who do not 'fit' into the framework totally defenceless and without representation, their right to subjectivity and to having a public voice having been further eroded.

This strongly suggests an ongoing need for social work research to be conceptualised and realised as communicative action, and hence the need to develop fully a hermeneutic approach in a research context. This is not to juxtapose a superior research *method* to the ones touched on so far, but rather to establish some *meta-theoretical criteria* which could guide the search for appropriate methods that might have to differ from situation to situation but which can be evaluated against criteria established by means of consensus-oriented communication. The existence of a diversity of possible methods necessitates communication; the imposition of one dogma – which essentially *is* positivism (Habermas, 1972) – but equally the 'anything goes' indifference to relativity which poses as postmodern (Fook, 2002) forecloses communication and thus understanding. It might therefore be less important to see social work as either a science or an art and to endorse the choice with the promotion of the corresponding research methods, than to recognise more fully the historical nature of social work in relation to the differentiation of modern societies.

In terms of social work's identity, the first two decades after the Second World War were a time when a unified, universal model of social work seemed achievable, based on the assumption, expressed in terms of ethical principles, that people had basically the same needs everywhere, regardless of culture and social and political context. Parsonian functionalist sociology, which prevailed not only in the US but also in large parts of Europe, provided the backdrop (and an explanation) for the way in which the social professions effected their task and status arrangements with the welfare states in whose rapid rise they played an increasingly central role. Universality and identity seemed to be secured even before the claims made to them had been empirically endorsed. This provided renewed evidence that once the link between social work's interest in being fully recognised as a profession and society's need for social work as a factor contributing to social stability and integration has been established, pragmatic/

functionalist interests in research and methodology will tend to outweigh those aimed at communicative differentiation of and engagement with lifeworld processes.

Where unease about the nature and function of research in social work emerged at all, it was explored from the perspective of whether social work needed its own approach to research or whether it should 'borrow' prevailing models from the social sciences. The 'traditional' instrument of research in social work had been the evaluation of case records, undertaken with a view to understanding the complexity of practice situations and thence improving intervention accordingly (Lyons, 2000; Walton, 1975). But increasingly this was seen as less respectable than the large-scale quantitative research approach which represented the contemporary social science standard but which could not at that time be replicated with the resources available to social work.

Research and the question of identity

One much-noted exception to conventional preferences, an example of qualitative research that received wide acclaim, was the study by Mayer and Timms (1970), *The Client Speaks*, although the self-critical implications of this research were seen immediately as handing arguments to a political lobby in Britain critical of social work's growing professional autonomy. The trend towards the dominance of positivist research standards was only halted, and that only temporarily perhaps, with the advent of new social movements in the 1970s and 1980s; these posed a profound challenge to the unifying and consolidating trend in the formation of social work's identity – a challenge encompassing but reaching beyond research methodology. Once the possibility of a plurality of fundamentally contrasting approaches to social work has been conceived, as demonstrated for instance by the emergence of feminist social work, and in its wake by the renewed interest in and valuing of personal experience over formal qualifications and expertise, the profession's position in society becomes insecure and contested. But precisely in this uncertainty, new stances on research can also form, leading in turn to a further differentiation of models of practice and a widening of the boundaries of social work overall.

In this situation a starker polarisation has set in between universalism and positivism-inspired empiricism on the one hand and a newly self-confident subjectivism and constructivism on the other. 'Experience' has come to be taken seriously again as a subject of and as a vehicle for welfare research, particularly in studies inspired by feminist ideas, which simultaneously challenge the alleged neutrality of conventional approaches. Hanmer and Hearn argue that 'Because gender-absence and gender-neutrality in social science is impossible to obtain, presentations in these traditions do not eliminate power relations between women and men, but rather only serve to obscure them' (1999, p. 107). Other social movements, notably those of black people, people with disability, psychiatric illness, social care users and trauma survivors, have added their voice to the critique of 'top-down research' and struggle to reclaim the right to authentic representation in research (Beresford and Evans, 1999).

With these challenges questions of identity have moved centre stage once more, not just in terms of the identities of service users, but also those of service providers, both individually and collectively. For the movements promoting emancipatory, user-led research have had a very distinct agenda of challenging the power of established professions, seeing this as maintained not least by means of 'authoritative' research. Here the interplay between intellectual, professional and political factors has come into play once again, for the shift in emphasis and orientation has really only become effective on the back of social policy changes aimed at altering fundamentally the role and structure of public social services (Gibbs, 2001).

It appears at first a curious and dangerous coincidence for social work that the issues of 'de-constructing' its power and structure are forced onto the agenda as it were from both directions, from neo-liberal policies and from user movements, and this makes it very difficult for social work to respond. The discipline and profession may well have considerable sympathy with the 'emancipatory' approach to research as it concurs with some of its own central values, but such sympathy is going to be short-lived if it results in the gradual abolition of social work's recognised place in society. However, once this conflict is seen in the light of social work's position straddling system and lifeworld, new, less defensive responses become possible, not least in terms of research strategies.

Similar problems and possibilities may pertain with regard to social work facing the dilemmas attendant upon the fundamental philosophical challenges posed to all 'truth claims' by poststructuralist and postmodern positions, which compound the uncertainty already long experienced by social work over its approach to research. Their programme has been to lay bare the power structures contained in all regimes of truth and has resulted in the destabilisation and decentring of all positions previously held to be authoritative. Identities can therefore no longer be taken as simply given, but only as constructed and transient. It must be stressed that this sobering realisation not only suspends the authority of empirical studies but also relativises the seeming authenticity of subjective accounts.

The sharp divisions over the function of research and the choice of research methods apparent in social work today are not new phenomena. However, they present themselves currently with unprecedented force, and this indicates not simply that social work *per se* is in a confused state but that the rupture between system and lifeworld and the processes of differentiation within each of those domains have become more acute. Social work is unavoidably caught up in these tensions and finds its role and identity threatened by the bewildering plurality of demands and of reference points in the associated debates. What seems to be more important than making decisions on whether to pursue this or that research methodology is to relate the discourse on research back to more fundamental reflections on the place and role of social work in society. Noting the plurality of forms of social work can serve as a heuristic device to provide a better understanding of the dilemmas it faces. On the one hand there are many parallel ways of interpreting social work's role on account of the nature of the discipline and profession in its historical context, and this means its dual mandate between system and lifeworld. On the other hand this perspective also provides a basic understanding for the shared themes connecting those different manifestations.

In its link to lifeworld processes, their often contradictory effects on both epistemology and practice notwithstanding, social work keeps open its potential for communicative action, action that engages with conflicting norms, wishes and aspirations in such a way that it creates the conditions for reaching a consensus. Social work research can ultimately only make sense as research that is congruent with the profession's social mandate, and this means that it needs to develop as communicative action, in Habermas's sense. The many attempts at framing social work research as a reflexive process which are currently under debate are hopeful signs in this direction. However, this discussion needs to be linked to a critical theory of society in order to prevent its function and its results from becoming absorbed into the system, with its pursuit of instrumental action, and thereby risking the unintended consequence of contributing to tighter and more powerful social control.

References

Beresford, P. and Evans, C. (1999) 'Research note: research and empowerment', *British Journal of Social Work*, 29 (5): 671–7.

Dillenburger, K. (1998) 'Evidencing effectiveness: The use of single-case designs in child care work', in D. Iwaniec. and J. Pinkerton (eds) *Making Research Work*, Chichester: Wiley, 71–91.

Fisher, M. (1999) 'Social work research, social work knowledge and the research assessment exercise', in B. Broad (ed.) *The Politics of Social Work Research and Evaluation*, Birmingham: Venture Press, 91–108.

Fook, J. (2002) 'Theorizing from practice: Towards an inclusive approach for social work research', *Qualitative Social Work*, 1 (1): 79–95.

Gibbs, B. (2001) 'The changing nature and context of social work research', *British Journal of Social Work*, 31: 689–701.

Habermas, J. (1972) *Knowledge and Human Interests*, trans. J.J. Shapiro, London: Heinemann.

—— (1987) *The Theory of Communicative Action Vol II*, trans. T. McCarthy, Cambridge: Polity.

—— (1990) *Moral Consciousness and Communicative Action*, trans. C. Lenhardt and S.W. Nicholsen, Cambridge: Polity.

Hanmer, J. and Hearn, J. (1999) 'Gender and welfare research', in F. Williams, J. Popay and A. Oakley (eds) *Welfare Research: A Critical Review*, London: UCL Press, 106–30.

Kazi, M.A.F. (1998) *Single-Case Evaluations by Social Workers*, Ashgate: Aldershot.

—— (2000) 'Contemporary perspectives in the evaluation of practice', *British Journal of Social Work*, 30 (6): 755–68.

Lyons, K. (2000) 'The place of research in social work education', *British Journal of Social Work*, 30 (4): 433–47.

MacDonald, G. (1994) 'Developing empirically-based practice in probation', *British Journal of Social Work*, 24 (4): 405–27.

Mayer, J.E. and Timms, N. (1970) *The Client Speaks: Working Class Impressions of Casework*, London: Routledge & Kegan Paul.

Pawson, R. and Tilley, N. (1997) *Realistic Evaluation*, Thousand Oaks, CA: Sage.

Powell, J. (2002) 'The changing conditions of social work research', *British Journal of Social Work*, 32 (1): 17–33.

Reid, W.J. (1994) 'The empirical practice movement', *Social Service Review*, 68 (2): 165–84.

Ruckdeschel, R.A. (1985) 'Qualitative research as a perspective', *Social Work Research and Abstracts*, 21 (2): 17–21.

Shaw, I. (1999) 'Evidence for practice', in I. Shaw and J. Lishman (eds) *Evaluation and Social Work Practice*, London: Sage, 14–40.

Sheppard, M. (1998) 'Practice validity, reflexivity and knowledge for social work', *British Journal of Social Work*, 28 (5): 763–81.

Sherman, E. and Reid, W.J. (eds) (1994) *Qualitative Research in Social Work*, New York: Columbia University Press.

Taylor, C. and White, S. (2001) 'Knowledge, truth and reflexivity: The problem of judgement in social work', *Journal of Social Work*, 1 (1): 37–59.

Trinder, L. (1996) 'Social work research: The state of the art (or science)', *Child and Family Social Work*, 1 (4): 233–42.

Walton, R. (1975) *Women in Social Work*, London: Routledge.

Webb, S. (2001) 'Some considerations on the validity of evidence-based practice in social work', *British Journal of Social Work*, 31 (1): 57–79.

White, S. (1998) 'Analysing the content of social work: Applying the lessons from qualitative research', in J. Cheetham. and M.A.F. Kazi (eds) *The Working of Social Work*, London: Jessica Kingsley, 153–69.

Further reading

Becker, S. and Bryman, A. (eds) (2004) *Understanding Research for Policy and Practice: Themes, Methods and Approaches*, Bristol: Policy Press.

Beresford, P. (2000) 'Service users' knowledges and social work theory', *British Journal of Social Work*, 30 (4): 489–503.

Butler, I. (2002) 'A code of ethics for social work and social care research', *British Journal of Social Work*, 32: 329–48.

Butler, I. and Pugh, S. (2004) 'The politics of social work research', in R. Lovelock, K. Lyons and J. Powell (eds) *Reflecting on Social Work: Discipline and Profession*, Aldershot: Ashgate, 55–71.

D'Cruz, H. and Jones, M. (2004) *Social Work Research: Ethical and Political Contexts*, London: Sage.

Dullea, K. and Mullender, A. (1999) 'Evaluation and empowerment', in I. Shaw and J. Lishman (eds) *Evaluation and Social Work Practice*, London: Sage.

Everitt, A. and Hardiker, P. (1996) *Evaluating for Good Practice*, Basingstoke: BASW/Macmillan.

Fisher, M. (2000) 'The role of service users in problem formulation and technical aspects of social research', *Social Work Education*, 21 (3): 305–12.

Gray, M., Plath, D. and Webb, S.A. (2009) *Evidence-based Social Work: A Critical Stance*, London: Routledge.

Hammersley, M. (2003) 'Social research today: Some dilemmas and distinctions', *Qualitative Social Work*, 2 (1): 25–44.

Holman, B. (1987) 'Research from the underside', *British Journal of Social Work*, 17 (6): 669–83.

Humphries, B. (2003) 'What else counts as evidence in evidence-based social work?' *Social Work Education*, 22 (1): 81–91.

—— (2008) *Social Work Researching for Social Justice*, Basingstoke: Palgrave Macmillan.

MacDonald, G. (1999) 'Social work and its evaluation: A methodological dilemma?', in F. Williams, J. Popay and A. Oakley (eds) *Welfare Research: A Critical Review*, London: UCL Press.

McLaughlin, H. (2007) *Understanding Social Work Research*, London: Sage.

Powell, J. (2009) 'Developing social work research', in R. Adams, L. Dominelli and M. Payne, *Practising Social Work in a Complex World*, 2nd edition, Basingstoke: Palgrave Macmillan, 321–30.

Rees, S. and Wallace, A. (1982) *Verdicts on Social Work*, London: Edward Arnold.

Reissman, C. and Quinney, L. (2005) 'Narrative in social work: A critical review', *Qualitative Social Work*, 4 (3): 391–412.

Shaw, I. and Norton, M. (2007) *The Kinds and Quality of Social Work Research in UK Universities*, London: SCIE.

Shaw, I., Briar-Lawson, K., Orme, J. and Ruckdeschel, R. (2010) *The SAGE Handbook of Social Work Research*, London: Sage.

Sheldon, B. (2001) 'The validity of evidence-based practice in social work: A reply to Stephen Webb', *British Journal of Social Work*, 31 (5): 801–9.

Smith, R. (2004) 'A matter of trust: Service users and researchers', *Qualitative Social Work*, 3 (3): 335–46.

Thyer, B. and Kazi, M. (eds) (2004) *International Perspectives on Evidence-based Practice in Social Work*, Birmingham: BASW.

Trevillion, S. (2000) 'Social work research: What kinds of knowledge/knowledges? An introduction to the papers', *British Journal of Social Work*, 30 (4): 429–32.

Trinder, L. (2000) 'Evidence-based practice in social work and probation', in L. Trinder and

S. Reynolds (eds) *Evidence-based Practice: A Critical Appraisal*, Oxford: Blackwell Science, 1–16.

Truman, C. (1999) 'User involvement in large-scale research: Bringing the gap between service users and service providers', in B. Broad (ed.) *The Politics of Social Work Research and Evaluation*, Birmingham: Venture Press.

Wallace, E. and Rees, S. (1988) 'The priority of client evaluations', in J. Lishman (ed.) *Evaluation*, 2nd edition, London: Jessica Kingsley, Research Highlights in Social Work 8.

Walters, I., Nutley, S., Percy-Smith, J. *et al.* (2004) *Improving the Use of Research in Social Care*, London: SCIE.

Whitmore, E. (2001) "'People listened to what we had to say": Reflections on an emancipatory qualitative evaluation', in I. Shaw and N. Gould (eds) *Qualitative Research in Social Work*, London: Sage, 83–99.

8 Social work and the changing face of the digital divide

Jan Steyaert and Nick Gould

Jan Steyaert is a social work academic based in the Netherlands and the UK; Nick Gould works in the UK. They have brought their combined experience together to produce an extremely detailed and full discussion of information technology and the digital divide. This extract focuses on two key aspects of the article: the overview of current thinking about information technology and social work's response to the digital divide.

From *British Journal of Social Work*, 39 (4): 740–53 (2009).

Introduction

During the last decade, it has become recognized in social work and social policy that information exchange and management are fundamental to the effective and equitable delivery of services. It is more than a desirable means of making administration more efficient; technology often structures the interface between those who use services and those who provide them. Deficiencies in the exchange of information are likely to obstruct access to services.

Social work commentators have often shown themselves reluctant to accept that information, and the technology that supports the management of information, play a defining role. Their critiques can be categorized under two headings: the humanist and the anti-humanist approaches. The humanist case is an objection to technology as representing an intrusion into the person-centred project of social work, displacing the authenticity of the encounter between worker and service user and replacing it with pre-occupations with accountability and bureaucratic efficiency (Burton and van den Broek, 2008). A corollary of this is the argument that human reasoning and the heuristics of human problem solving cannot be reduced to algorithms and depend on tacit knowledge (Sapey, 1997). The latter position overlaps with the anti-humanist case, so called because it derives from the poststructuralist and related Foucaultian analyses of social work (Webb and McBeath, 1989). It focuses on the role of technology in regulating the subjectivity of the person, extending the capillaries of power between actors. This line of critique returned recently in the social work literature in Parton's (2008) assertion that social work is being transformed from the 'social' to the 'informational'. His argument is that there has been 'a shift from a narrative to a database way of thinking and operating' (Parton, 2008,

p. 253) within which the close relationship with individuals is replaced by a more distant concern with subjects reconstituted as the aggregation of the data held about them.

Much of this literature is characterized by an implicit pessimism about the potentiality of technology, and an implicit contention that a form of practice could exist that stands outside the sordid business of using technology to collate and disseminate information. It is difficult to locate this alternative reality given social work's historical background as a bureauprofession. As the authors have commented elsewhere, social work arguably lies within a historical tradition that goes back to sixteenth-century poor law administration. Indeed, Parton acknowledges that the 'informational' character of social work is not new, but has become more dominant with the arrival of information and communication technologies. The recent modernization of social services is made possible and shaped by information technologies. The proliferation of activities such as care management, commissioning, contracting and regulation required by these innovations necessitate the assembly and manipulation of large amounts of data (Steyaert and Gould, 1999).

Nevertheless, this is emphatically not to argue that the operation of technology is neutral in its impacts on users of services, even though there is probably no going back in terms of the deployment of information technology. An emergent risk is that differential access to familiarity with technology can reinforce social inequalities and add to the vulnerabilities of individuals and social groups that are most in need of social work intervention. Connected citizens are getting better services, within both the private and the public sector. For example, UK citizens who buy their train tickets online are said to save on average a third of the costs (see *www.thetrainline.com*) and citizens who have internet accounts receive a higher interest rate from their banks. Similar examples can be found in public services, including social work (e.g. by finding online information about topics like debt, addiction, divorce, etc. or by getting quicker online support such as counselling.

Social work's interventions

. . . analysing and describing the problem of the digital divide are one thing: finding solutions to it and developing 'remedies' another. Social work has been one of the actors developing and implementing such remedies. Over the past decade, several social interventions have been trialled, evaluated and implemented. But as the nature of the digital divide has changed, so the nature of these interventions changed.

When the digital divide was first identified as a new challenge in social policy, initiatives emerged to provide public access for those not having access at work or at home. Public libraries were among the first to offer such opportunities, but were not the only organizational framework for public access points. Other frameworks were local schools, community technology centres (CTCs) and the commercial sector (cybercafés). While the commercial public access points tend to cluster in rich and tourist areas, others focus on low-income neighbourhoods, the first of which was probably the Playing to Win project in Manhattan, as early as 1983.

The majority of these initiatives did not limit their intervention to providing access to computers and internet connections, but expanded their services to include computer training and awareness raising. CTCs, in particular, became hubs for acquiring the information skills so necessary in the information age. The shift from providing access to digital skills was not the end of developments. As these basic building blocks for social 'e-inclusion' became established, the aims and activities moved towards applying information tools and skills for enhancing labour market participation and building social capital in low-income neighbourhoods. Technology became a tool for community development, in both an economic and a social sense. Using the internet is no longer an end in itself, but equally a tool for working on social inclusion.

Not all social interventions tackling the digital divide are geared towards public access. Another strategy recognizes the differences between gaining access at a public place versus access in the household. The aim consequently became to provide low-income households with computers for home use, sometimes geared specifically towards households with school-aged children, so as to enable both parents and children to benefit from technology. Some initiatives rely on fiscal regimes to make the purchase of a computer more attractive. As market prices for technologies drop (and most likely also because of the changed economic situation), these tax programmes have been cut in some countries.

Another approach to providing home access for low-income households involves recycled or refurbished computers, involving vocational training of less-educated staff to improve their labour market position. Interestingly, the biggest Dutch initiative in this area stopped its work in late 2003 as mainstream computers became cheaper and the economic recession limited the availability of second-hand computers. Also, users of refurbished computers were not always able to make use of the latest software. These same issues are also relevant to the discussion about shipping old computers from Western companies to developing countries.

In addition to initiatives geared towards public access or getting computers into households, some strategies focused on changing technology and its diffusion patterns. For instance, some argue that the monopoly of Microsoft is a threat to a cohesive information society, as their software is too expensive. They consequently argue that open-source software is a good alternative to lower the 'cost of operation' of new technology and increased usage of such open-source software can contribute to bridging the digital divide. However, working with open-source software currently relies on users having strong digital skills and confidence, which are two elements citizens on the wrong side of the digital divide seldom have.

Another strategy focuses specifically on the position of disabled citizens in the digital divide and the lack of accessibility of technology (Steyaert, 2005). In many Western countries, this led to the emergence of policy action and a legal framework that called on technology providers (hardware, software and content) to construct their products and services so as to maximize accessibility. The 1998 update of the US Rehabilitation Act (see *www.section508.gov*) indicates that government agencies in their procurement of products and services need to take into account accessibility. This and similar laws have resulted in companies like Microsoft and Adobe making a real investment in improving the accessibility of their software.

. . . some spatial differential access patterns are not so much related to choices of consumers as those of companies. As indicated earlier, when it comes to deployment of new infrastructure, there is a tendency for companies to 'cherry pick'. Again, in some countries, there has been some policy action and a legal framework to enforce universal access.

Within this landscape of social interventions tackling the divide, the observation can be made that the digital divide has not only changed as a result of social interventions, but equally as a result of changing technology. Software has become more reliable and user-friendly: hardware has become cheaper and easier to handle to the point of being sold at low-cost supermarkets. Subscribing to an internet service provider is nowadays a smooth process compared to the struggle it took to get an internet connection a decade ago. The infrastructure of the information society has matured considerably.

Part of this changing technology is the development from work tools (word processing, number crunching, databases) to multi-purpose tools. Laptops are now marketed as 'entertainment centres'. Leisure applications such as watching films, downloading music or playing games are probably more common usages of new media than 'serious' applications. Within this context, social work faces the challenge to develop new social interventions, new 'remedies' to tackle the 'content preferences' version of the divide. If it is no longer variations in access to technology or digital skills that are the basis for social exclusion, but the type of applications people use the technology for, providing low-cost computers and the IT skills to use them are no longer appropriate as the sole strategies.

Other remedies are needed. From a technological perspective, it would be possible to use internet filtering and, for example, limit publicly subsidized computer and internet access to 'good content' and exclude gaming and entertainment content. From a social work perspective, however, such an approach would raise discussions about censorship and paternalism. Outside social work, the use of 'persuasive technology' (technology that guides and changes the behaviour of citizens in ways that are good for them and society) is less disputed. We are all familiar with applications of persuasive technology, such as the car that beeps intrusively if the driver does not wear a seatbelt.

Health care has been faced with a similar challenge of finding new interventions, when it became clear human behaviour had become an important factor in endangering health. Smoking, drinking alcohol and lack of physical activity became as problematic for health as germs and accidents. Traditional health care (GPs, hospitals, pharmacies, etc.) consequently has been expanded, with public health initiatives geared towards behavioural changes that promote healthy lifestyles. Citizens are now subject to a whole range of initiatives that dissuade them from smoking or excessive drinking, from becoming overweight. Such approaches raise issues both relating to 'what works' in terms of changing behaviour, as well as 'what is allowed', in terms of where personal freedom allows people to act foolishly (Leichter, 1991).

Tackling the digital divide will need a similar approach to that of 'public social work' so that not only internet access is promoted and digital skills are enhanced, but also that people are encouraged to use the internet in ways that positively contribute to their social quality of life.

Conclusion: implications for social work

Over the last decade, we have seen a growing interest in fighting the digital divide and preventing technology from becoming a new platform for social exclusion. In an unusual coalition, this movement united governments at all levels, profit as well as non-profit organizations and community development workers. There was a great sense of urgency, resulting in a myriad of social interventions. Lately, in many countries, the interest has weakened considerably. One could be sceptical and suggest that government/business were only interested in the digital divide issue up to the point at which a sufficient critical mass of e-consumers was established.

While interest decreases, complexity increases. It is now clear that solving the digital divide is more complex than 'providing the kit' and several layers of complexity need to be added to our understanding of the digital divide. Additionally, digital exclusion cannot be separated from more general social exclusion patterns, as both reinforce each other, as this paper has argued. As we begin to see the growth of social work services online (Waldman and Rafferty, 2006), these issues will become increasingly in the fore front of social work's everyday practice.

While social interventions aimed at reducing the digital divide have expanded from their original focus of providing access to include enhancing digital skills and inviting citizens to become information producers (the so-called Web 2.0), they have yet to address the challenge posed by the expanding entertainment nature of the internet and the differences in content preferences across socio-economic groups. As part of its overall concern with reducing social exclusion, social work needs to ensure that the wide availability of the information opportunities of the internet does not only benefit the already information-rich. If not, the work of Neil Postman becomes relevant again, but this time with a social exclusion element added to it: will socially vulnerable citizens be amusing themselves to death?

References

Burton, J. and van den Broek, D. (2008) 'Accountable and countable: Information management systems and the bureaucratization of social work', *British Journal of Social Work*, 38 (3): 493–506.

Leichter, H. (1991) *Free to Be Foolish: Politics and Health Promotion in the United States and Great Britain*, Princeton, NJ: Princeton University Press.

Parton, N. (2008) 'Changes in the form of knowledge in social work: From the "social" to the "informational"?', *British Journal of Social Work*, 38: 253–69.

Sapey, B. (1997) 'Social work tomorrow: Towards a critical understanding of technology in social work', *British Journal of Social Work*, 27(6): 803–14.

Steyaert, J. (2005) 'Web based higher education, the inclusion/exclusion paradox', *Journal of Technology in Human Services*, 23 (1/2): 67–78.

Steyaert, J. and Gould, N. (1999) 'Social services, social work and information management, some European perspectives', *European Journal of Social Work*, 2 (2): 165–75.

Waldman, J. and Rafferty, J. (2006) 'Experience from virtual social work practice: Implications for education', *Journal of Evidence Based Social Work*, 3 (3/4): 127–48.

Webb, S. and McBeath, G. (1989) 'A political critique of Kantian ethics in social work', *British Journal of Social Work*, 19: 491–506.

Further reading

Horgan, P. (2009) *Interrogating the Ethics of Telecare Services: A Conceptual Framework for Dementia Home Care Professionals*, unpublished MPhil thesis, Edinburgh: University of Edinburgh.

Hudson, J. (2002) 'Community care in the information age', in B. Bytheway, V. Bacigalup, J. Bornat, J. Johnson and S. Spurr (eds) *Understanding Care, Welfare and Community: A Reader*, London: Routledge and Open University, 265–73.

Peckover, S., White, S. and Hall, C. (2008) 'Making and managing electronic children: E-assessment and child welfare', *Information, Communication & Society*, 11 (3): 375–94.

Rafferty, J. and Steyaert, J. (2007) 'Social work in a digital society', in M. Lymbery and K. Postle (eds) *Social Work: A Companion to Learning*, London: Sage, 165–76.

Reeves, S. and Freeth, D. (2003) 'New forms of technology, new forms of collaboration?', in A. Leathard (ed.) *Interprofessional Collaboration: From Policy to Practice in Health and Social Care*, London: Brunner-Routledge, 79–92.

9 Addressing barriers to participation

Service user involvement in social work training

Gina Tyler

Gina Tyler writes this article from the perspective of her experience as a service user and social work trainer. Her article is drawn from a journal issue which was produced and edited by service users; this was a first for social work education. The article is re-produced almost in total; all that is missing is a letter and some acknowledgements at the end of the article. Readers are urged to go to issue 25(4) of this journal for more insight into service user involvement, as well as to the additional reading at the end of this chapter.

From *Social Work Education*, 25 (4): 385–92 (2006).

Being termed a 'service user' is meaningless to anyone if it does not consider the person behind the label. Although I am proud of who I am, what I have achieved and enjoy being me, it is important that people see the 'bigger picture' of who I am. The label 'service user' applies to us all, and in many cases is only a very small part of everyday life. However, for some, it is a huge part of life, especially if services are not being provided as well as they could be. After becoming disabled later in life, I discovered what it meant to be a 'service user' in terms of health and social care. I could see gaps in service provision, and how some workers did not appear to see why they needed to involve service users at every possible level of the decision making process. Some workers often offered tokenistic gestures to involve people, but this was not real involvement, and made me more determined to challenge this. Involving service users in a tokenistic way achieves nothing other than ticking boxes and fabricating figures, which are then used to measure counterfeit involvement.

I use community care services and I use Direct Payments to pay for the assistance I need in order to lead a full and independent life (as I always have). I did not see why my independence should be compromised just because I was now physically limited in what I can and cannot do for myself. I employ five personal assistants, and deal with the day-to-day management of staff. I embrace the 'social model of disability', which identifies people as being disabled by society, attitudes, and poor design to our physical environment. This model places the ownership of disability with society and not with an individual's impairment.

I first became involved in the education of social work students in 2002. I was approached by a tutor from the University of Lincoln who co-ordinated and taught the community care unit. She asked if I would be willing to facilitate a seminar group for a semester. Although I had been a trainer in healthcare for many years before becoming disabled, I did not think I would be able to teach students at degree level. Despite my personal fears, it did seem a good opportunity for me to learn new skills, whilst teaching social work students from my own previous secular experience of social care, and that of being a service user. I could see the value in how the service user/carer perspective could enrich and qualify students' learning. It was also a good opportunity to teach as many people who would listen about Direct Payments, and the freedom it could offer. This of course meant that students were being taught by a person actually using the services, which would one day employ the student.

Students who are taught from the outset that service users are an integral part of care planning and service provision, soon identify and address barriers to participation, far more readily than their peers who have not had the same type of education within their establishment. Universities who are not involving service users in their social work programmes are not providing a balanced education to potential practitioners, and could well be stunting the growth, development and improvement of future service provision. This in turn presents a possible barrier in terms' of workforce development (workers being trained to meet the demand of more localised service provision in communities).

'Barriers to participation' has become such a common phrase to both service users and professionals alike that it is easy to miss the point of what participation is really about and why. It is almost as if the phrase is used at every opportunity to quantify and substantiate good practice. However, unless service users are involved at a meaningful level, which is of benefit to all parties, the exercise is futile and unfulfilling. The exercise may be regarded as a tokenistic gesture on the part of the worker, and can create a barrier in its own right.

Service users have been involved with many consultation meetings, questionnaires, evaluation and feedback exercises, but seen little or no change in the way services are provided. Furthermore, they have seen no difference in the way that workers engage with them. It is because service users do not see change, or receive constructive feedback on their involvement, that they see little incentive in taking any further part in future participation 'opportunities'.

The term 'opportunity' is often a word that is used to *sell* service user involvement. It has in the past been common practice for agencies and their workers to involve service users simply so they can tick the relevant boxes needed to evaluate their service provision, or appear to be meeting the recommended benchmarks and targets. It is also commonplace to use service user participation as a means to secure funding for employment posts. The downfall of this type of practice is that, although service user involvement is encouraged and promoted, albeit with good intentions, little education or training is given to agencies and their workers to explain *why* they need to promote 'meaningful' service user and carer involvement. As a result, the principles that underpin the importance of service user and carer involvement are misplaced or lost. Good practice is about involving service users at a level that changes the way services are provided and improves the way that workers engage with service users. Services can, in turn, begin to be shaped to suit the needs of the service user or carer, rather than expecting people to fit the service provision. Indeed, meaningful service user involvement should determine how a service user or carer can have the choice to look at various options, and tailor individual services that actually meet all, not part, of their individual needs.

This is not to say that all workers and agencies do not promote meaningful participation of their service users as this is simply not true. Many agencies are working very hard to strengthen partnerships with service user led organisations and proactive individuals who want to work at improving service provision. Indeed, it would not be a true partnership between workers who want to move service provision forward, and bring it out of the dark ages, unless they are consulting with service users who are able to easily fill the gaps in knowledge, albeit with or without support.

Meaningful participation is indeed a difficult objective to achieve in its fullest terms, but not impossible. Consultation needs to take place with a range of service users in order to reflect a range of personal experience and skills. There are many barriers which exist that prevent service users from becoming involved in educating students. Common barriers are often created by the internal logistics and structural organisation of the university. Barriers such as providing transport to and from the venue, paying for childcare costs, organising or paying for a carer to sit with a person who is usually looked after by the person getting involved, producing information in a variety of formats to suit individual requirement or even offering a form of payment which will not interfere with the person's ability to claim benefits. These may seem relatively small issues, but to some service users they are incredibly large barriers that seem impossible to bypass. This discourages service users and carers from getting involved, and a vicious cycle is created by the very organisation who is trying to encourage participation. Not all service users want to attend large meetings and events. They may feel intimidated by the environment or the type of language being used. If someone cannot understand what is being said, how then can they contribute at a meaningful level? There is no place for jargon when promoting meaningful involvement of service users, as this leaves many people who have lots to offer feeling excluded and frustrated at not being able to understand what is being discussed.

Professionals need to move away from their own environment and comfort zone, and meet service users in an environment they feel most relaxed in. One-to-one consultation work is prolific, but can be costly. These additional costs need to be met to allow a non-discriminative approach to involving all service users. There is also the issue of times when meetings can be held. These times are often predetermined to comply with professionals' working typical working patterns. This is not practical for many service users who may also have work commitments, appointments, and responsibilities. Agencies and workers must be willing to be flexible in their approach to working to include all service users. Some service users are excluded because of agencies not being flexible enough in their approach. If an agency is not willing to show flexibility in terms of involving service users in consultation, then chances are they will continue to provide inflexible services too.

There are, of course, many barriers to participation and we have only looked at a very few of them. The question of how these barriers can be overcome lies entirely with both parties being willing to give and take, but this must be done on equal terms. For example, involving young people in social care education programmes can be difficult due to students studying at the same times as the young people are attending school.

At the University of Lincoln we held consultation sessions with some young care leavers from the Young People's Support Service (YPSS). The initial consultation session took place over a meal at a local Chinese restaurant, which was a nice event for all of us. Furthermore, we all got the opportunity to get to know each other in an informal way, and indeed learned quite a lot from one another. This session was productive because we were able to discuss various ideas that the young people had, and we were able to explore ways that we could help put the ideas into action. We all had a great time and were very excited about working together.

Subsequent meetings were held in the familiar surroundings of the YPSS centre (the young people told us this was more convenient for them). All our meetings took place during the early evening so that as many young people as possible were able to be included (workers claimed lieu time from their employers, and this turned the emphasis on the workers having to make childcare and transport arrangements rather than the service users). We asked the young people to tell us ways in which they could get their personal experiences across to social work students without needing to come into the university. The young people decided that they could write letters to the social work students. This was a good idea, but we really wanted their letters to make a difference to the students in terms of the learning experience, and for students to think about them for a long time to come.

The young people decided to write a letter to the students to tell them about the things a social worker should know when working with young people. Three young people produced three quite different letters, with three totally different perspectives on what they thought was important for students to learn. To give added power and emphasis to the letters, and to ensure that the content was taken as seriously as possible, we recorded the young person reading their letter onto audio cassette. It was at this point that we all realised the potentially powerful teaching tool we had created. Little did we know that the students would later comment on the powerful effect this was to have on them as individuals and as social work trainees.

Service user involvement does not have to be complex and strategically planned. Often some general group rules and guidelines are enough to get you started. Workers need to be willing to take ownership of the barriers that prevent service user participation and focus clearly on ways to overcome them. Service users and workers alike need the time, tools and resources to move towards changing the way services are provided as well as the way workers involve service users in decision making.

Working together and reviewing current position, as well as consistently planning ways to improve partnerships between agencies and service users, will be a starting block of enhancing and sustaining relationships between experts. Service user/carer knowledge needs recognising as expert knowledge, since the foundations of promoting good practice starts with professional equality, and appreciation of what service users and carers bring to education and training. The benefits of involving service users at a meaningful level, creates a 'win-win' situation, and the rewards can be reaped for years to come as we see service provision being tailored to meet the individual needs of the people who use services.

Further reading

Advocacy in Action (2007) 'Why bother? The truth about service user involvement', in M. Lymbery and K. Postle (eds) *Social Work: A Companion to Learning*, London: Sage, 51–62.

Beresford, P. (2007) *The Changing Roles and Tasks of Social Work from Service Users' Perspectives: A Literature Informed Discussion Paper*, London: Shaping Our Lives.

——— (2007) 'User involvement, research and health inequalities: Developing new directions', *Health and Social Care in the Community*, 15 (4): 306–12.

Beresford, P., Adshead, L. and Croft, S. (2006) *Palliative Care, Social Work and Service Users: Making Life Possible*, London: Jessica Kingsley.

Beresford, P., Croft, S. and Adshead, L. (2008) " 'We don't see her as a social worker": A service user case study of the importance of the social worker's relationship and humanity', *British Journal of Social Work*, 38 (7):1388–407.

Branfield, F. and Beresford, P. (2006) *Making User Involvement Work: Supporting Service User Networking and Knowledge*, York: Joseph Rowntree Foundation.

Charnley, H., Roddam, G. and Wistow, J. (2009) 'Working with service users and carers', in R. Adams, L. Dominelli and M. Payne (eds) *Themes Issues and Critical Debates*, 3rd edition, Basingstoke: Palgrave Macmillan, 193–208.

Clark, M., Davis, A., Fisher, A., Glynn, T. and Jefferies, J. (2008) *Transforming Services, Changing Lives: Working with User Involvement in the Mental Health Services*, Birmingham: CEIMH and Suresearch, The University of Birmingham.

Cree, V.E. and Davis, A. (2007) *Social Work: Voices from the Inside*, London, Routledge.

Croft, S. and Beresford, P. (2008) 'Service users' perspectives', in M. Davies (ed.) *The Blackwell Companion to Social Work*, 3rd edition, Oxford: Blackwell, 393–401.

Davis, A. (2009) 'Addressing health inequalities: The role of service user and people's health movements', in P. Bywaters, E. McLeod and L. Napier (eds) *Social Work and Global Health Inequalities: Practice and Policy Development*, Bristol: Policy Press, 265–74.

Doel, M. and Best, L. (2008) *Experiencing Social Work: Learning from Service Users*, London: Sage.

Postle, K., Beresford, P. and Hardy, S. (2008) 'Assessing research and involving people using health and social care services: Addressing the tensions', *Evidence and Policy*, 4 (3): 251–62.

Part II

Knowledge and values for social work

Commentary 2

This section of the book moves beyond the profession of social work to consider the knowledge and values which underpin social work practice. As briefly discussed in the Introduction, I have chosen to use the word 'knowledge' in preference to that of 'theory' because I see this as a broader and more inclusive term. There has, in truth, been a lot of debate within social work over the years about theory. Some have gone so far as to argue that social work does not have any theories at all, or at least, not in the sense of formal scientific theories, because it is almost impossible in social work to be sufficiently sure that 'a' caused 'b', or that 'd' is the likely consequence of 'c'. Of course, this is also the case for other enabling professions including medicine and education. This intellectual tangle has been ably explored by Howe (1992 and 2009), Thompson (1995), Payne (2005), Beckett (2006) and Gray and Webb (2009). Suffice to say that my own position supports that of Taylor and White (2006), who argue that a position of 'respectful uncertainty' is preferable to making professional judgements on the basis of theory or knowledge which is always, by its very nature, likely to be incomplete, changing and contested. This should not, however, lead anyone to assume that there is no useful knowledge in social work. On the contrary, as this section of the reader will demonstrate, social workers have much to learn.

So what do social workers need to know? That is a huge question which cannot be fully answered in these short chapters. But it is also, paradoxically, an easy question to answer, if we have the courage to take it back to its most basic. Social workers need to know about people, about society and about themselves. Let us consider each in turn.

- Social workers need to know about people. They need to know what makes people tick; what allows them to be full human beings; what gets in the way of this and what promotes this; what makes people a problem to themselves and others; and what is most helpful to those in difficulty. Social workers also need to know how to communicate with people, and how to relate to others.
- They need to know about society. Social work is, as its name suggests, a 'social' profession. It is about the relationship between the individual and society, and students therefore need to know about society and about the role of social work within society.
- Social workers need to know about themselves. This has been a central notion within social work since its early days, often couched in the term 'use of self'. The

adage 'know thyself' is a saying which dates back to ancient Greece, where it was inscribed at the temple of Apollo at Delphi and central to the teachings of Greek philosophers. This went out of fashion for a while in social work education, as task-centred and systems approaches overtook psychodynamic ways of thinking. A focus on 'use of self' is now back on the agenda (see Cree 2003; Cree and Davis 2007; Harrison and Ruch 2007; O'Connor *et al.* 2006), emanating from two rather different, but at times overlapping, bodies of knowledge. The first is the notion of reflexivity, sometimes called 'critical reflection' (see Gould and Baldwin 2004; White *et al.* 2006; Schon 1987), drawn from a sociological perspective and particularly evident in feminist and research literature (see Alvesson and Sköldberg 2000; Finlay and Gough 2003; Hertz 1997; May and Williams 1998). The second is the idea of 'emotional intelligence', drawn from a psychological tradition, but also owing allegiance to feminist and social psychological writing (see Howe 2008).

The extracts I have chosen for this part of the book are not all written by social workers. This is because the ideas presented here are those which I believe are of key significance *for* social work, not *by* social work. This means that some of the texts and authors may be unfamiliar to social work readers, while others are the much-loved 'usual suspects' whose work appears in most of the social work education textbooks. Some of the extracts are very recent, and others were written some time ago but have enduring importance for social work. The language in these extracts is, at times, rather dated (for example, using the word 'man' to mean 'person' or 'human kind'). This demonstrates that ideas are bigger than terminology. Although language-use may change over time, insight has the capacity to transcend this again and again.

Key questions

1   How have ideas drawn from psychology contributed to social work's theory and knowledge base?
2   What other kinds of knowledge does and should social work draw on?
3   To what extent might social work be called a 'social' profession?
4   How do ethics and values come together in social work?

References

Alvesson, M. and Sköldberg, K. (2000) *Reflexive Methodology*, Sage: London.
Beckett, C. (2006) *Essential Theory for Social Work Practice*, London: Sage.
Cree, V.E. (ed.) (2003) *Becoming a Social Worker*, London: Routledge.
Cree, V.E. and Davis, A. (2007) *Social Work: Voices from the Inside*, London: Routledge.
Finlay, L. and Gough, B. (eds) (2003) *Reflexivity: A Practical Guide for Researchers in Health and Social Sciences*, Oxford: Blackwell.
Gould, N. and Baldwin, M. (eds) (2004) *Social Work, Critical Reflection and the Learning Organization*, Aldershot: Ashgate.
Gray, M. and Webb, S. (2009) *Social Work Theories and Methods*, London: Sage.
Harrison, K. and Ruch, G. (2007) 'Social work and the use of self: On becoming and being a social worker', in *Social Work: A Companion to Learning*, London: Sage.
Hertz, R. (ed.) (1997) *Reflexivity and Voice*, London: Sage.
Howe, D. (1992) *An Introduction to Social Work Theory*, Aldershot: Ashgate.

—— (2008) *The Emotionally Intelligent Social Worker*, Basingstoke: Palgrave Macmillan.

—— (2009) *A Brief Introduction to Social Work Theory*, Basingstoke: Palgrave.

May, T. and Williams, M. (eds) (1998) *Knowing the Social World*, Buckingham: Open University Press.

O'Connor, I., Hughes, M., Turney, D., Wilson, J. and Setterlund, D. (2006) *Social Work and Social Care Practice*, London: Sage.

Payne, M. (2005) *Modern Social Work Theory*, 3rd edition, Basingstoke: Palgrave Macmillan.

Schon, D. (1987) *Educating the Reflective Practitioner: Toward a New Design for Teaching and Learning in the Professions*, San Francisco, CA: Jossey-Bass.

Taylor, C. and White, S. (2006) 'Educating and reasoning in social work: Educating for humane judgement', *British Journal of Social Work*, 36: 937–54.

Thompson, N. (1995) *Theory and Practice in Health and Social Welfare*, Buckingham: Open University Press.

White, S., Fook, J. and Gardner, F. (2006) *Critical Reflection in Health and Social Care*, Maidenhead: Open University Press.

Further reading

Oko, J. (2008) *Understanding and Using Theory in Social Work*, Exeter: Learning Matters.

10 Attachment theory and social relationships

David Howe

David Howe is a social work academic in the UK who has written and researched for many years on psychodynamic approaches and attachment theory. In this extract, he introduces the work of the British psychoanalyst, John Bowlby (1907–1990), who made a huge contribution to our understanding of the importance of attachment for children and their later emotional and physical well-being. Bowlby's research began with disturbed children in child guidance clinics and residential nurseries during and after the Second World War. As the extract shows, Bowlby continued to focus on attachment throughout his life, and many others have picked up and developed his ideas further.

From *Attachment Theory for Social Work Practice*, Basingstoke: Macmillan (1995): 45–57.

Maternal deprivation

. . . for the developing infant, social relationships are both the problem and the solution. If the child is to develop social competence, he or she needs to become fully engaged in good quality social relationships. The maturing child will be exposed to a range of significant relationships, each of which will be capable of influencing the developmental pathway followed by that child. Forming a close attachment to a caregiving figure is still regarded as perhaps the most important early social relationship, but others, described as 'beyond attachment', become increasingly important, particularly as the child grows older. The child is part of a social network and if attachment relationships are weak with, say, the mother, it might be that the father, an older sister or a grandparent serves equally well as that child's selective attachment figure. Rutter (1991: 341) notes the growing recognition that developmentalists now give to the quality and character of social relationships in understanding the formation of the self and the structuring of personality:

> Attention has shifted from 'mother-love' as such to the growth of social relationships. However, within the latter topic, the concept of attachment has come to dominate both theory and empirical research. The basic idea is that children have a natural propensity to maintain proximity with a mother figure, that this leads to an attachment relationship and that the quality of this relationship in terms of security/insecurity serves the basis of later relationships.

Throughout the late 1930s and 1940s John Bowlby had been investigating and reflecting upon the nature and purpose of the close relationships we form with people throughout our lives, and particularly those we forge in childhood. 'The making and breaking of affectional bonds' as he was later to call his subject of enquiry loomed ever larger in his attempts to understand the psychological behaviour and development of human beings. A trained psychoanalyst, he became increasingly dissatisfied with the ability of psychoanalytical theory on its own to explain many of the psychological phenomenon with which he was working. His discovery of the work of ethologists in the early 1950s revolutionised his thinking about early child development and was eventually to lead to his formulation of 'attachment theory'.

In his work with people like James Robertson, Bowlby recognised and described the upset and pain that children experience when they are separated from their parents. The mixture of tears, protest and anger observed by the researchers was both impressive and, they thought, in need of explanation. Such effects were witnessed when children were temporarily separated from their parents, but they could also be observed in cases where the separation was both more profound and traumatic. It was in these latter cases that Bowlby saw some of the longer-term effects of 'maternal deprivation' – neurotic and delinquent behaviour in the children when they grew older, and possible mental illness in adults. He needed a theory to explain why the serious disruption of particular childhood relationships seemed to cause such havoc in the psychological wellbeing and social behaviour of the deprived individuals.

Bowlby submitted his review of the research evidence to the World Health Organisation in 1951 under the title *Maternal Care and Mental Health*. It appeared to him that children who had been deprived of their mothers, particularly those brought up in institutions, suffered in terms of their emotional, intellectual, verbal, social and even physical development. By the time they had reached adolescence, these children had problems in forming steady or stable social relationships. They tended to be rather shallow and promiscuous in their dealings with others. Delinquent behaviour and personality problems appeared to be the fate of those who had experienced long-term separations from their mothers or mother substitutes during the first few years of life. It seemed that the lack of a warm, intimate and continuous relationship with the mother during infancy, rather than middle or later childhood, was likely to lead to a person with a disturbed personality who might also suffer cognitive impairment, anxiety and depression (Rutter 1991: 332).

However, not only were these claims soon to be qualified by Bowlby himself, but others began to subject them to critical scrutiny. Rutter (1981) observed that 'maternal deprivation' in fact conflated and therefore confused two categories of disturbed infant relationship. Bowlby, in his controversial and groundbreaking 1951 report to the World Health Organisation, was writing about maternal *privation* (children who had *never* had maternal care and were raised in institutions) and not maternal *deprivation* (children who had had a relationship with their mother but who had then lost or been removed from her). While the child who has had no maternal care or who has not received constant care by a substitute caretaker almost invariably displays long-term psychological disturbance, the developmental consequences are more complex and difficult to predict in the case of maternal deprivation.

Looking back, it now seems that in the early 1950s the case was somewhat overstated. It was simply too sweeping to argue that babies needed full-time and exclusive mothering if they were to develop into psychologically health adults. Certainly short separations from mother (illness, holidays, work), although temporarily upsetting, had no long-term adverse consequences. Indeed, research began to show that it was remaining in prolonged disturbed relationships that was more likely to lead to impaired development rather than simply losing a relationship. For example, the discord and emotional conflict surrounding parental divorce was shown to be much more damaging to a child's psychological development than parental death. However, this is not to say that losing a parent, whether by death or separation, is not disturbing. It clearly does cause emotional upset and even damage. Many children suffer a double blow: a history of conflict between parents often preceded their separation.

Nevertheless, it does seem that there are risks for the child when relationships are not sustained on a regular and long-term basis. According to Rutter (1991: 341 and 361), 'it seems that the postulate that a lack of continuity in loving committed parent-child relationships is central has received substantial support', and that 'What has stood the test of time most of all has been the proposition that the qualities of parent-child relationships constitute a central aspect of parenting, that the development of social relationships occupies a crucial role in personality growth, and that abnormalities in relationships are important in many types of psychopathology.' What has been qualified is that the mother–child relationship is the only important relationship in a child's development.

In the earliest formulations, there was the strong implication that no-one else but the mother was sufficiently important or would do. Feminist critiques were particularly fierce throughout the 1970s and 1980s. They argued that what was important for the child was not exclusive and concentrated care by one woman but stable, regular and shared care by a reliable number of adults and older children. The mother is clearly a very important member of this social environment, but fathers, grandparents and older brothers and sisters might also play a regular and significant role in that child's experience of social relationships.

The emergence of attachment theory

Bowlby himself continued to develop and refine his ideas right up until his death in 1990 at the age of 83, but perhaps his greatest achievement was to respond to some of the critics of the concept of maternal deprivation by vigorously developing the original theoretical perspective into what we now know as attachment theory.

Like many original thinkers, Bowlby recognised that there were fundamentally important issues and potentially deep insights lying behind the seemingly obvious answers to the somewhat fatuous questions being asked about childhood experiences and psychological development. Why should children be upset when they are separated from their mothers? Why do children who are loved and cared for in a consistent and stable manner nearly always grow up into well-adjusted adults? Why do children who have never had a constant mother-figure find social life and relationships so difficult? It is only when you to stop to think about these questions that you realise that it is not at all obvious how they should be answered other than to say something like 'of course a loved child will grow up into a socially competent adult and an unloved child will not'. This answer tells us nothing about how these psychological states work or might come about.

Psychoanalysis's 'drive theory' attempted to explain these phenomena in terms of the child's 'libido', the psychic energy that builds up and demands release and gratification and which is the direct mental counterpart of the physiological needs that cause tensions in our body. In the case of young babies, the need to feed brings the infant into a close and powerful relationship with, usually, the mother. The mother, or her breast, can discharge the baby's libido by feeding the child. Any delay or failure to reduce libido is experienced as anxiety. The ability to feed and thereby gratify her infant is the basis of the baby's love for her – the 'cupboard love' theory of relationships according to Bowlby.

Taking this line of thought a stage further allowed Freud to suggest that it was not the mere loss of the food supply that caused anxiety but the actual or possible loss of the food *supplier* – the mother and her breast as the objects to which the child and his or her love were relating. Any prolonged separation from the mother threatens gratification of physiological needs. There is therefore a build-up in libido and anxiety.

Within this theoretical outlook, any relationship or attachment with the mother that happens to develop is simply the result of the infant's physiological needs being met. Such needs are generally concerned with food or the infant's sexuality defined in the broad sense of finding satisfaction and pleasure in responding to the environment for purpose of growth and development. Psychoanalytic theory reduced attachment behaviour to a by-product of the traditional instincts.

Bowlby comprehensively rejected this analysis and saw attachment as a primary, biologically sponsored behaviour in its own right. The need to be close to a parent-figure, to seek comfort, love and attention from that person, is every bit as basic as the desire for food and warmth. In other words, there is a biological predisposition to relate with particular human beings irrespective of anything else. 'The young child's hunger for his mother's love and presence is as great as his hunger for food . . . Attachment is a "primary motivational system" with its own workings and interface with other motivational systems' (Bowlby 1973).

The work of the ethologists

However, Bowlby's development of attachment theory was not just in response to his criticisms of psychoanalysis. In the 1950s he became more and interested in the work and ideas of ethologists – scientists who study animals and their behaviour both under laboratory conditions and in their natural habitat. There seemed every reason to consider aspects of human behaviour in exactly the same way that ethologists were studying animal behaviour. Human beings and their behaviour are as much a product of evolution as are monkeys, cats and their behaviour. The science of ethology stimulated new and interesting answers to the old questions about why and how human infants become attached to certain adults. In fact, 'The distinguishing characteristic of the theory of attachment that we have jointly developed,' write Ainsworth and Bowlby (1991: 333), 'is that it is an ethological approach to personality development.'

Lorenz was showing how newly hatched geese followed their mother and became anxious if they lost sight of her. Harlow was experimenting with monkeys, discovering that under laboratory conditions infant primates preferred to spend most of their day clinging to a surrogate monkey covered in soft, furry towelling even though 'she' did not provide any milk. The surrogate wire-mesh monkey that did provide milk was only visited when the baby was hungry. It seemed that there was a biological need to relate to a mother-figure whether or not she supplied food.

These observations appeared to demonstrate that attachment behaviour is not derived from other primary behaviours such as feeding. 'Geese demonstrate bonding without feeding; rhesus monkeys show feeding without bonding. Thus, argues Bowlby, we must postulate an attachment system unrelated to feeding, which, adopting a biological approach from which psychoanalysis had increasingly become divorced, makes sound evolutionary sense' (Holmes 1993: 64). Attachment, as a class of behaviours, is therefore conceived as distinct from feeding behaviour and sexual behaviour and remains highly significant throughout life (Bowlby 1991: 305).

Attachment behaviour

Attachment behaviour becomes activated when an individual experiences stress. Stress is felt when the individual (i) has pressing physical needs (hunger, pain, illness, fatigue); (ii) is subject to environmental threats (a frightening event or attack): or (iii) experiences a relationship problem (long-term separation from attachment figure or rejection by attachment figure) (Simpson and Rholes 1994: 185). Three basic characteristics are associated with attachment behaviour (Weiss 1991: 66):

1   *Proximity seeking.* The child will attempt to remain within protective range of his parents. The protective range is reduced in strange threatening situations.
2   *Secure base effect.* The presence of an attachment figure fosters security in the child. This results in inattention to attachment considerations and encourages confident exploration and play.
3   *Separation protest.* Threat to the continued accessibility of the attachment figure gives rise to protest and to active attempts to ward off the separation.

Many developmental psychologists believe that babies are biologically programmed to become psychologically *attached* to their parents or other significant caretakers. Many also believe that parents, too, are biologically predisposed to *bond* with their child although the instinctual drive here is much less predictable and is often modified by the parent's own attachment experience. Furthermore, women are more likely, through evolutionary pressures and necessity, to show a biological aptitude for bonding and forming close, co-operative relationships (Ainsworth 1991: 35).

Premature birth involving the mother's immediate separation from her baby interferes with the natural expression of maternal responsiveness (Klaus and Kennel 1982). There is some evidence that a mother's ability to bond quickly with her baby is upset if the infant is immediately removed, for whatever reason. And although most adoptive mothers show maternal behaviour from the start, they report that it takes several weeks for full motivation and responsiveness to become established with their baby.

Lack of attachment relationships means that children's physical and psychological needs are less likely to be met. Evolution has therefore contrived to ensure that the inclination to form attachment relationships, along with sexual behaviour, eating behaviour and exploratory behaviour, is built into our natural make-up. 'To leave their development solely to the caprices of individual learning,' exclaims Bowlby (1988: 5), 'would be the height of biological folly.' And although most researchers have concentrated on the mother–child relationship as the axis along which attachment behaviour might be observed and assessed, there is increasing recognition that babies possess a general biological predisposition to relate with other human beings and that a selective attachment might preferentially develop with, say, a father or grandparent if the mother is emotionally or physically unavailable (Nash and Hay 1993).

A secure base

Attachment – along with the seeking of food, fear and wariness, sociability and the exploration of new experiences – is one of a number of genetically based behaviours designed to engage the infant with the social and physical world whilst at the same time ensuring his or her safety. Attachment behaviour is triggered not by internal physiological needs, but by external threats and dangers. Attachment's prime biological function is to ensure that the vulnerable infant seeks protection when it feels anxious. In evolutionary terms this makes perfect sense. When anxiety levels are low, the infant is free to let his or her attention wander elsewhere, and in the case of older babies, the child can physically leave the mother's immediate vicinity and *explore* the environment of other people and things. The relaxed child can concentrate on exploring and learning about how things look, work and react. In Ainsworth's terms, the mother to whom the child is attached provides a *secure base*: a place of safety, comfort and warmth when anxiety levels rise (Ainsworth and Wittig 1969).

The primary developmental task, therefore, during a child's first year of life is for his or her parents to provide a social environment which promotes feelings of security and trust. Fahlberg (1991: 69) sees parents meeting the child's dependency needs and, quoting Hymes, she advises: 'During the first year when a parent wonders "What should I do when . . .?" the guideline for deciding should be, "What will help my child learn to trust me?"'

During their second year of life, toddlers are beginning to separate from their parents and develop a stronger concept of self. The words *me, mine* and *no* as well as *you* and *me* are prominent in the child's vocabulary. Fahlberg (1991: 74), again quoting Hymes, advises that 'When parents are faced with a "What should I do when . . .?" question about toddlers, the standard for deciding is "What will make my child feel more capable?"'

Exploration of the environment and learning are necessary if the child is to become socially and physically competent, but in situations of threat and danger there comes a point when feelings of adaptive anxiety and the display of attachment behaviour must override the wish to play. Attachment behaviour ensures that the child lives to learn another day. We might say that attachment behaviour and exploratory behaviour are mutually exclusive (Bowlby 1979: 132–3).

In general, young children appear to play and talk more when their mothers are present. Securely attached children who know that there is a secure base to which to return if things get difficult approach new situations with greater confidence. For example, a toddler can leave her mother sitting on a park bench while she plays anywhere up to eighty metres away (Anderson 1972). From time to time the child will return to tell her mother something or receive some physical contact before she runs off again.

The insecurely attached child finds it more difficult to relax, play and explore. If this child runs into difficulties, she is less certain that there is a safe, welcoming, sympathetic and secure base to which to return. She spends more of her energies on keeping a wary eye on what is happening and not on learning about the world of things, people and relationships.

So, if the human infant is to survive physically and become socially competent, it is necessary for him or her to be in close contact with and have access to others who are able to provide both protection as well as useful social experiences. An infant's caretakers must offer the developing child a combination of safety and stimulation. One without the other is not sufficient. If the child receives physical nourishment and protection but does not experience consistent and warm dealings with other people who also offer conversation, interest and understanding, then the child grows physically but not socially, emotionally or linguistically. He or she will not be able to cope adequately with the everyday demands of social life.

To this extent, attachment is a biological mechanism which helps ensure that the infant survives into adulthood so that he or she can, in turn, have children and so perpetuate the species. When a child is threatened, experiences uncertainty, is tired or feels upset, the level of anxiety rises, particularly if the child is some distance from his or her parents. Anxiety activates attachment behaviour and the infant seeks his or her attachment figure for safety and comfort. Rutter and Rutter (1993: 114) note that even when a child is punished or mal-treated by a parent, there is still the inclination to cling to and show attachment towards that person if there is no-one else available.

Loss and separation anxiety

Anxiety is at root an adaptive evolutionary response. It must also be emphasised that attachment is *not* the same as dependency. Indeed, the more securely attached a child feels the greater confidence and autonomy he or she displays throughout childhood. When we are feeling anxious or distressed, we tend to make particular demands on those relationships which are important to us. Although the frequency and intensity of attachment behaviour usually decreases with age, it still plays a part throughout the life cycle. It is particularly likely to appear when we feel distressed, afraid or ill.

Throughout his writings, Bowlby was keen to emphasise the importance of loss and separation in understanding people's pain, anger and depression. Whereas loss and separation increase feelings of vulnerability and fear, grief requires expression and acknowledgement. Whenever a love relationship breaks down or is lost, we experience separation anxiety and grief (Bowlby 1973). The way other people react to those who have experienced a loss is important to the success of the grieving process. Any significant disruption in a meaningful relationship is experienced as a loss. We see it in its simplest and perhaps most direct form in young children who are separated from their prime caregiver.

In his studies with James Robertson, Bowlby observed the effects of temporary separation on young children who were admitted to hospital or residential nursery. The research was carried out in the days when hospitalised children did not see their parents and were looked after by a rota of nurses.

The researchers recognised three phases in the child's reactions to the separation: (i) protest, (ii) withdrawal, and (iii) detachment. Immediate separation from the parents resulted in unconsolable crying. There would be a general restlessness with regression to more babyish behaviours, including loss of bladder control. This was followed by a phase of apathy and listlessness with the young child showing no interest in anything or anybody. The final stage, after a few days or sometimes weeks, saw some settling down, recovery and a return to play but relationships remained shallow and uncommitted.

Upon reunion with their parents, the children exhibited a mixture of extreme clinging, crying, anger and even temporary rejection in which the parent would be ignored. If the period in hospital was not too long, these effects were not prolonged and the child would return to normal levels of behaviour.

This separation and loss sequence was seen to be the direct corollary of attachment behaviour. The loss of an attachment figure represents a double blow. Having lost the mother or caregiver, the child feels insecure. Feeling insecure normally activates attachment behaviour and a return to the attachment figure, but she, of course, is not available. This is a particularly distressing experience. The combination of separation from the key attachment figure *and* a lack of personalised caregiving during the separation produce the greatest upset (Rutter and Rutter 1993: 127).

If it is also remembered that the young child's personality and emerging sense of self form within relationships, it will be appreciated that any disruption to that relationship is not simply just a loss but a threat to the integrity of the self. This has major implications for children placed with new caregivers, including adopters or foster parents. They need to understand that they are dealing with a young personality that was still in the process of forming within the now disrupted attachment relationship.

References

Ainsworth, M.D.S. (1991) 'Attachments and other affectional bonds across the life cycle', in C.M. Parkes, J. Stevenson-Hinde and P. Marris (eds) *Attachment across the Life Cycle*, London: Tavistock/Routledge, 33–51.

Ainsworth, M.D.S. and Bowlby, J. (1991) 'An ethological approach to personality development', *American Psychologist*, April: 333–41.

Ainsworth, M.D.S. and Wittig, B. (1969) 'Attachment and exploratory behaviour of one year olds in a strange situation', in B.M. Foss (ed.) *Determinants of Infant Behaviour, Volume 4*, New York: Wiley, 111–36.

Anderson, J. (1972) 'Attachment out of doors', in N. Blurton-Jones (ed.) *Ethological Studies of Child Behaviour*, Cambridge: Cambridge University Press.

Bowlby, J. (1951) *Maternal Care and Maternal Health*, Geneva: World Health Organization.

—— (1969) *Attachment and Loss, Volume 1: Attachment*, London: Hogarth Press.

—— (1973) *Attachment and Loss, Volume 2: Separation, Anxiety and Anger*, London: Hogarth Press.

—— (1979) *The Making and Breaking of Affectional Bonds*, London: Tavistock.

—— (1988) *A Secure Base: Clinical Applications of Attachment Theory*, London: Routledge.

—— (1991) 'Postscript', in C.M. Parkes, J. Stevenson-Hinde and Marris (eds) *Attachment across the Life Cycle*, London: Tavistock/Routledge, 293–7.

Fahlberg, V.I. (1991) *A Child's Journey through Placement*, Indianapolis, IN: Perspectives Press.

Holmes, J. (1993) *John Bowlby and Attachment Theory*, London: Routledge.

Klaus, M.H. and Kennel, J.H. (1982) *Maternal–Infant Bonding*, 2nd edition, St Louis, MI: Mosby.

Nash, A. and Hay, D.F. (1993) 'Relationships in infancy as precursors and causes of later relationships and psychopathology', in D.F. Hay and A. Angold (eds) *Precursors and Causes in Development and Psychopathology*, Chichester: John Wiley, 198–232.

Rutter, M. (1981) *Maternal Deprivation Reassessed,* 2nd edition, Harmondsworth: Penguin.

—— (1991) 'A fresh look at maternal deprivation', in P. Bateson (ed.) *The Development and Integration of Behaviour*, Cambridge: Cambridge University Press, 331–76.

Rutter, M. and Rutter, M. (1993) *Developing Minds: Challenge and Continuity across the Life Span*, Harmondsworth: Penguin.

Simpson, J.A. and Rholes, W.S. (1994) 'Stress and secure base relationships in adulthood', in K. Bartholomew and D. Perlman (eds) *Attachment Processes in Adulthood, Volume 5: Advances in Personal Relationships*, London: Jessica Kingsley, 181–204.

Weiss, R.S. (1991) 'The attachment bond in childhood and adulthood', in C.M. Parkes, J. Stevenson-Hinde and Marris (eds) *Attachment across the Life Cycle*, London: Tavistock/ Routledge, 66–76.

Further reading

Howe, D., Brandon, M., Hinings, D. and Schofield, G. (1999) *Attachment Theory, Child Maltreatment and Family Support: A Practice and Assessment Model*, Basingstoke: Palgrave.

Mooney, G.C. (2009) *Theories of Attachment: An Introduction to Bowlby, Ainsworth, Gerber, Brazelton, Kennell, and Klause*, St Paul, MN: Redleaf Press.

Prior, V. and Glaser, D. (2006) *Understanding Attachment and Attachment Disorders: Theory, Evidence and Practice*, London: Jessica Kingsley.

11 On death and dying

Elisabeth Kubler-Ross

Elisabeth Kubler-Ross (1926–2004), a Swiss-born psychiatrist who spent most of her life working with dying and bereaved people in the United States, has had a major influence on the knowledge which underpins social work practice. She observed that dying people went through five stages of adjustment, not necessarily in sequence, and sometimes at the same point in time. Her ideas continue to be helpful in understanding reactions to loss and change of all kinds, not just those associated with death and dying. The extract is heavily edited, omitting all practice examples. Please go to the original to get much more flavour of Kubler-Ross's rich understanding of people at a time of change.

From *On Death and Dying*, London: Tavistock (1970): 37–123.

First stage: Denial and isolation

. . . , the patient's first reaction may be a temporary state of shock from which he recuperates gradually. When his initial feeling of numbness begins to disappear and he can collect himself again, man's usual response is 'No, it cannot be me.' Since in our unconscious mind we are all immortal, it is almost inconceivable for us to acknowledge that we too have to face death. Depending very much on how a patient is told, how much time he has to gradually acknowledge the inevitable happening, and how he has been prepared throughout life to cope with stressful situations, he will gradually drop his denial and use less radical defense mechanisms.

We have also found that many of our patients have used denial when faced with hospital staff members who had to use this form of coping for their own reasons. Such patients can be quite elective in choosing different people among family members or staff with whom they discuss matters of their illness or impending death while pretending to get well with those who cannot tolerate the thought of their demise. It is possible that this is the reason for the discrepancy of opinions in regard of the patient's needs to know about a fatal illness.

Second stage: Anger

If our first reaction to catastrophic news is, 'No, it's not true, no, it cannot involve me,' this has to give way to a new reaction, when it finally dawns on us: 'Oh, yes, it is me, it was not a mistake.' Fortunately or unfortunately very few patients are able to maintain a make-believe world in which they are healthy and well until they die.

When the first stage of denial cannot be maintained any longer, it is replaced by feelings of anger, rage, envy, and resentment. The logical next question becomes: 'Why me?' As one of our patients, Dr. G., put it, 'I suppose most anybody in my position would look at somebody else and say, "Well, why couldn't it have been him?" and this has crossed my mind several times. . . . An old man whom I have known ever since I was a little kid came down the street. He was eighty-two years old, and he is of no earthly use as far as we mortals can tell. He's rheumatic, he's a cripple, he's dirty, just not the type of a person you would like to be. And the thought hit me strongly, now why couldn't it have been old George instead of me?'

In contrast to the stage of denial, this stage of anger is very difficult to cope with from the point of view of family and staff. The reason for this is the fact that this anger is displaced in all directions and projected onto the environment at times almost at random. The doctors are just no good, they don't know what tests to require and what diet to prescribe. They keep the patients too long in the hospital or don't respect their wishes in regards to special privileges. They allow a miserably sick roommate to be brought into their room when they pay so much money for some privacy and rest, etc. The nurses are even more often a target of their anger. Whatever they touch is not right. The moment they have left the room, the bell rings. The light is on the very minute they start their report for the next shifts of nurses. When they do shake the pillows and straighten out the bed, they are blamed for never leaving the patients alone. When they do leave the patients alone, the light goes on with the request to have the bed arranged more comfortably. The visiting family is received with little cheerfulness and anticipation, which makes the encounter a painful event. They then either respond with grief and tears, guilt or shame, or avoid future visits, which only increases the patient's discomfort and anger.

The problem here is that few people place themselves in the patient's position and wonder where this anger might come from. Maybe we too would be angry if all our life activities were interrupted so prematurely; if all the buildings we started were to go unfinished, to be completed by someone else; if we had put some hard-earned money aside to enjoy a few years of rest and enjoyment, for travel and pursuing hobbies, only to be confronted with the fact that 'this is not for me.' What else would we do with our anger, but let it out on the people who are most likely to enjoy all these things? People who rush busily around only to remind us that we cannot even stand on our two feet anymore. People who order unpleasant tests and prolonged hospitalization with all its limitations, restrictions, and costs, while at the end of the day they can go home and enjoy life. People who tell us to lie still so that the infusion or transfusion does not have to be restarted, when we feel like jumping out of our skin to be doing something in order to know that we are still functioning on some level!

Third stage: Bargaining

The third stage, the stage of bargaining, is less well known but equally helpful to the patient, though only for brief periods of time. If we have been unable to face the sad facts in the first period and have been angry at people and God in the second phase, maybe we can succeed in entering into some sort of an agreement which may postpone the inevitable happening: 'If God has decided to take us from this earth and he did not respond to my angry pleas, he may be more favorable if I ask nicely.' We are all familiar with this reaction when we observe our children first demanding, then asking for a favor. They may not accept our 'No' when they want to spend a night in a friend's house. They may be angry and stamp their foot. They may lock themselves in their bedroom and temporarily express their anger by rejecting us. But they will also have second thoughts. They may consider another approach. They will come out eventually, volunteer to do some tasks around the house, which under normal circumstances we never succeeded in getting them to do, and then tell us, 'If I am very good all week and wash the dishes every evening, then will you let me go?' There is a slight chance naturally that we will accept the bargain and the child will get what was previously denied.

The terminally ill patient uses the same maneuvers. He knows, from past experiences, that there is a slim chance that he may be rewarded for good behavior and be granted a wish for special services. His wish is most always an extension of life, followed by the wish for a few days without pain or physical discomfort. A patient who was an opera singer, with a distorting malignancy of her jaw and face who could no longer perform on the stage, asked 'to perform just one more time.' When she became aware that this was impossible, she gave the most touching performance perhaps of her life-time. She asked to come to the seminar and to speak in front of the audience, not behind a one-way mirror. She unfolded her life story, her success, and her tragedy in front of the class until a telephone call summoned her to return to her room. Doctor and dentist were ready to pull all her teeth in order to proceed with the radiation treatment. She had asked to sing once more – to us – before she had to hide her face forever.

Another patient was in utmost pain and discomfort, unable to go home because of her dependence on injections for pain relief. She had a son who proceeded with his plans to get married, as the patient had wished. She was very sad to think that she would be unable to attend this big day, for he was her oldest and favorite child. With combined efforts, we were able to teach her self-hypnosis which enabled her to be quite comfortable for several hours. She had made all sorts of promises if she could only live long enough to attend this marriage. The day preceding the wedding she left the hospital as an elegant lady. Nobody would have believed her real condition. She was 'the happiest person in the whole world' and looked radiant. I wondered what her reaction would be when the time was up for which she had bargained.

The bargaining is really an attempt to postpone; it has to include a prize offered 'for good behavior,' it also sets a self-imposed 'deadline' (e.g., one more performance, the son's wedding), and it includes an implicit promise that the patient will not ask for more if this one postponement is granted. None of our patients have 'kept their promise'; in other words, they are like children who say, 'I will never fight my sister again if you let me go.' Needless to add, the little boy will fight his sister again, just as the opera singer will try to perform once more.

Most bargains are made with God and are usually kept a secret or mentioned between the lines or in a chaplain's private office. In our individual interviews without an audience we have been impressed by the number of patients who promise 'a life dedicated to God' or 'a life in the service of the church' in exchange for some additional time. Many of our patients also promised to give parts of or their whole body 'to science' (if the doctors use their knowledge of science to extend their life).

Fourth stage: Depression

When the terminally ill patient can no longer deny his illness, when he is forced to undergo more surgery or hospitalization, when he begins to have more symptoms or becomes weaker and thinner, he cannot smile it off anymore. His numbness or stoicism, his anger and rage will soon be replaced with a sense of great loss. This loss may have many facets: a woman with a breast cancer may react to the loss of her figure; a woman with a cancer of the uterus may feel that she is no longer a woman. Our opera singer responded to the required surgery of her face and the removal of her teeth with shock, dismay, and the deepest depression. But this is only one of the many losses that such a patient has to endure.

All these reasons for depressions are well known to everybody who deals with patients. What we often tend to forget, however, is the preparatory grief that the terminally ill patient has to undergo in order to prepare himself for his final separation from this world. If I were to attempt to differentiate these two kinds of depressions, I would regard the first one a reactive depression, the second one a preparatory depression. The first one is different in nature and should be dealt with quite differently from the latter.

The second type of depression is one which does not occur as a result of a past loss but is taking into account impending losses. Our initial reaction to sad people is usually to try to cheer them up, to tell them not to look at things so grimly or so hopelessly. We encourage them to look at the bright side of life, at all the colorful, positive things around them. This is often an expression of our own needs, our own inability to tolerate a long face over any extended period of time. This can be a useful approach when dealing with the first type of depression in terminally ill patients. It will help such a mother to know that the children play quite happily in the neighbor's garden since they stay there while their father is at work. It may help a mother to know that they continue to laugh and joke, go to parties, and bring good report cards home from school – all expressions that they function in spite of mother's absence.

When the depression is a tool to prepare for the impending loss of all the love objects, in order to facilitate the state of acceptance, then encouragements and reassurances are not as meaningful. The patient should not be encouraged to look at the sunny side of things, as this would mean he should not contemplate his impending death. It would be contraindicated to tell him not to be sad, since all of us are tremendously sad when we lose one beloved person. The patient is in the process of losing everything and everybody he loves. If he is allowed to express his sorrow he will find a final acceptance much easier, and he will be grateful to those who can sit with him during this stage of depression without constantly telling him not to be sad. This second type of depression is usually a silent one in contrast to the first type, during which the patient has much to share and requires many verbal interactions and often active interventions on the part of people in many disciplines. In the preparatory grief there is no or little need for words. It is much more a feeling that can be mutually expressed and is often done better with a touch of a hand, a stroking of the hair, or just a silent sitting together. This is the time when the patient may just ask for a prayer, when he begins to occupy himself with things ahead rather than behind. It is a time when too much interference from visitors who try to cheer him up hinders his emotional preparation rather than enhances it.

Fifth stage: Acceptance

If a patient has had enough time (i.e., not a sudden, unexpected death) and has been given some help in working through the previously described stages, he will reach a stage during which he is neither depressed nor angry about his 'fate.' He will have been able to express his previous feelings, his envy for the living and the healthy, his anger at those who do not have to face their end so soon. He will have mourned the impending loss of so many meaningful people and places and he will contemplate his coming end with a certain degree of quiet expectation. He will be tired and, in most cases, quite weak. He will also have a need to doze off or to sleep often and in brief intervals, which is different from the need to sleep during the times of depression. This is not a sleep of avoidance or a period of rest to get relief from pain, discomfort, or itching. It is a gradually increasing need to extend the hours of sleep very similar to that of the newborn child but in reverse order. It is not a resigned and hopeless 'giving up,' a sense of 'what's the use' or 'I just cannot fight it any longer,' though we hear such statements too. (They also indicate the beginning of the end of the struggle, but the latter are not indications of acceptance.)

Acceptance should not be mistaken for a happy stage. It is almost void of feelings. It is as if the pain had gone, the struggle is over, and there comes a time for 'the final rest before the long journey' as one patient phrased it. This is also the time during which the family needs usually more help, understanding, and support than the patient himself. While the dying patient has found some peace and acceptance, his circle of interest diminishes. He wishes to be left alone or at least not stirred up by news and problems of the outside world. Visitors are often not desired and if they come, the patient is no longer in a talkative mood. He often requests limitation on the number of people and prefers short visits. This is the time when the television is off. Our communications then become more nonverbal than verbal. The patient may just make a gesture of the hand to invite us to sit down for a while. He may just hold our hand and ask us to sit in silence. Such moments of silence may be the most meaningful communications for people who are not uncomfortable in the presence of a dying person. We may together listen to the song of a bird from the outside. Our presence may just confirm that we are going to be around until the end. We may just let him know that it is all right to say nothing when the important things are taken care of and it is only a question of time until he can close his eyes forever. It may reassure him that he is not left alone when he is no longer talking and a pressure of the hand, a look, a leaning back in the pillows may say more than many 'noisy' words.

There are a few patients who fight to the end, who struggle and keep a hope that makes it almost impossible to reach this stage of acceptance. They are the ones who will say one day, 'I just cannot make it anymore,' the day they stop fighting, the fight is over. In other words, the harder they struggle to avoid the inevitable death, the more they try to deny it, the more difficult it will be for them to reach this final stage of acceptance with peace and dignity. The family and staff may consider these patients tough and strong, they may encourage the fight for life to the end, and they may implicitly communicate that accepting one's end is regarded as a cowardly giving up, as a deceit or, worse yet, a rejection of the family.

Hope

We have discussed so far the different stages that people go through when they are faced with tragic news – defense mechanisms in psychiatric terms, coping mechanisms to deal with extremely difficult situations. These means will last for different periods of time and will replace each other or exist at times side by side.

In listening to our terminally ill patients we were always impressed that even the most accepting, the most realistic patients left the possibility open for some cure, for the discovery of a new drug or the 'last-minute success in a research project,' as Mr. J. expressed it. It is this glimpse of hope which maintains them through days, weeks, or months of suffering. It is the feeling that all this must have some meaning, will pay off eventually if they can only endure it for a little while longer. It is the hope that occasionally sneaks in, that all this is just like a nightmare and not true; that they will wake up one morning to be told that the doctors are ready to try out a new drug which seems promising, that they will use it on him and that he may be the chosen, special patient, just as the first heart transplant patient must have felt that he was chosen to play a very special role in life. It gives the terminally ill a sense of a special mission in life which helps them maintain their spirits, will enable them to endure-more tests when everything becomes such a strain – in a sense it is a rationalization for their suffering at times; for others it remains a form of temporary but needed denial.

No matter what we call it, we found that all our patients maintained a little bit of it and were nourished by it in especially difficult times. They showed the greatest confidence in the doctors who allowed for such hope – realistic or not – and appreciated it when hope was offered in spite of bad news. This does not mean that doctors have to tell them a lie; it merely means that we share with them the hope that something unforeseen may happen, that they may have a remission, that they will live longer than is expected. If a patient stops expressing hope, it is usually a sign of imminent death.

Further reading

Machin, L. (2008) *Working with Loss and Grief: A New Model for Practitioners*, London: Sage.

Marris, P. (1986) *Loss and Change*, revised edition, London: Routledge & Kegan Paul.

Parkes, C.M. (1996) *Bereavement: Studies of Grief in Adult Life*, 3rd edition, London: Routledge.

Parkes, C.M. and Markus, A. (eds) (1998) *Coping with Loss: Helping Patients and their Families*, London: BMJ.

Weinstein, J.A. (2007) *Working with Loss, Death and Bereavement: A Guide for Social Workers*, London: Sage.

Weston, R., Martin, T. and Anderson, Y. (eds) (1998) *Loss and Bereavement: Managing Change*, Oxford: Blackwell Science.

Wimpenny, P. and Costello, J. (2010) *Grief, Loss and Bereavement Care*, London: Routledge.

12 Parent, adult and child

Thomas A. Harris

Unlike those of the two previous chapters, this book is not currently part of social work's usual canon of literature. Nevertheless, I believe that the ideas in it deserve a revisiting, because it is a book which literally changed the way I thought about the world, and I would like to share this 'light-bulb' moment with others. The book is now out of print but, as the extract shows, it has within it wisdom about human beings and about our relationships with others, developed from an interactionist approach to psychology (also called transactional analysis, or TA). Thomas A. Harris (1910–1995) was a psychiatrist, originally from Texas in the Unites States. He is widely acknowledged as having simplified TA for a popular audience. The chosen extract introduces some of the fundamental ideas in TA.

From *I'm OK – You're OK*, London: Pan Books (1973): 16–34.

Early in his work in the development of Transactional Analysis, Berne observed that as you watch and listen to people you can see them change before your eyes. It is a total kind of change. There are simultaneous changes in facial expression, vocabulary, gestures, posture, and body functions, which may cause the face to flush, the heart to pound, or the breathing to become rapid.

Continual observation has supported the assumption that . . . three states exist in all people. It is as if in each person there is the same little person he was when he was three years old. There are also within him his own parents. These are recordings in the brain of actual experiences of internal and external events, the most significant of which happened during the first five years of life. There is a third state, different from these two. The first two are called Parent and Child, and the third, Adult. (See Figure 12.1.)

These states of being are not roles but psychological realities. Berne says that 'Parent, Adult, and Child are not concepts like Superego, Ego, and Id . . . but phenomenological realities' (Berne, 1961, 24). The state is produced by the playback of recorded data of events in the past, involving real people, real times, real places, real decisions, and real feelings.

The Parent

The Parent is a huge collection of recordings in the brain of unquestioned or imposed external events perceived by a person in his early years, a period which we have designated roughly as the first five years of life. This is the period before the social birth

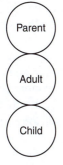

Figure 12.1 The Personality.

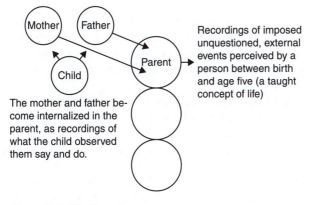

Figure 12.2 The Parent.

of the individual, before he leaves home in response to the demands of society and enters school. (See Figure 12.2.) The name Parent is most descriptive of this data inasmuch as the most significant 'tapes' are those provided by the example and pronouncements of his own real parents or parent substitutes. Everything the child saw his parents do and everything he heard them say is recorded in the Parent. Everyone has a Parent in that everyone experienced external stimuli in the first five years of life. Parent is specific for every person, being the recording of that set of early experiences unique to him.

The data in the Parent was taken in and recorded 'straight' without editing. The situation of the little child, his dependency, and his inability to construct meanings with words made it impossible for him to modify, correct, or explain. Therefore, if the parents were hostile and constantly battling each other, a fight was recorded with the terror produced by seeing the two persons on whom the child depended for survival about to destroy each other. There was no way of including in this recording the fact that the father was inebriated because his business had just gone down the drain or that the mother was at her wits' end because she had just found she was pregnant again.

In the Parent are recorded all the admonitions and rules and laws that the child heard from his parents and saw in their living. They range all the way from the earliest parental communications, interpreted nonverbally through tone of voice, facial expression, cuddling, or noncuddling, to the more elaborate verbal rules and regulations espoused by the parents as the little person became able to understand words. In this set of recordings are the thousands of 'no's' directed at the toddler, the repeated 'don'ts' that bombarded him, the looks of pain and horror in mother's face when his clumsiness brought shame on the family in the form of Aunt Ethel's broken antique vase.

Likewise are recorded the coos of pleasure of a happy mother and the looks of delight of a proud father. When we consider that the recorder is on all the time we begin to comprehend the immense amount of data in the Parent. Later come the more complicated pronouncements: Remember, Son, wherever you go in the world you will always find the best people are Methodists; never tell a lie; pay your bills; you are judged by the company you keep; you are a good boy if you clean your plate; waste is the original sin; you can never trust a man; you can never trust a woman; you're damned if you do and damned if you don't; you can never trust a cop; busy hands are happy hands; don't walk under ladders; do unto others as you would have them do unto you; do others in that they don't do you in.

The significant point is that whether these rules are good or bad in the light of a reasonable ethic, they are recorded as *truth* from the source of all security, the people who are 'six feet tall' at a time when it is important to the two-foot-tall child that he please and obey them. It is a permanent recording. A person cannot erase it. It is available for replay throughout life.

This replay is a powerful influence throughout life. These examples – coercing, forcing, sometimes permissive but more often restrictive – are rigidly internalized as a voluminous set of data essential to the individual's survival in the setting of a group, beginning with the family and extending throughout life in a succession of groups necessary to life.

Another characteristic of the Parent is the fidelity of the recordings of inconsistency. Parents say one thing and do another. Parents say, 'Don't lie,' but tell lies. They tell children that smoking is bad for their health but smoke themselves. They proclaim adherence to a religious ethic but do not live by it. It is not safe for the little child to question this inconsistency, and so he is confused. Because this data causes confusion and fear, he defends himself by turning off the recording.

Much Parent data appears in current living in the 'how-to' category: how to hit a nail, how to make a bed, how to eat soup, how to blow your nose, how to thank the hostess, how to shake hands, how to pretend no one's at home, how to fold the bath towels, or how to dress the Christmas tree. The *how to* comprises a vast body of data acquired by watching the parents. It is largely useful data which makes it possible for the little person to learn to get along by himself. Later (as his Adult becomes more skilful and free to examine Parent data) these early ways of doing things may be updated and replaced by better ways that are more suited to a changed reality. A person whose early instructions were accompanied by stern intensity may find it more difficult to examine the old ways and may hang on to them long after they are useful, having developed a compulsion to do it 'this way and no other'.

When we realize that thousands of these simple rules of living are recorded in the brain of every person, we begin to appreciate what a comprehensive vast store of data the Parent includes. Many of these edicts are fortified with such additional imperatives as 'never' and 'always' and 'never forget that' and, we may assume, pre-empt certain primary neurone pathways that supply ready data for today's transactions. These rules are the origins of compulsions and quirks and eccentricities that appear in later behaviour. Whether Parent data is a burden or a boon depends on how appropriate it is to the present, on whether or not it has been updated by the Adult, the function of which we shall discuss in this chapter.

There are sources of Parent data other than the physical parents. A three-year-old who sits before a television set many hours a day is recording what he sees. The programmes he watches are a 'taught' concept of life. If he watches programmes of violence, I believe he records violence in his Parent. That's how it is. That is life! This conclusion is certain if his parents do not express opposition by switching the channel. If they enjoy violent programmes the youngster gets a double sanction – the set and the folks – and he assumes permission to be violent provided he collects the required amount of injustices. The little person collects his own reasons to shoot up the place, just as the sheriff does; three nights of cattle rustlers, a stage holdup, and a stranger foolin' with Miss Kitty can be easily matched in the life of the little person. Much of what is experienced at the hands of older siblings or other authority figures also is recorded in the Parent. Any external situation in which the little person feels himself to be dependent to the extent that he is not free to question or to explore produces data which is stored in the Parent. (There is another type of external experience of the very small child which is not recorded in the Parent, and which we shall examine when we describe the Adult.)

The Child

While external events are being recorded as that body of data we call the Parent, there is another recording being made simultaneously. This is the recording of *internal* events, the responses of the little person to what he sees and hears. (Figure 12.3.)

It is this 'seeing and hearing and feeling and understanding' body of data which we define as the Child. Since the little person has no vocabulary during the most critical of his early experiences, most of his reactions are *feelings*. We must keep in mind his situation in these early years. He is small, he is dependent, he is inept, he is clumsy, he has no words with which to construct meanings. Emerson said we 'must know how to estimate a sour look'. The child does not know how to do this. A sour look turned in his direction can only produce feelings that add to his reservoir of negative data about himself. *It's my fault. Again. Always is. Ever will be. World without end.*

During this time of helplessness there are an infinite number of total and uncompromising demands on the child. On the one hand, he has the urges (genetic recordings) to empty his bowels ad lib., to explore, to know, to crush and to bang, to

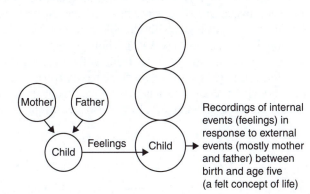

Figure 12.3 The Child.

express feelings, and to experience all of the pleasant sensations associated with move-ment and discovery. On the other hand, there is the constant demand from the environment, essentially the parents, that he give up these basic satisfactions for the reward of parental approval. This approval, which can disappear as fast as it appears, is an unfathomable mystery to the child, who has not yet made any certain connexion between cause and effect.

The predominant by-product of the frustrating, civilizing process is negative feelings. On the basis of these feelings the little person early concludes, 'I'm not OK.' We call this comprehensive self-estimate the NOT OK, or the NOT OK Child. This conclusion and the continual experiencing of the unhappy feelings which led to it and confirm it are recorded permanently in the brain and cannot be erased. This permanent recording is the residue of having been a child. Any child. Even the child of kind, loving, well-meaning parents. It is the *situation of childhood* and *not* the intention of the parents which produces the problem.

As in the case of the Parent, the Child is a state into which a person may be trans-ferred at almost any time in his current transactions. There are many things that can happen to us today which recreate the situation of childhood and bring on the same feelings we felt then. Frequently we may find ourselves in situations where we are faced with impossible alternatives, where we find ourselves in a corner, either actually, or in the way we see it. These 'hook the Child', as we say, and cause a replay of the original feelings of frustration, rejection, or abandonment, and we relive a latter-day version of the small child's primary depression. Therefore, when a person is in the grip of feelings, we say his Child has taken over. When his anger dominates his reason, we say his Child is in command.

There is a bright side, too! In the Child is also a vast store of positive data. In the Child reside creativity, curiosity, the desire to explore and know, the urges to touch and feel and experience, and the recordings of the glorious, pristine feelings of first discover-ies. In the Child are recorded the countless, grand *a-ha* experiences, the firsts in the life of the small person, the first drinking from the garden hose, the first stroking of the soft kitten, the first sure hold on mother's nipple, the first time the lights go on in response to his flicking the switch, the first submarine chase of the bar of soap, the repetitious going back to do these glorious things again and again. The feelings of these delights are recorded, too. With all the NOT OK recordings, there is a counterpoint, the rhythmic OK of mother's rocking, the sentient softness of the favourite blanket, a continuing good response to favourable external events (if this is indeed a favoured child), which also is available for replay in today's transactions. This is the flip side, the happy child, the carefree, butterfly-chasing little boy, the little girl with chocolate on her face. This comes on in today's transactions, too. However, our observations both of small children and of ourselves as grownups convince us that the NOT OK feelings far outweigh the good. This is why we believe it is a fair estimate to say that everyone has a NOT OK Child.

If, then, we emerge from childhood with a set of experiences which are recorded in an inerasable Parent and Child, what is our hope for change? How can we get off the hook of the past?

The Adult

At about ten months of age a remarkable thing begins to happen to the child. Until that time his life has consisted mainly of helpless or unthinking responses to the demands and stimulations by those around him. He has had a Parent and a Child. What he has not had is the ability either to choose his responses or to manipulate his surroundings. He has had no self-direction, no ability to move out to meet life. He has simply taken what has come his way.

At ten months, however, he begins to experience the power of locomotion. He can manipulate objects and begins to move out, freeing himself from the prison of immobility. It is true that earlier, as at eight months, the infant may frequently cry and need help in getting out of some awkward position, but he is unable to get out of it by himself. At ten months he concentrates on inspection and exploitation of toys.

The ten-month-old has found he is able to do something which grows from his own awareness and original thought. This self-actualization is the beginning of the Adult. (Figure 12.4.) Adult data accumulates as a result of the child's ability to find out for himself what is different about life from the 'taught concept' of life in his Parent and the 'felt concept' of life in his Child. The Adult develops a 'thought concept' of life based on data gathering and data processing.

The motility which gives birth to the Adult becomes reassuring in later life when a person is in distress. He goes for a walk to 'clear his mind'. Pacing is seen similarly as a relief from anxiety. There is a recording that movement is good, that it has a separating quality, that it helps him see more clearly what his problem is.

The Adult, during these early years, is fragile and tentative. It is easily 'knocked out' by commands from the Parent and fear in the Child. Mother says about the crystal goblet, 'No, no! Don't touch that!' The child may pull back and cry, but at the first opportunity he will touch it anyway to see what it is all about. In most persons the Adult, despite all the obstacles thrown in its way, survives and continues to function more and more effectively as the maturation process goes on.

The Adult is 'principally concerned with transforming stimuli into pieces of information, and processing and filing that information on the basis of previous experience' (Berne, 1961). It is different from the Parent, which is 'judgemental in an imitative way and seeks to enforce sets of borrowed standards, and from the Child, which tends to react more abruptly on the basis of prelogical thinking and poorly differentiated or distorted perceptions'. Through the Adult the little person can begin to tell the difference between life as it was taught and demonstrated to him (Parent), life as he felt it or wished it or fantasied it (Child), and life as he figures it out by himself (Adult).

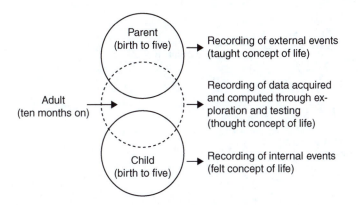

Figure 12.4 Gradual emergence of the Adult beginning at ten months.

The Adult is a data-processing computer, which grinds out decisions after computing the information from three sources: the Parent, the Child, and the data which the Adult has gathered and is gathering (Figure 12.5). One of the important functions of the Adult is to examine the data in the Parent, to see whether or not it is true and still applicable today, and then to accept it or reject it: and to examine the Child to see whether or not the feelings there are appropriate to the present or are archaic and in response to archaic Parent data. The goal is not to do away with the Parent and Child but to be free to examine these bodies of data. The Adult, in the words of Emerson, 'must not be hindered by the name of goodness, but must examine if it be goodness'; or badness, for that matter, as in the early decision, 'I'm not OK'.

    . . . *We cannot erase the recording, but we can choose to turn it off!*

In the same way that the Adult updates Parent data to determine what is valid and what is not, it updates Child data to determine which feelings may be expressed safely. In our society it is considered appropriate for a woman to cry at a wedding, but it is not considered appropriate for that woman to scream at her husband afterwards at the reception. Yet both crying and screaming are emotions in the Child. The Adult keeps emotional expression appropriate. The Adult's function in updating the Parent and Child is diagrammed in Figure 12.6. The Adult within the Adult in this figure refers to updated reality data. (The evidence once told me space travel was only fantasy; now I know it is reality.)

Another of the Adult's functions is *probability estimating*. This function is slow in developing in the small child and, apparently, for most of us, has a hard time catching up throughout life. The little person is constantly confronted with unpleasant alternatives (either you eat your spinach or you go without ice cream), offering little incentive for examining probabilities. Unexamined probabilities can underlie many of our transactional failures, and unexpected danger signals can cause more Adult 'decay', or delay,

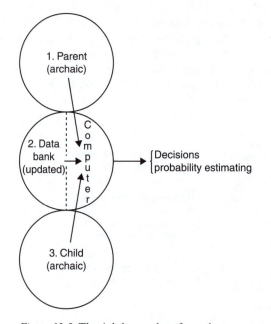

Figure 12.5 The Adult gets data from three sources.

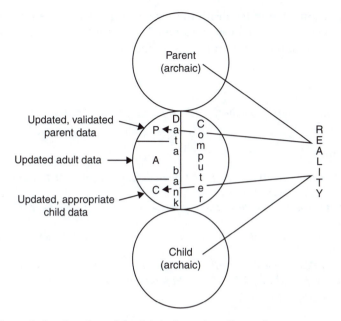

Figure 12.6 The updating function of the Adult through reality testing.

than expected ones. There are similarities here to the stock ticker in investment concerns, which may run many hours behind on very active trading days. We sometimes refer to this delay as 'computer lag', a remedy for which is the old, familiar practice of 'counting to ten'.

The capacity for probability estimating can be increased by conscious effort. Like a muscle in the body, the Adult grows and increases in efficiency through training and use. If the Adult is alert to the possibility of trouble, through probability estimating, it can also devise solutions to meet the trouble if and when it comes.

Under sufficient stress, however, the Adult can be impaired to the point where emotions take over inappropriately. The boundaries between Parent, Adult, and Child are fragile, sometimes indistinct, and vulnerable to those incoming signals which tend to recreate situations we experienced in the helpless, dependent days of childhood. The Adult sometimes is flooded by signals of the 'bad news' variety so overwhelming that the Adult is reduced to an 'onlooker' in the transaction. An individual in this situation might say. 'I knew what I was doing was wrong, but I couldn't help myself.'

The ongoing work of the Adult consists, then, of checking out old data, validating or invalidating it, and refiling it for future use. If this business goes on smoothly and there is a relative absence of conflict between what has been taught and what is real, the computer is free for important new business, *creativity*. Creativity is born from curiosity in the Child, as is the Adult. The Child provides the 'want to' and the Adult provides the 'how to'. The essential requirement for creativity is computer time. If the computer is cluttered with old business there is little time for new business. Once checked out, many Parent directives become automatic and thus free the computer for creativity. Many of our decisions in day-to-day transactions are automatic. For instance, when we see an arrow pointing down a one-way street, we automatically refrain from going the opposite way. We do not involve our computer in lengthy data processing about highway engineering, the traffic death toll, or how signs are painted. Were we to start from scratch in every decision or operate entirely without the data that was supplied by our parents, our computer would rarely have time for the creative process.

References

Berne, E. (1961) *Transactional Analysis in Psychotherapy*, New York: Grove Press.

Further reading

Berger, J. and Luckman, T. (1967) *The Social Construction of Reality: A Treatise in the Sociology of Knowledge*, Harmondsworth: Penguin.
Berne, E. (1968) *Games People Play: The Psychology of Human Relationships*, Harmondsworth: Penguin.
—— (2001) *Transactional Analysis in Psychotherapy: The Classic Handbook to Its Principles*, London: Souvenir Press.
Stewart, I. (2007) *Transactional Analysis Counselling in Action*, 3rd revised edition, London: Sage.
Stewart, I. and Joines, V. (1987) *TA Today: A New Introduction to Transactional Analysis*, Melton Mowbray: Lifespace Publishing

13 The promise

C. Wright Mills

It is my great privilege to introduce the work of C. Wright Mills (1916–1962), the American sociologist who reminds us that the problems which social work often confronts as personal problems (as failings in the individual, their upbringing or their personality) are in fact social problems; their remedies lie in society, and not within individuals or even within families. This is a message which should be remembered throughout social work practice, as we work with individuals and families who are struggling to deal with the impact of poverty, poor housing, educational disadvantage, social exclusion and discrimination of all kinds. *The Sociological Imagination* has been hugely influential on the thinking of generations of sociologists, feminists, radicals, policy-makers and, of course, social workers. The chosen extract is from the first chapter in the book.

From *The Sociological Imagination*, Oxford: Oxford University Press (1959): 8–11.

2

Perhaps the most fruitful distinction with which the sociological imagination works is between 'the personal troubles of milieu' and 'the public issues of social structure.' This distinction is an essential tool of the sociological imagination and a feature of all classic work in social science.

Troubles occur within the character of the individual and within the range of his immediate relations with others; they have to do with his self and with those limited areas of social life of which he is directly and personally aware. Accordingly, the statement and the resolution of troubles properly lie within the individual as a biographical entity and within the scope of his immediate milieu – the social setting that is directly open to his personal experience and to some extent his willful activity. A trouble is a private matter: values cherished by an individual are felt by him to be threatened.

Issues have to do with matters that transcend these local environments of the individual and the range of his inner life. They have to do with the organization of many such milieux into the institutions of an historical society as a whole, with the ways in which various milieux overlap and interpenetrate to form the larger structure of social and historical life. An issue is a public matter: some value cherished by publics is felt to be threatened. Often there is a debate about what that value really is and about what it is that really threatens it. This debate is often without focus if only because it is the very nature of an issue, unlike even widespread trouble, that it cannot very well be defined in terms of the immediate and everyday environments of ordinary men. An issue, in fact, often involves a crisis in institutional arrangements, and often too it involves what Marxists call 'contradictions' or 'antagonisms.'

In these terms, consider unemployment. When, in a city of 100,000, only one man is unemployed, that is his personal trouble, and for its relief we properly look to the character of the man, his skills, and his immediate opportunities. But when in a nation of 50 million employees, 15 million men are unemployed, that is an issue, and we may not hope to find its solution within the range of opportunities open to any one individual. The very structure of opportunities has collapsed. Both the correct statement of the problem and the range of possible solutions require us to consider the economic and political institutions of the society, and not merely the personal situation and character of a scatter of individuals.

Consider war. The personal problem of war, when it occurs, may be how to survive it or how to die in it with honor; how to make money out of it; how to climb into the higher safety of the military apparatus; or how to contribute to the war's termination. In short, according to one's values, to find a set of milieux and within it to survive the war or make one's death in it meaningful. But the structural issues of war have to do with its causes; with what types of men it throws up into command; with its effects upon economic and political, family and religious institutions, with the unorganized irresponsibility of a world of nation-states.

Consider marriage. Inside a marriage a man and a woman may experience personal troubles, but when the divorce rate during the first four years of marriage is 250 out of every 1,000 attempts, this is an indication of a structural issue having to do with the institutions of marriage and the family and other institutions that bear upon them.

Or consider the metropolis – the horrible, beautiful, ugly, magnificent sprawl of the great city. For many upper-class people, the personal solution to 'the problem of the city' is to have an apartment with private garage under it in the heart of the city, and forty miles out, a house by Henry Hill, garden by Garrett Eckbo, on a hundred acres of private land. In these two controlled environments – with a small staff at each end and a private helicopter connection – most people could solve many of the problems of personal milieux caused by the facts of the city. But all this, however splendid, does not solve the public issues that the structural fact of the city poses. What should be done with this wonderful monstrosity? Break it all up into scattered units, combining residence and work? Refurbish it as it stands? Or, after evacuation, dynamite it and build new cities according to new plans in new places? What should those plans be? And who is to decide and to accomplish whatever choice is made? These are structural issues; to confront them and to solve them requires us to consider political and economic issues that affect innumerable milieux.

In so far as an economy is so arranged that slumps occur, the problem of unemployment becomes incapable of personal solution. In so far as war is inherent in the nation-state system and in the uneven industrialization of the world, the ordinary individual in his restricted milieu will be powerless – with or without psychiatric aid – to solve the troubles this system or lack of system imposes upon him. In so far as the family as an institution turns women into darling little slaves and men into their chief providers and unweaned dependents, the problem of a satisfactory marriage remains incapable of purely private solution. In so far as the overdeveloped megalopolis and the overdeveloped automobile are built-in features of the overdeveloped society, the issues of urban living will not be solved by personal ingenuity and private wealth.

What we experience in various and specific milieux, I have noted, is often caused by structural changes. Accordingly, to understand the changes of many personal milieux we are required to look beyond them. And the number and variety of such structural changes increase as the institutions within which we live become more embracing and more intricately connected with one another. To be aware of the idea of social structure and to use it with sensibility is to be capable of tracing such linkages among a great variety of milieux. To be able to do that is to possess the sociological imagination.

Further reading

Becker, S. (1997) *Responding to Poverty: The Politics of Cash and Care*, London: Longman.

Beresford, P., Green, D., Lister, R. and Woodard, K. (2002) 'The effects of poverty', in B. Bytheway, V. Bacigalup, J. Bornat, J. Johnson and S. Spurr (eds) *Understanding Care, Welfare and Community: A Reader*, London: Routledge and Open University, 20–8.

Cree, V.E. (2010) *Sociology for Social Workers and Probation Officers*, 2nd revised edition, London: Routledge.

Davis, A. and Garrett, P.M. (2004) 'Progressive practice for tough times: Social work, poverty and division in the twenty-first century', in M. Lymbery and S. Butler (eds) *Social Work Ideals and Practice Realities*, Basingstoke: Macmillan.

Drakeford, M. (2002) 'Poverty and the social services', in B. Bytheway, V. Bacigalupo, J. Bornat, J. Johnson and S. Spurr (eds) *Understanding Care, Welfare and Community: A Reader*, London: Routledge and Open University Press, 29–37.

Ferguson, I., Lavalette, M. and Mooney, G. (2002) *Rethinking Welfare: A Critical Perspective*, London: Sage.

Holman, B. (1988) *Faith in the Poor*, London: Lion Hudson.

Jordan, B. (1996) *A Theory of Poverty and Social Exclusion*, Cambridge: Polity Press.

Walker, C. and Walker, A. (2009) 'Social policy, poverty and social work', in R. Adams, L. Dominelli and M. Payne (eds) *Social Work: Themes, Issues and Critical Debates*, 3rd edition, London: Palgrave Macmillan, 74–89.

14 Developing anti-discriminatory practice

Neil Thompson

One of the most persistent criticisms targeted at mainstream social work practice in the past and in the present day is that it is too focused on individual problems (see Chapter 13). It is important, therefore, that we now take time to consider the impact of social divisions on individuals and society, and explore how social work might seek to develop an anti-discriminatory and anti-oppressive kind of practice. It should be acknowledged that there is a massive amount of literature which examines each of the social divisions which are touched on only briefly here, as well as a complex and, at times, difficult literature on discrimination and oppression. I have chosen Neil Thompson to introduce this subject because he writes in a straightforward way, and his work offers a useful, basic introduction to the subject. Readers are encouraged to see this as a launch-pad to more advanced texts, as well as taking forward the ideas already explored in the previous chapter. Neil Thomson works as an independent consultant and trainer in social and occupational welfare in the UK.

From D.R. Tomlinson and W. Trew (eds) *Equalising Opportunities, Minimising Oppression: A Critical Review of Anti-discriminatory Policies in Health and Social Welfare*, London: Routledge (2002): 41–54.

What is anti-discriminatory practice?

The basis of anti-discriminatory practice can be understood in terms of a sequence, with each of the following four terms linked to the next one in the 'chain': from diversity to difference through to discrimination and oppression. I shall explain each in turn.

Diversity

I use this term in its quite literal sense to refer to the fact that society is characterised by immence variation. Although there are many similarities and commonalities that can be identified, it remains the case that there are huge differences to be found not only across social groups but also within them. Society reflects this diversity in so far as social groups tend continually to form and reform around aspects of identity they have in common such as: religion or creed; 'community' or identification with a locality; occupation or vocation; and a wide array of leisure and recreational lifestyles. The range of these identities is extensive, and innumerable subtle distinctions can be drawn both between and within the social groups that are formed. Diversity is to be found as much among, say, 'travellers' – people who do not follow sedentary, settled living patterns, as among the 'domiciled' – people who do. It is distinctions such as these that provide a starting point for investigating this topic.

The contemporary emphasis on promoting, affirming or even celebrating diversity – the 'diversity approach', as it has come to be known – is, in part, a recognition of the changes in British culture that are associated with the development of what Rex (1996) has called 'moderate multiculturalism'. As Bonnett (2000) has shown, at other points in history such diversity was construed unequivocally as presenting, in its own right, a threat to political and social unity, to the feeling of togetherness or of national community. By contrast, the emphasis of the promoting diversity approach is that the existence of a diverse population is, in itself, seen as an asset, rather than a problem requiring a solution. Diversity is seen as the basis of a society enriched by the variety of differences across the population. Anti-discriminatory practice therefore involves recognising and promoting the value of diversity.

Difference

Diversity is based on difference – that is, it is the range of differences in society that add up to form the backcloth of diversity. Such differences can be conceptualised in two important ways in relation to diversity. First, difference can be seen in terms of the classic social divisions of class, gender, race, ethnicity, disability, sexual orientation and so on, as well as other less well-documented social categories and boundaries. Second, it can be understood in terms of social reality being in a constant state of flux, such perpetual change reflecting the ways in which people continually adapt to circumstances. That is, a recognition of difference as an important issue involves a move away from 'essentialism' – the view of individuals as fixed and immutable identities. I shall return to this point below.

The notion of difference as an important issue is closely associated with post-structuralist and postmodernist thought in which social differences are recognised as fundamental elements of the social order and the nature of social reality (Stewart, 2001).

Discrimination

The point that should be emphasised here is that, wherever there is difference, there is the potential for discrimination. In its literal sense, the word 'discriminate' means to delineate or identify a difference. That is, to discriminate, in its general sense, is an essential part of social interaction, and indeed of making sense of our lives. While it may seem a simple and obvious point to grasp, it should be made clear that it is therefore a particular type of discrimination that is being specified when we look at anti-discriminatory practice – a quite specific and negative type of unfair, oppressive discrimination. What is in question here, then, are those forms of discrimination that lead to particular individuals and/or groups being discriminated against and thus suffering a disadvantage – or, to use the legal term, a detriment. This is where the fourth term, that of oppression, comes in, as it is through being disadvantaged and discriminated against that people experience oppression.

Oppression

What is at issue here is the range of situations where discrimination takes place in unfair, inappropriate, and destructive ways which have oppressive consequences for the people who are discriminated against. This involves recognising that discrimination is not simply unfair, in a narrow, ethical sense, but also a major source of disadvantage, pain, suffering and degradation – in short, oppression.

It is unfortunately the case that those people who see anti-discriminatory practice as a threat to their own position of power and privilege will often attempt to counter it by deploying the 'positive' aspects of the term discrimination. Thus it will be argued that people are of course different, and are going to be discriminated between and against – that is reality, it is part of human nature. However, this is to oversimplify the relationship between discrimination and oppression.

As Mishra (1995) points out, although, in many senses, the arguments against discrimination on the basis of gender, disability and ethnicity, have been accepted by UK and other European governments, the arguments for equality have not. The acceptance of inequality means that it is considered fair to discriminate against, for example, those who do not fit in with the economic imperative of a flexible labour market because they are unable, or unwilling to be flexible in finding and keeping work – indeed, such discrimination is endorsed. This can lead to a 'naturalising' of social inequality, in which such discrimination is presented as natural and indeed necessary for social and economic stability. It is part of the conservative and liberal traditions of social thought for it to be regarded as legitimate for social groups to engage in discriminatory actions within circumscribed areas, such as work, health and personal relationships, within certain limits, and by legal means (Thompson and Thompson, 1993). The process and act of negative discrimination are masked, and even justified, by the ideology of competitive individualism which supports this oppression and is presented as a positive facet of society.

It is important to note that some commentators, such as Phillipson (1992), make a distinction between anti-discriminatory and anti-oppressive practice, reserving the former for relatively narrow, legalistic approaches to these issues. I regard the two terms as referring to the same thing. Whether attempts are made to stop the discrimination that leads to the oppression, or to deal with the resulting oppression, the primary objective in practice remains broadly the same. One of my concerns is that it is very easy for people who are part of the same anti-oppressive movement to end up fighting each other over terminology. We do, of course have to be clear about what we mean, and so care needs to be taken to present our ideas with as much clarity as possible.

In sum, then, my answer to the question of 'what is anti-discriminatory practice?' is that it is any form of practice that tries to prevent the recognition of difference being used as the basis of unfair discrimination, leading to oppressive consequences for people. The starting point is the recognition of diversity as an asset, a positive advantage rather than a problem, and difference, equally, as something that can bestow benefits. From this point, the legitimate need to discriminate between people can be separated from processes of unfair, unjust or destructive comparison, so that we do not reach the position of oppression.

Unless we take seriously the dangers of unfair discrimination being allowed to lead to oppression, we run the risk of failing in our duty of care, with the possible outcome that our interventions do more harm than good. It is therefore important to have at least a basic grasp of the complexities of making anti-discriminatory practice a reality, and so it is to this that we now turn.

How do we make anti-discriminatory practice a reality?

To address this question, I shall draw on what I refer to as 'PCS analysis' (Thompson, 2001). Put succinctly, PCS analysis is a framework which breaks down the complex issues of discrimination into three separate but inter-related levels: Personal, Cultural and Structural. The basis of PCS analysis is that any approaches to the questions of discrimination and oppression which do not take account of all three of these levels, and their inter-relationships, is in danger of oversimplifying a very complex set of issues. I shall explain, in turn, what is meant by each of the three terms, personal, cultural and structural.

Personal

A key objective of developing a multidimensional approach is to address the problem that so often occurs where people see only the personal aspects of discrimination: a person is seen as being a 'racist', or a 'chauvinist', for example – as if it were simply a matter of personal qualities. Discrimination is very often represented simply as the manifestation of a set of personal prejudices, attitudes of bigotry that are seen as part of the individual's psychological make-up. Of course, for some people, discriminatory views are indeed a significant part of their personal identity – members of extremist racialist organisations, for example. But the limitation of such an approach to the issue of discrimination is that it often leads other people to rely on statements such as: 'I'm not prejudiced, so this is not an issue for me', as if there is nothing more to consider than personal prejudice or personal views on the subject.

The key point is that the cultural and structural levels always operate in tandem with the personal level. Even if racism is not a significant part of a particular individual's persona or attitudes on a personal level, it will nonetheless remain an issue to be addressed at the cultural and structural levels with which we all engage, on a continuous basis, whether or not we are aware of it. We are all part of the networks of shared meanings and discourses that form the cultural level and the networks of power and social standing that form the structural level. Personal prejudice is, therefore, part of the complex web of discrimination, but we should be wary of overestimating its importance and thus underestimating the significance of cultural and structural factors

Cultural

In describing the cultural level, I use culture in an anthropological sense to apply to the entire set of belief systems of a society. That is, I am not confining my idea of culture to that of specific sets of moral beliefs and values. PCS analysis does not relate only to culture in the sense of religious, national or ethnic background. I use the term, rather, to refer to a set of shared meanings, where people use language and imagery in a particular way to produce a 'discourse' – a set of ideas and meanings that come as a package. Embedded within these sets of ideas and meanings are images of what certain groups in society are like, and how they are expected to behave. These images are often inaccurate and carry discriminatory connotations about those that they represent.

Stereotypes are an important feature of the cultural level. Righton (1990) makes a useful distinction between 'typifications' and 'stereotypes' in respect of the images of people that are presented within discourse. A typification is a set of expectations that we have about a person, a group or a thing. As long as these expectations are provisional, and provide us with a guide which we change and update with experience, then our typifications are a helpful means of breaking down the complexity of social reality. But, when we are dealing with a stereotype, on the other hand, problems of discrimination come to the fore. A stereotype is a fixed and unchanging set of expect-ations we hold on to because our sense of personal security may be threatened if they are thrown into question.

One relevant example of a stereotype is that of the 'immigrant community' which figured strongly in the political and cultural discourse of the 1950s and 1960s in Britain (Abbott, 1971). The counterposing of the 'immigrant' to the 'host' commu-nity in language played a key role in defining the status of the respective parties involved. The white majority community was the host, and the black and Asian immigrant, minority communities were the guests. An implication of this termi-nology was that the immigrant did not have a right to belong in the host society and was, rather, a temporary visitor who should not abuse the hospitality offered. The white community was portrayed as 'settled' and characterised by togetherness and belonging. Immigrants, on the other hand, were presented as having problems of adapting to this settled community on account of their different backgrounds and expectations. Divisions within the host community were thus obscured within this discourse.

The 'host community' was, throughout this period, itself highly stratified and characterised by very significant inequalities of wealth, power and status between social classes. As Crompton (1993: 193) comments, all of the various 'heuristic maps' of sociological analysis have identified a 'persisting concentration of economic, organ-isational and political power within an "upper class" which comprises only a small minority of the population'. This 'majority' problem of difference is generally and conveniently forgotten in the discourse of ethnic difference at the cultural level, a tendency which is still apparent even in the more socially 'inclusive' policy which holds at the time of writing (Burden and Hamm, 2000).

Language use is also an important aspect of the cultural level. For example, language is important in reinforcing attitudes to, and beliefs about, older people. Fennell *et al.* (1988: 7) comment that they try, as teachers and writers, to avoid using terms such as 'the elderly', 'geriatrics, 'the elderly mentally infirm', 'the old' or 'the confused'. This is not in an attempt to deny that there are physical and mental changes in old age, but rather 'to try, linguistically, to remind ourselves constantly of human variety in the groups we are categorising and to underline the "people status" (people like us in other words) of elderly people as opposed to the "thing status" (objects inferior to us) of "the elderly"'. Thus they regard 'older people' and 'people in old age' as preferable terms to 'the elderly'.

The use of terminology is very important in constructing social identities as Foucault (1977, 1979) has shown. Language is not an inert container of words that we pick up and use as the occasion demands, but something that is active and dynamic within the social world.

Structural

It is no coincidence that there are so many powerful assumptions, sets of meanings and images operating at the cultural level to reinforce power relations in society. Discrimination operates at that level in terms of institutionalised power relationships. Taking gender and sexism, as one important example, it is recognised that positions of power in organisations are predominantly held by men (Abbott and Wallace, 1997). Equally, in respect of racism, the cultural cues for racial discrimination to take place are associated with the fact that powerful positions in society are overwhelmingly held by white people (Small, 1994).

Power, at a structural level, can be seen to follow the 'fault lines' of society that is, to reflect the social divisions of class, race, ethnicity, gender, age, disability and so on. Power is not equally distributed across the structure of society, and indeed the structured nature of society gives some groups more power at the expense of others (for example, in relation to class and poverty – Jones and Novak, 1999).

The cultural factors both reflect and reinforce the structural basis of society – the power relations that underpin it. Recognising discrimination is therefore not simply a matter of identifying a specific piece of behaviour or action, it is more a matter of appreciating the continuous interplay of all three levels. PCS analysis is a dynamic model of this interaction, and that is one of the reasons why it is so complex, and why one of the dangers is that of oversimplification, as I shall discuss below.

Within PCS analysis, ideology can be seen as the glue that binds the levels together: it is transmitted from the cultural level to the personal level, from where it is reflected back again, and it is transmitted to the structural level to underpin social divisions and the distribution of power in society. In this process, the effect of ideology is to allow the structural divisions to appear 'normal' and for people thus routinely to accept them without great question. For example, at the structural level, the 'feminisation of poverty' (Millar, 1989), a process characterised by the salience of women's employment profile in poorly paid, insecure, part-time work, is considered to be a consequence of females, especially in their roles as mothers, *naturally* having less interest in the world of work outside the home.

Developing anti-discriminatory practice is not a simple matter, nor is it something that can be done in a short period of time. What is required is a commitment to wrestling with the complexities, learning the difficult lessons and being prepared to take the necessary steps over an extended period of time. This is a major undertaking, but one that is necessary if we are serious about not allowing discrimination and oppression to undermine our efforts to support people through the problems and challenges they face.

References

Abbott, P. and Wallace, C. (1997) *An Introduction to Sociology: Feminist Perspectives*, London: Routledge.

Abbott, S. (1971) *The Prevention of Racial Discrimination in Britain*, London: Oxford University Press.

Bonnett, A. (2000) *White Identities*, Harlow: Pearson.

Burden, T. and Hamm, T. (2000) 'Responding to socially excluded groups', in J. Percy-Smith (ed.) *Policy Responses to Social Exclusion: Towards Inclusion?*, Buckingham: Open University Press.

Crompton, R. (1993) *Class and Stratification: An Introduction to Current Debates*, Cambridge: Polity Press.

Fennell, G., Phillipson, C. and Evers, H. (1988) *The Sociology of Old Age*, Milton Keynes: Open University Press.

Foucault, M. (1977) *Discipline and Punish*, London: Allen Lane.

—— (1979) *The History of Sexuality, Volume 1: An Introduction*, London: Allen Lane.

Jones, C. and Novak, T. (1999) *Poverty, Welfare and the Disciplinary State*, London; Routledge.

Millar, J. (1989) 'Social security, equality and women in the UK', *Policy and Politics*, 17 (4): 311–19.

Mishra, R. (1995) 'Social policy after socialism', in J. Baldock. and M. May (eds) *Social Policy Review 7*, Canterbury: Social Policy Association.

Phillipson, J. (1992) *Practising Equality: Women, Men and Social Work*, London: Central Council for Education and Training in Social Work.

Rex, J. (1996) 'National identity in the democratic multi-cultural state', *Sociological Research Online*, 1(2), www.socresonline.org.uk/socresonline/1/2 (accessed 23 April 2001).

Righton, P. (1990) 'Orientating ourselves', Prologue to Open University K254 *Working with Children and Young People*, Milton Keynes: Open University.

Small, S. (1994) *The Black Experience in the United States and England in the 1980s*, London: Routledge.

Stewart, A. (2001) *Theories of Power and Domination: The Politics of Empowerment in Late Modernity*, London: Sage.

Thompson, N. (2001) *Anti-discriminatory Practice*, 3rd edition, Basingstoke: Palgrave.

Thompson, S. and Thompson, N. (1993) *Perspectives on Ageing*, Social Work Monograph no. 122, Norwich: University of East Anglia.

Further reading

Clifford, D. and Burke, B. (2009) *Anti-oppressive Ethics and Values in Social Work*, Basingstoke: Palgrave Macmillan.

Dalrymple, J. and Burke, B. (2006) *Anti-oppressive Practice: Social Care and the Law*, Maidenhead: Open University Press.

Dominelli, L. (2002) *Anti-oppressive Social Work Theory and Practice*, Basingstoke: Palgrave.

—— (2002) *Feminist Social Work Theory and Practice*, Basingstoke: Palgrave.

—— (2008) *Anti-racist Social Work*, 3rd edition, Basingstoke: Palgrave Macmillan.

—— (2009) 'Anti-oppressive practice: The challenges of the twenty-first century', in R. Adams, L. Dominelli and M. Payne (eds) *Social Work: Themes, Issues and Critical Debates*, 3rd edition, Basingstoke: Palgrave Macmillan, 49–64.

McDonald, P. and Coleman, M. (1999) 'Deconstructing hierarchies of oppression and adopting a "multiple model" approach to anti-oppressive practice', *Social Work Education*, 18 (1) 19–33.

Payne, G. (ed.) (2006) *Social Divisions*, 2nd edition, Basingstoke: Palgrave.

Thompson, N. (2006) *Anti-discriminatory Practice*, 4th edition, Basingstoke: Palgrave Macmillan.

Williams, C. (1999) 'Connecting anti-racist and anti-oppressive theory and practice: Retrenchment or reappraisal?', *British Journal of Social Work*, 29: 211–30.

Wilson, A. and Beresford, P. (2000) 'Anti-oppressive practice: Emancipation or appropriation?', *British Journal of Social Work*, 2 (30): 553–73.

15 Black feminist epistemology and toward a politics of empowerment

Patricia Hill Collins

Continuing the theme of social divisions, this is a hugely important book written by an African-American feminist sociologist. I include this, not just because of its original contribution, but because it brings together important debates about the nature of knowledge, oppression, social justice and change. Hill Collins writes from a particular standpoint, but her ideas are widely applicable in helping us to think positively about the individual and society, and about social work and social justice. The extract has been drawn from the final two chapters in this book. I hope that students will be encouraged to get hold of the book and read more.

From *Black Feminist Thought: Knowledge, Consciousness and the Politics of Empowerment*, 2nd edition, London: Routledge (2000), 251–90.

Chapter 11 Black Feminist Epistemology

Toward truth

The existence of Black feminist thought suggests another path to the universal truths that might accompany the 'truthful identity of what is.' In this volume I place Black women's subjectivity in the center of analysis and examine the inter-dependence of the everyday, taken-for-granted knowledge shared by African-American women as a group, the more specialized knowledge produced by Black women intellectuals, and the social conditions shaping both types of thought. This approach allows me to describe the creative tension linking how social conditions influenced a Black women's standpoint and how the power of the ideas themselves gave many African-American women the strength to shape those same social conditions. I approach Black feminist thought as situated in a context of domination and not as a system of ideas divorced from political and economic reality. Moreover, I present Black feminist thought as subjugated knowledge in that African-American women have long struggled to find alternative locations and epistemologies for validating our own self-definitions. In brief, I examine the situated, subjugated standpoint of African-American women in order to understand Black feminist thought as a partial perspective on domination.

Because U.S. Black women have access to the experiences that accrue to being both Black and female, an alternative epistemology used to rearticulate a Black women's standpoint should reflect the convergence of both sets of experiences. Race and gender may be analytically distinct, but in Black women's everyday lives, they work together.

The search for the distinguishing features of an alternative epistemology used by African-American women reveals that some ideas that Africanist scholars identify as characteristically 'Black' often bear remarkable resemblance to similar ideas claimed by feminist scholars as characteristically 'female.' This similarity suggests that the actual contours of intersecting oppressions can vary dramatically and yet generate some uniformity in the epistemologies used by subordinate groups. Just as U.S. Black women and African women encountered diverse patterns of intersecting oppressions yet generated similar agendas concerning what mattered in their feminisms, a similar process may be at work regarding the epistemologies of oppressed groups. Thus the significance of a Black feminist epistemology may lie in its ability to enrich our understanding of how subordinate groups create knowledge that fosters both their empowerment and social justice.

This approach to Black feminist thought allows African-American women to explore the epistemological implications of transversal politics. Eventually this approach may get us to a point at which, claims Elsa Barkley Brown, 'all people can learn to center in another experience, validate it, and judge it by its own standards without need of comparison or need to adopt that framework as their own' (1989, 922). In such politics, 'one has no need to "decenter" anyone in order to center someone else: one has only to constantly, appropriately, "pivot the center"' (p. 922).

Rather than emphasizing how a Black women's standpoint and its accompanying epistemology differ from those of White women, Black men, and other collectivities. Black women's experiences serve as one specific social location for examining points of connection among multiple epistemologies. Viewing Black feminist epistemology in this way challenges additive analyses of oppression claiming that Black women have a more accurate view of oppression than do other groups. Such approaches suggest that oppression can be quantified and compared and that adding layers of oppression produces a potentially clearer standpoint (Spelman 1988). One implication of some uses of standpoint theory is that the more subordinated the group, the purer the vision available to them. This is an outcome of the origins of standpoint approaches in Marxist social theory, itself reflecting the binary thinking of its Western origins. Ironically, by quantifying and ranking human oppressions, standpoint theorists invoke criteria for methodological adequacy that resemble those of positivism. Although it is tempting to claim that Black women are more oppressed than everyone else and therefore have the best standpoint from which to understand the mechanisms, processes, and effects of oppression, this is not the case.

Instead, those ideas that are validated as true by African-American women, African-American men, Latina lesbians, Asian-American women, Puerto Rican men, and other groups with distinctive standpoints, with each group using the epistemological approaches growing from its unique standpoint, become the most 'objective' truths. Each group speaks from its own standpoint and shares its own partial, situated knowledge. But because each group perceives its own truth as partial, its knowledge is unfinished. Each group becomes better able to consider other groups' standpoints without relinquishing the uniqueness of its own standpoint or suppressing other groups' partial perspectives. 'What is always needed in the appreciation of art, or life,' maintains Alice Walker, 'is the larger perspective. Connections made, or at least attempted, where none existed before, the straining to encompass in one's glance at the varied world the common thread, the unifying theme through immense diversity' (1983, 5). Partiality, and not universality, is the condition of being heard; individuals and groups forwarding knowledge claims without owning their position are deemed less credible than those who do.

Alternative knowledge claims in and of themselves are rarely threatening to conventional knowledge. Such claims are routinely ignored, discredited, or simply absorbed and marginalized in existing paradigms. Much more threatening is the challenge that alternative epistemologies offer to the basic process used by the powerful to legitimate knowledge claims that in turn justify their right to rule. If the epistemology used to validate knowledge comes into question, then all prior knowledge claims validated under the dominant model become suspect. Alternative epistemologies challenge all certified knowledge and open up the question of whether what has been taken to be true can stand the test of alternative ways of validating truth. The existence of a self-defined Black women's standpoint using Black feminist epistemology calls into question the content of what currently passes as truth and simultaneously challenges the process of arriving at that truth.

Chapter 12 Toward a Politics of Empowerment

. . . Black feminist thought offers two important contributions concerning the significance of knowledge for a politics of empowerment. First, Black feminist thought fosters a fundamental paradigmatic shift in how we think about unjust power relations. By embracing a paradigm of intersecting oppressions of race, class, gender, sexuality, and nation, as well as Black women's individual and collective agency within them. Black feminist thought reconceptualizes the social relations of domination and resistance. Second, Black feminist thought addresses ongoing epistemological debates concerning the power dynamics that underlie what counts as knowledge. Offering U.S. Black women new knowledge about our own experiences can be empowering. But activating epistemologies that criticize prevailing knowledge and that enable us to define our own realities *on our own terms* has far greater implications.

Thus far, this volume has synthesized two main approaches to power. One way of approaching power concerns the dialectical relationship linking oppression and activism, where groups with greater power oppress those with lesser amounts. Rather than seeing social change or lack of it as preordained and outside the realm of human action, the notion of a dialectical relationship suggests that change results from human agency. Because African-American women remain relegated to the bottom of the social hierarchy from one generation to the next, U.S. Black women have a vested interest in opposing oppression. This is not an intellectual issue for most African-American women – it is a lived reality. As long as Black women's oppression persists, so will the need for Black women's activism. Moreover, dialectical analyses of power point out that when it comes to social injustice, groups have competing interests that often generate conflict. Even when groups understand the need for the type of transversal politics they often find themselves on opposite sides of social issues. Oppression and resistance remain intricately linked such that the shape of one influences that of the other. At the same time, this relationship is far more complex than a simple model of permanent oppressors and perpetual victims.

Another way of approaching power views it not as something that groups possess, but as an intangible entity that circulates within a particular matrix of domination and to which individuals stand in varying relationships. These approaches emphasize how individual subjectivity frames human actions within a matrix of domination. U.S.

Black women's efforts to grapple with the effects of domination in everyday life are evident in our creation of safe spaces that enable us to resist oppression, and in our struggles to form fully human love relations with one another, and with children, fathers, and brothers, as well as with individuals who do not see Black women as worthwhile. Oppression is not simply understood in the mind – it is felt in the body in myriad ways. Moreover, because oppression is constantly changing, different aspects of an individual U.S. Black woman's self-definitions intermingle and become more salient: Her gender may be more prominent when she becomes a mother, her race when she searches for housing, her social class when she applies for credit, her sexual orientation when she is walking with her lover, and her citizenship status when she applies for a job. In all of these contexts, her position in relation to and within intersecting oppressions shifts.

Together, these two approaches to power point to two important uses of knowledge for African-American women and other social groups engaged in social justice projects. Dialectical approaches emphasize the significance of knowledge in developing self-defined, group-based standpoints that, in turn, can foster the type of group solidarity necessary for resisting oppressions. In contrast, subjectivity approaches emphasize how domination and resistance shape and are shaped by individual agency. Issues of consciousness link the two. In the former, group-based consciousness emerges through developing oppositional knowledges such as Black feminist thought. In the latter, individual self-definitions and behaviors shift in tandem with a changed consciousness concerning everyday lived experience. Black feminist thought encompasses both meanings of consciousness – neither is sufficient without the other. Together, both approaches to power also highlight the significance of multiplicity in shaping consciousness. For example, viewing domination itself as encompassing intersecting oppressions of race, class, gender, sexuality, and nation points to the significance of these oppressions in shaping the overall organization of a particular matrix of domination. Similarly, personal identities constructed around individual understandings of race, class, gender, sexuality, and nation define each individual's unique biography.

Both of these approaches remain theoretically useful because they each provide partial and different perspectives on empowerment. Unfortunately, these two views are often presented as *competing* rather than potentially *complementary* approaches. As a result, each provides a useful starting point for thinking through African-American women's empowerment in the context of constantly changing power relations, but neither is sufficient. Black feminism and other social justice projects require a language of power that is grounded within yet transcends these approaches. Social justice projects need a common, functional vocabulary that furthers their understanding of the politics of empowerment.

Thus far, using African-American women's experiences as a lens, this volume has examined race, gender, class, sexuality, and nation as forms of oppression that work together in distinctive ways to produce a distinctive U.S. matrix of domination. But earlier chapters have said much less about *how* these and other oppressions are organized. In response, this chapter sketches out a preliminary, vocabulary of power and empowerment that emerges from these seemingly competing approaches to power. Whether viewed through the lens of a single system of power, or through that of intersecting oppressions, any particular matrix of domination is organized via four interrelated domains of power, namely, the structural, disciplinary, hegemonic, and interpersonal domains. Each domain serves a particular purpose. The structural domain organizes oppression, whereas the disciplinary domain manages it. The hegemonic domain justifies oppression, and the interpersonal domain influences everyday lived experiences and the individual consciousness that ensues.

It is important to remember that although the following argument is developed from the standpoint of U.S. Black women, its significance is much greater. Recall that Black feminist thought views Black women's struggles as part of a wider struggle for human dignity and social justice. When coupled with the Black feminist epistemological tenet that dialogue remain central to assessing knowledge claims, the domains-of-power argument presented here should serve to stimulate dialogues about empowerment.

In the United States the particular contours of each domain of power illustrates how intersecting oppressions of race, class, gender, sexuality, and nation are organized in unique ways. Black women are incorporated in each domain of power in particular ways that while exhibiting patterns of common differences with women of African descent transnationally, remain quintessentially American. For example, the structural domain regulates citizenship rights, and much of African-American women's struggles have centered on gaining rights routinely granted to other American citizens. U.S. Black women have long recognized that the absence of usable citizenship rights limited Black women's ability to oppose the mammy, matriarch, jezebel and other controlling images routinely advanced within the hegemonic domain. Citizenship rights enable African-American women to pursue focused educations and challenge these portrayals of U.S. Black women. These moves toward empowerment are important, yet they remain dependent on ideas about American citizenship and therefore American national identity.

At the same time, as individuals and as part of groups who oppose U.S. social injustices, African-American women's resistance strategies reflect their placement both within each domain and within the U.S. matrix of domination. For example, through its reliance on rules, the disciplinary domain manages domination. African-American women rule breakers and rule benders and, upon occasion, Black women who capture positions of authority so that they can change the rules themselves become empowered within the disciplinary domain. Thus US Black women's experiences and ideas illustrate how these four domains of power shape domination. But they also illustrate how these same domains have been and can be used as sites of Black women's empowerment.

The politics of empowerment

Rethinking Black feminism as a social justice project involves developing a complex notion of empowerment. Shifting the analysis to investigating how the matrix of domination is structured along certain axes – race, gender, class, sexuality, and nation – as well as how it operates through interconnected domains of power – structural, interpersonal, disciplinary, and hegemonic – reveals that the dialectical relationship linking oppression and activism is far more complex than simple models of oppressors and oppressed would suggest. This inclusive perspective enables African-American women to avoid labeling one form of oppression as more important than others, or one expression of activism as more radical than another. It also creates conceptual space to identify some new linkages. Just as oppression is complex, so must resistance aimed at fostering empowerment demonstrate a similar complexity.

When it comes to power, the challenges raised by the synergistic relationship among domains of power generate new opportunities and constraints for African-American women who now desegregate schools and workplaces, as well as those who do not. On the one hand, entering places that denied access to our mothers provides new opportunities for fostering social justice. Depending on the setting, using the insights gained via outsider-within status can be a stimulus to creativity that helps both African-American women and our new organizational homes. On the other hand, the commodification of outsider-within status whereby African-American women's value to an organization lies solely in our ability to market a seemingly permanent marginal status can suppress Black women's empowerment. Being a permanent outsider within can never lead to power because the category, by definition, requires marginality. Each individual must find her own way, recognizing that her personal biography, while unique, is never as unique as she thinks.

When it comes to knowledge, Black women's empowerment involves rejecting the dimensions of knowledge that perpetuate objectification, commodification, and exploitation. African-American women and others like us become empowered when we understand and use those dimensions of our individual, group, and formal educational ways of knowing that foster our humanity. When Black women value our self-definitions, participate in Black women's domestic and transnational activist traditions, view the skills gained in schools as part of a focused education for Black community development, and invoke Black feminist epistemologies as central to our worldviews, we empower ourselves. C. Wright Mills's (1959) concept of the 'sociological imagination' identifies its task and its promise as a way of knowing that enables individuals to grasp the relations between history and biography within society. Resembling the holistic epistemology required by Black feminism, using one's point of view to engage the sociological imagination can empower the individual. 'My fullest concentration of energy is available to me,' Audre Lorde maintains, 'only when I integrate all the parts of who I am, openly, allowing power from particular sources of my living to flow back and forth freely through all my different selves, without the restriction of externally imposed definition' (1984, 120–1). Developing a Black women's standpoint to engage a collective Black feminist imagination can empower the group.

Black women's empowerment involves revitalizing U.S. Black feminism as a social justice project organized around the dual goals of empowering African-American women and fostering social justice in a transnational context. Black feminist thought's emphasis on the ongoing interplay between Black women's oppression and Black women's activism presents the matrix of domination and its interrelated domains of power as responsive to human agency. Such thought views the world as a dynamic place where the goal is not merely to survive or to fit in or to cope; rather, it becomes a place where we feel ownership and accountability. The existence of Black feminist thought suggests that there is always choice, and power to act, no matter how bleak the situation may appear to be. Viewing the world as one in the making raises the issue of individual responsibility for bringing about change. It also shows that while individual empowerment is key, only collective action can effectively generate the lasting institutional transformation required for social justice.

References

Brown, E.B. (1989) 'African-American women's quilting: A framework for conceptualizing and teaching African-American women's history', *Signs*, 14 (4): 921–9.
Lorde, A. (1984) *Sister Outsider*, Trumansberg, NY: Crossing Press.

Mills, C.W. (1959) *The Sociological Imagination*, Oxford: Oxford University Press.
Spelman, E.V. (1988) *Inessential Woman: Problems of Exclusion in Feminist Thought*, Boston, MA: Beacon.
Walker, A. (1983) *In Search of Our Mother's Gardens*, New York: Harcourt Brace Jovanovich.

Further reading

Barry, B. (2005) *Why Social Justice Matters*, Cambridge: Polity Press.
Craig, G., Burchardt, T. and Gordon, D. (eds) (2008) *Social Justice and Public Policy: Seeking Fairness in Diverse Societies*, Bristol: Policy Press.
Cree, V.E. (2010) *Sociology for Social Workers and Probation Officers*, 2nd revised edition, London: Routledge.
Ferguson, I. (2007) *Reclaiming Social Work: Challenging Neo-liberalism and Promoting Social Justice*, London: Sage.
Ferguson, I. and Woodward, R. (2009) *Radical Social Work in Practice: Making a Difference*, Bristol: Policy Press.
McDonald, P. and Coelamn, M. (1999) 'Deconstructing hierarchies of oppression and adopting a "multiple model" approach to anti-oppressive practice', *Social Work Education*, 18 (1): 19–33.
Price, V. and Simpson, G. (2007) *Transforming Society?: Social Work and Sociology*, Bristol: Policy Press.

16 Pedagogy of the oppressed

Paulo Freire

Paulo Freire (1921–1997) was a radical educator in Brazil. His book is a standard text on community education courses, but is less well-known on social work programmes. But if we think about what social workers do as a kind of social education, then Freire's notion of 'conscientization' has much to offer social work, just as his analysis of power and oppression, and his call for the need for critical reflection, are central to current ideas in social work theory and practice. Freire has also much to pass on to social work educators and trainers, as students are forced to leap-frog through an increasingly demanding and cluttered curriculum. The extracts can only offer a way in – again, I hope students will read more.

From *Pedagogy of the Oppressed*, 2nd edition, Harmondsworth: Penguin
(1996): 45–58.

A careful analysis of the teacher–student relationship at any level, inside or outside the school, reveals its fundamentally *narrative* character. This relationship involves a narrating Subject (the teacher) and patient, listening objects (the students). The contents, whether values or empirical dimensions of reality, tend in the process of being narrated to become lifeless and petrified. Education is suffering from narration sickness.

The teacher talks about reality as if it were motionless, static, compartmentalized and predictable. Or else he expounds on a topic completely alien to the existential experience of the students. His task is to 'fill' the students with the contents of his narration – contents which are detached from reality, disconnected from the totality that engendered them and could give them significance. Words are emptied of their concreteness and become a hollow, alienated and alienating verbosity.

Narration (with the teacher as narrator) leads the students to memorize mechanically the narrated content. Worse still, it turns them into 'containers', into receptacles to be filled by the teacher. The more completely he fills the receptacles, the better a teacher he is. The more meekly the receptacles permit themselves to be filled, the better students they are.

Education thus becomes an act of depositing, in which the students are the depositories and the teacher is the depositor. Instead of communicating, the teacher issues communiqués and 'makes deposits' which the students patiently receive, memorize, and repeat. This is the 'banking' concept of education, in which the scope of action allowed to the students extends only as far as receiving, filling, and storing the deposits. They do, it is true, have the opportunity to become collectors or cataloguers of the things they store. But in the last analysis, it is men themselves who are filed away through the lack of creativity, transformation, and knowledge in this (at best) misguided system. For apart from inquiry, apart from the praxis, men cannot be truly human. Knowledge emerges only through invention and re-invention, through the restless, impatient, continuing, hopeful inquiry men pursue in the world, with the world, and with each other.

In the banking concept of education, knowledge is a gift bestowed by those who consider themselves knowledgeable upon those whom they consider to know nothing. Projecting an absolute ignorance onto others, a characteristic of the ideology of oppression, negates education and knowledge as processes of inquiry. The teacher presents himself to his students as their necessary opposite; by considering their ignorance absolute, he justifies his own existence. The students, alienated like the slave in the Hegelian dialectic, accept their ignorance as justifying the teacher's existence – but, unlike the slave, they never discover that they educate the teacher.

The *raison d'être* of libertarian education, on the other hand, lies in its drive towards reconciliation. Education must begin with the solution of the teacher–student contradiction, by reconciling the poles of the contradiction so that both are simultaneously teachers *and* students.

This solution is not (nor can it be) found in the banking concept. On the contrary, banking education maintains and even stimulates the contradiction through the following attitudes and practices, which mirror oppressive society as a whole:

1 The teacher teaches and the students are taught.
2 The teacher knows everything and the students know nothing.
3 The teacher thinks and the students are thought about.
4 The teacher talks and the students listen – meekly.
5 The teacher disciplines and the students are disciplined.
6 The teacher chooses and enforces his choice, and the students comply.
7 The teacher acts and the students have the illusion of acting through the action of the teacher.
8 The teacher chooses the programme content, and the students (who were not consulted) adapt to it.
9 The teacher confuses the authority of knowledge with his own professional authority, which he sets in opposition to the freedom of the students.
10 The teacher is the subject of the learning process, while the pupils are mere objects.

It is not surprising that the banking concept of education regards men as adaptable, manageable beings. The more students work at storing the deposits entrusted to them, the less they develop the critical consciousness which would result from their intervention in the world as transformers of that world. The more completely they accept the passive role imposed on them, the more they tend simply to adapt to the world as it is and to the fragmented view of reality deposited in them.

The capacity of banking education to minimize or annul the students' creative power and to stimulate their credulity serves the interests of the oppressors, who care neither to have the world revealed nor to see it transformed. The oppressors use their 'humanitarianism' to preserve a profitable situation. Thus they react almost instinctively against any experiment in education which stimulates the critical faculties and is not content with a partial view of reality but is always seeking out the ties which link one point to another and one problem to another.

Indeed, the interests of the oppressors lie in 'changing the consciousness of the oppressed, not the situation which oppresses them' (Simone de Beauvoir in *La Pensée de Droite Aujourd'hui*) for the more the oppressed can be led to adapt to that situation, the more easily they can be dominated. To achieve this end, the oppressors use the banking concept of education in conjunction with a paternalistic social action apparatus, within which the oppressed receive the euphemistic title of 'welfare recipients'. They are treated as individual cases, as marginal men who deviate from the general configuration of a 'good, organized, and just' society. The oppressed are regarded as the pathology of the healthy society, which must therefore adjust these 'incompetent and lazy' folk to its own patterns by changing their mentality. These marginals need to be 'integrated', 'incorporated' into the healthy society that they have 'forsaken'.

The truth is, however, that the oppressed are not marginals, are not men living 'outside' society. They have always been inside – inside the structure which made them 'beings for others'. The solution is not to 'integrate' them into the structure of oppression, but to transform that structure so that they can become 'beings for themselves'. Such transformation, of course, would undermine the oppressors' purposes; hence their utilization of the banking concept of education to avoid the threat of student conscientization.

The 'humanism' of the banking approach masks the effort to turn men into automatons – the very negation of their ontological vocation to be more fully human.

Those who use the banking approach, knowingly or unknowingly (for there are innumerable well-intentioned bank-clerk teachers who do not realize that they are serving only to dehumanize), fail to perceive that the deposits themselves contain contradictions about reality. But, sooner or later, these contradictions may lead formerly passive students to turn against their domestication and the attempt to domesticate reality. They may discover through existential experience that their present way of life is irreconcilable with their vocation to become fully human. They may perceive through their relations with reality that reality is really a *process*, undergoing constant transformation. If men are searchers and their ontological vocation is humanization, sooner or later they may perceive the contradiction in which banking education seeks to maintain them, and then engage themselves in the struggle for their liberation.

But the humanist, revolutionary educator cannot wait for this possibility to materialize. From the outset, his efforts must coincide with those of the students to engage in critical thinking and the quest for mutual humanization. His efforts must be imbued with a profound trust in men and their creative power. To achieve this, he must be a partner of the students in his relations with them.

The banking concept does not admit to such a partnership – and necessarily so. To resolve the teacher–student contradiction, to exchange the role of depositor, prescriber, domesticator, for the role of student among students would be to undermine the power of oppression and to serve the cause of liberation.

Implicit in the banking concept is the assumption of a dichotomy between man and the world: man is merely *in* the world, not *with* the world or with others; man is spectator, not re-creator. In this view, man is not a conscious being (*corpo consciente*); he is rather the possessor of a consciousness; an empty 'mind' passively open to the reception of deposits of reality from the world outside. For example, my desk, my books, my coffee cup, all the objects before me – as bits of the world which surrounds me – would be 'inside' me, exactly as I am inside my study right now. This view makes no distinction between being accessible to consciousness and entering consciousness. The distinction, however, is essential: the objects which surround me are simply accessible to my consciousness, not located within it. I am aware of them, but they are not inside me.

It follows logically from the banking notion of consciousness that the educator's role is to regulate the way the world 'enters into' the students. His task is to organize a process which already happens spontaneously, to 'fill' the students by making deposits of information which he considers constitute true knowledge. And since men 'receive' the world as passive entities, education should make them more passive still, and adapt them to the world. The educated man is the adapted man, because he is more 'fit' for the world. Translated into practice, this concept is well suited to the purposes of the oppressors, whose tranquillity rests on how well men fit the world the oppressors have created, and how little they question it.

The more completely the majority adapt to the purposes which the dominant minority prescribe for them (thereby depriving them of the right to their own purposes), the more easily the minority can continue to prescribe. The theory and practice of banking education serve this end quite efficiently. Verbalistic lessons, reading requirements,[1] the methods for evaluating 'knowledge', the distance between the teacher and the taught, the criteria for promotion: everything in this ready-to-wear approach serves to obviate thinking.

Yet only through communication can human life hold meaning. The teacher's thinking is authenticated only by the authenticity of the students' thinking. The teacher cannot think for his students, nor can he impose his thought on them. Authentic thinking, thinking that is concerned about *reality*, does not take place in ivory-tower isolation, but only in communication. If it is true that thought has meaning only when generated by action upon the world, the subordination of students to teachers becomes impossible.

Education as the exercise of domination stimulates the credulity of students, with the ideological intent (often not perceived by educators) of indoctrinating them to adapt to the world of oppression. This accusation is not made in the naïve hope that the dominant elites will thereby simply abandon the practice. Its objective is to call the attention of true humanists to the fact that they cannot use the methods of banking education in the pursuit of liberation, as they would only negate that pursuit itself. Nor may a revolutionary society inherit these methods from an oppressor society. The revolutionary society which practises banking education is either misguided or mistrustful of men. In either event, it is threatened by the spectre of reaction.

Unfortunately, those who espouse the cause of liberation are themselves surrounded and influenced by the climate which generates the banking concept, and often do not perceive its true significance or its dehumanizing power. Paradoxically, then, they utilize this very instrument of alienation in what they consider an effort to liberate. Indeed, some 'revolutionaries' brand as innocents, dreamers, or even reactionaries those who would challenge this educational practice. But one does not liberate men by alienating them. Authentic liberation – the process of humanization – is not another 'deposit' to be made in men. Liberation is a praxis: the action and reflection of men upon their world in order to transform it. Those truly committed to the cause of liberation can accept neither the mechanistic concept of consciousness as an empty vessel to be filled, nor the use of banking methods of domination (propaganda, slogans – deposits) in the name of liberation.

The truly committed must reject the banking concept in its entirety, adopting instead a concept of men as conscious beings, and consciousness as consciousness directed towards the world. They must abandon the educational goal of deposit-making and replace it with the posing of the problems of men in their relations with the world. 'Problem-posing' education, responding to the essence of consciousness – *intentionality* – rejects communiqués and embodies communication. It epitomizes the special characteristic of consciousness: being *conscious of*, not only as intent on objects but as turned in upon itself in a Jasperian 'split' – consciousness as consciousness *of* consciousness.

Liberating education consists in acts of cognition, not transferrals of information. It is a learning situation in which the cognizable object (far from being the end of the cognitive act) intermediates the cognitive actors – teacher on the one hand and students on the other. Accordingly, the practice of problem-posing education first of all demands a resolution of the teacher–student contradiction. Dialogical relations – indispensable to the capacity of cognitive actors to cooperate in perceiving the same cognizable object – are otherwise impossible.

Indeed, problem-posing education, breaking the vertical patterns characteristic of banking education, can fulfill its function of being the practice of freedom only if it can overcome the above contradiction. Through dialogue, the teacher-of-the-students and the students-of-the-teacher cease to exist and a new term emerges: teacher-student with students-teachers. The teacher is no longer merely the-one-who-teaches, but one who is himself taught in dialogue with the students, who in their turn while being taught also teach. They become jointly responsible for a process in which all grow. In this process, arguments based on 'authority' are no longer valid; in order to function, authority must be *on the side of* freedom, not *against* it. Here, no one teaches another, nor is anyone self-taught. Men teach each other, mediated by the world, by the cognizable objects which in banking education are 'owned' by the teacher.

Students, as they are increasingly faced with problems relating to themselves in the world and with the world, will feel increasingly challenged and obliged to respond to that challenge. Because they apprehend the challenge as interrelated to other problems within a total context, not as a theoretical question, the resulting comprehension tends to be increasingly critical and thus constantly less alienated. Their response to the challenge evokes new challenges, followed by new understandings; and gradually the students come to regard themselves as committed.

Education as the practice of freedom – as opposed to education as the practice of domination – denies that man is abstract, isolated, independent, and unattached to the world; it also denies that the world exists as a reality apart from men. Authentic reflection considers neither abstract man nor the world without men, but men in their relations with the world. In these relations consciousness and world are simultaneous: consciousness neither precedes the world nor follows it. '*La conscience et le monde sont dormés d'un même coup; extérieur par essence à la conscience, le monde est, par essence relatif à elle*', writes Sartre.

That which had existed objectively but had not been perceived in its deeper implications (if indeed it was perceived at all) begins to 'stand out', assuming the character of a problem and therefore of challenge. Thus, men begin to single out elements from their 'background awarenesses' and to reflect upon them. These elements are now objects of men's consideration, and, as such, objects of their action and cognition.

In problem-posing education, men develop their power to perceive critically *the way they exist* in the world *with which* and *in which* they find themselves; they come to see the world not as a static reality, but as a reality in process, in transformation. Although the dialectical relations of men with the world exist independently of how these relations are perceived (or whether or not they are perceived at all), it is also true that the form of action men adopt is to a large extent a function of how they perceive themselves in the world. Hence, the teacher-student and the students-teachers reflect simultaneously on themselves and the world without dichotomizing this reflection from action, and thus establish an authentic form of thought and action.

Problem-posing education affirms men as beings in the process of *becoming* – as unfinished, uncompleted beings in and with a likewise unfinished reality. Indeed, in contrast to other animals who are unfinished, but not historical, men know themselves to be unfinished; they are aware of their incompleteness. In this incompleteness and this awareness lie the very roots of education as an exclusively human manifestation. The unfinished character of men and the transformational character of reality necessitate that education be an ongoing activity.

The point of departure of the movement lies in men themselves. But since men do not exist apart from the world, apart from reality, the movement must begin with the men-world relationship. Accordingly, the point of departure must always be with men in the 'here and now', which constitutes the situation within which they are submerged, from which they emerge, and in which they intervene. Only by starting from this situation – which determines their perception of it – can they begin to move. To do this authentically they must perceive their state not as fated and unalterable, but merely as limiting – and therefore challenging.

A deepened consciousness of their situation leads men to apprehend that situation as an historical reality susceptible of transformation. Resignation gives way to the drive for transformation and inquiry, over which men feel themselves in control. If men, as historical beings necessarily engaged with other men in a movement of inquiry, did not control that movement, it would be (and is) a violation of men's humanity. Any situation in which some men prevent others from engaging in the process of inquiry is one of violence. The means used are not important; to alienate men from their own decision-making is to change them into objects.

This movement of inquiry must be directed towards humanization – man's historical vocation. The pursuit of full humanity, however, cannot be carried out in isolation or individualism, but only in fellowship and solidarity; therefore it cannot unfold in the antagonistic relations between oppressors and oppressed. No one can be authentically human while he prevents others from being so. The attempt *to be more* human, individualistically, leads to *having more*, egotistically: a form of dehumanization. Not that it is not fundamental *to have* in order *to be* human. Precisely because it *is* necessary, some men's *having* must not be allowed to constitute an obstacle to others' *having*, to consolidate the power of the former to crush the latter.

Problem-posing education, as a humanist and liberating praxis, posits as fundamental that men subjected to domination must fight for their emancipation. To that end, it enables teachers and students to become subjects of the educational process by overcoming authoritarianism and an alienating intellectualism; it also enables men to overcome their false perception of reality. The world – no longer something to be described with deceptive words – becomes the object of that transforming action by men which results in their humanization.

Note

1 For example, some teachers specify in their reading lists that a book should be read from pages 10 to 15 – and do this to 'help' their students!

Further reading

Baldwin, M. and Teater, B. (2011) *Social Work in the Community: Making a Difference*, Bristol: Policy Press.

Brake, M. and Bailey, R. (eds) (1980) *Radical Social Work and Practice*, London: Edward Arnold.

Ferguson, I. and Woodward, R. (2009) *Radical Social Work in Practice: Making a Difference*, Bristol: Policy Press.

Fook, J. and Askeland, G.A. (2007) 'Challenges of critical reflection: "Nothing ventured, nothing gained"', *Social Work Education*, 26 (5): 520–33.

Langan, M. (2002) 'The legacy of radical social work', in R. Adams, L. Dominelli and M. Payne (eds) *Social Work: Themes, Issues and Critical Debates*, 2nd edition, London: Palgrave Macmillan.

Ledwith, M. (2005) *Community Development: A Critical Approach*, Bristol: Policy Press.

McLaughlin, K. (2008) *Social Work, Politics and Society: From Radicalism to Orthodoxy*, Bristol: Policy Press.

Solomon, B.B. (1987) 'Empowerment: Social work in oppressed communities', *Journal of Social Work Practice*, 2 (4): 79–91.

Specht, H. and Courtney, M. (1994) *Unfaithful Angels: How Social Work Has Abandoned Its Mission*, New York: Free Press.

Stepney, P. (2006) 'Mission impossible? Critical practice in social work', *British Journal of Social Work*, 36: 1289–307.

White, S., Fook, J. and Gardner, F. (eds) (2006) *Critical Reflection in Health and Social Care*, Maidenhead: Open University Press.

17 The role of the law in welfare reform

Critical perspectives on the relationship between law and social work practice

Suzy Braye and Michael Preston-Shoot

The law is another large and ever-increasing body of knowledge with which social workers must be familiar and confident. Suzy Braye and Michael Preston-Shoot are UK social work academics who have written about the law and social work for many years. This extract teases out differing approaches to the law, using an entertaining metaphor of maps, roads and paths to provide an informative analysis of the relationship between the law and social work practice.

From *International Journal of Social Welfare*, 15: 19–26 (2006).

Beliefs about law and practice

It is possible to identify a number of beliefs or assumptions about the relationship between law and social work practice, assumptions that are not necessarily helpful in the context of the search for robust and reliable frameworks for welfare provision. These assumptions will be explored and challenged, and an argument made for more realistic ways forward.

The belief that law provides a clear map for welfare practice

This assumption is displayed when things go wrong in practice and people, usually children, get hurt. It underpinned the harsh criticisms of social workers' legal knowledge in the UK in the 1980s, and is perhaps most graphically illustrated recently in the report of the enquiry into the death of Victoria Climbié. Beneath the criticisms of individual professional practice (Beckford Report, 1985; Butler-Sloss, 1988; Carlisle Report, 1987), management mechanisms (Laming, 2003) and collaborative inter-agency practice (Reder, et al., 1993) lies an unquestioned assumption that the legal framework for protecting children is in itself sound. There are a number of problems with this position.

There is in fact no one legal map relating to professional practice, but a series of maps. Law is drawn from a range of sources – statute, court decisions, codes of practice, policy and practice guidance. Practitioners need a whole bag of legal maps, because no one alone shows the whole legal framework. Statute, as one legal map, is constantly being redrawn, either by itself as when one act repeals or develops another, or by judicial decisions and government guidance. For example, in the UK, judicial concern that local authorities were insufficiently accountable for how they delivered care plans for young people resulted in the Adoption and Children Act 2002, amending the Children Act 1989 to create a route back to court to review the outcome of care orders. Courts have caused mental health law to be redrawn so that it is compatible with the European Convention on Human Rights and Fundamental Freedoms in respect of when a same gender partner may act as a nearest relative[1] and when an approved social worker must consult a nearest relative.[2] Government guidance on assessment of children in need (Department of Health, 2000) and disabled people (Department of Health, 1990, 1991, 2002) is essential for finding direction in childcare and community care practice.

Equally, courts can find a mandate that does not exist in statute. They may use their inherent jurisdiction, and social workers may use the doctrine of necessity in the short term, to safeguard and promote the welfare of an adult who lacks capacity.[3] Yet judicial influence on welfare policy and practice is often ignored, at the expense of statutory and executive influences (Alexander, 2003). This is a serious omission, when law can be a powerful tool with which to hold the state accountable for its actions towards its citizens, and can support practitioners in challenging oppressive state interventions towards service users or claiming rights that are being denied.

Not only are there multiple maps, they also sometimes contradict each other. For example, Preston-Shoot and Vernon (2002) illustrate how youth justice law in the UK is internally inconsistent and superimposed upon, rather than dovetailed with, welfare provision for children in need. Similarly, young people of sufficient age and understanding may refuse assessment under the Children Act 1989. However, they may not themselves exercise choice of school or challenge decisions under education law about what services they should receive in response to any special educational needs.

The arrival of new maps will have significant impact on how practitioners and their managers journey across the terrain. Registration of social workers in the UK (Care Standards Act 2000) and New Zealand (Social Workers Registration Act 2003) will impact on the employer/employee relationship and may enable practitioners to resist unlawful and/or unethical practice within their agencies (Preston-Shoot, 2000). The Human Rights Act 1998 has begun to hold social work decision-making in the UK accountable in a legal sense to a degree familiar to practitioners in the USA (Jankovic and Green, 1981) and Australia (Charlesworth *et al.*, 2000).

Lastly, the clarity of the map is also compromised because some features, some aspects of law, are more detailed than others. The main roads may be clearly drawn, but the mountain tracks less well defined. Practitioners in the UK may be able easily to locate a list of factors to be taken into account by courts when making decisions about children's welfare (s.1(3) Children Act 1989); they will struggle to find a legal answer to questions of how they should handle information given to them in confidence by a child. They might find a clear definition of unlawful discrimination on grounds of race (s.I Race Relations Act 1976), but until recently will have struggled to locate a legal framework for challenging discrimination on grounds of sexuality, or age.

The belief that the legal map is the only one practitioners need

This assumption also underpinned the 1980s' criticisms of social work's lack of legal awareness, and can be seen in the current rush to law to overcome the concerns relating to children's protection identified earlier in the UK context. But there are problems here too.

The legal map is not the only one in the backpack. Tucked into another pocket is the 'ethical duty of care' map, showing professional values that may contradict what is legally mandated, or at least be tangential to it (Alexander, 2003). Where the legal map shows a mountain, here may be a valley, or an opposing contour. In respect of asylum and immigration policies, for example, social workers may wish actively to oppose legal rules that deny people access to such fundamentals as housing and social security (Humphries, 2004).

Other factors intervene in the map-reading process. In an adversarial court system such as in the UK, the principle of welfare can become secondary to the quality of evidence and the quality of advocacy that is entered. Writers in both the UK (King and Trowell, 1992) and the USA (Madden and Wayne, 2003) point to how legal processes can lead to harmful or anti-therapeutic outcomes, with social workers having to weigh this in the balance when considering intervention in people's lives.

Moreover, some territory has not been mapped at all. The profile of law differs between practice contexts. A practitioner charged with the responsibility of compulsorily detaining a distressed person in psychiatric hospital will identify without any difficulty their mandate in law. A practitioner in post-adoption counselling may not look to law at all for theirs.

Lastly, the map is not always available when it is needed. Even if practitioners are exceptionally well-equipped with the latest version, the weather can change, the mist comes down, it gets dark, the torch runs out, and the expedition loses its bearings. It is unwise to be without back up equipment – compasses, flares, wet weather gear, energy food, survival kit and other ways of staying safe. Thus practitioners must have principles and practice wisdom to help navigate the challenges of the unexpected. As Kennedy with Richards (2004) points out, practice is located within interacting layers of contextual and often contradictory factors, of which law is only one.

The belief that if the map is accurate enough (i.e. that the law is sound), it will lead safely to the destination

This assumption is found in uncritical calls for evidence-based practice that assume a formula can be applied in professional interventions that will produce the desired effect each time. It is found in the haste with which law can be formulated to respond to political imperatives, for something to be seen to be done, to respond to single, albeit shocking, incidents. But this assumption is problematic too.

The map is not the territory, it is only a map. It gives a bird's-eye view from afar, enabling travellers to see how features on the ground might relate to one another, what direction they might pursue, and what they might meet in the way. Out there in the 'swampy lowlands' of practice (Schön, 1983) some of the features on the map are not recognisable on the ground. There are new features that do not appear on the map, and changes in the landscape that can confuse and challenge certainty. This applies tolegal practitioners as much as to social workers (Charlesworth *et al.*, 2000). The process is not as simple as the client entering, gathering facts and applying a (legal) solution. Emotional dynamics may affect the process and outcome of the encounter. The issue may be unclear. There may be several people whose interests must be considered and weighed in the balance. Central to this recognition is the growing emphasis on service-user participation in the definition of 'problems' that are to be the focus of professional intervention, and in the devising of 'solutions' to those problems.

Mapping is not just a question of contours. It also requires understanding of how a landscape is formed and changes. For example, in relation to counteracting discrimination on grounds of 'race' or disability, the failure of anti-discriminatory legislation to tackle oppression (Brophy and Smart, 1985; Cockburn, 1991) provides evidence that mapping that captures the contours (legal definitions and rules) without the landscape (attitudes) is likely to prove ineffective as a guide towards equality.

Indeed, the belief that the legal rules are the best place to start is arguably based on only one view of the relationship between individuals, communities and the state. Arguably, it could be inappropriate to begin with the state moving into people's private lives but more appropriate to engage with mandates within communities and move out towards the state (Mafile'o, 2004).

The belief in accurate maps leading to reliable destinations is also compromised by activity on the ground. Travellers are sometimes encouraged to dispense with the map in favour of following a set of less technical and clearer directions that minimise uncertainty. Agencies commonly produce sets of procedures – sets of instructions for employees to follow in going about their daily practice. Procedures are intended to standardise practice, to ensure that essential components are observed, that the organisation can fulfil its accountability. They are problematic when they require a predetermined decision to be made whenever certain circumstances pertain – for example in blanket statements that an authority does not provide night-sitting for disabled people[4] or that domiciliary care packages above a certain weekly cost cannot be provided and residential care must be offered.[5] They fetter discretion under the legal framework and can result in unlawful action.

How do practitioners use the law?

If such beliefs and assumptions are ill-founded, what then might constitute a more robust foundation for a positive relationship between law and practice? The way forward lies arguably in exploring and understanding how practitioners use the law to achieve goals that take account both of professional and service user priorities, and ensuring that law provides tools that are fit for that purpose.

From research recently conducted, it is possible to identify a useful model for conceptualising the different forms of relationship between law and practice. The model emerges from an international review of approaches to law teaching on social work qualification programmes. The review comprised both a review of international published and unpublished research and a UK-based survey of education practice, and is reported in detail elsewhere (Braye and Preston-Shoot, 2005). The emerging model reflects some of the myths and assumptions about the relationship between law and social work identified above, and points a way forward in the search for a more robust conceptual framework within which to locate professional practice.

In the centre of the diagram (Figure 17.1) lie the knowledge, skills and values that inform and drive practice. These may be profiled and configured in different ways, giving rise to three patterns of thinking and decision-making represented by the points of the triangle.

In the approach characterised by technical rationality, legal knowledge is the driving

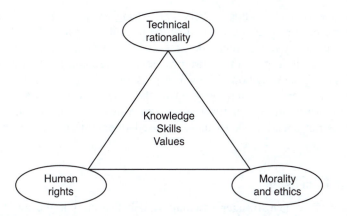

Figure 17.1 Rationality, ethics and human rights as patterns of organisation for knowledge, skills and values in the application of law to social work practice.

force for practice. Emphasis is placed on practitioners having technical knowledge of the 'nuts and bolts' of the legal framework, of the powers and duties that are contained therein. The skills prioritised are those of applying that knowledge deductively to situations encountered in practice. From the starting point of knowing, for example, that there exists a duty to protect children, the question is what then does this mean for any particular child? What features exist within the child's circumstances that fit the legal map? Does any harm or damage sustained by the child fit any legal definition that triggers a duty to act?[6] Procedural guidance in the form of assessment checklists for practitioners to aid decision-making is located within this model. Values are implicit rather than explicit here, and are likely to be construed as broad principles that underpin practice, such as 'working in partnership with parents', 'listening to children' or 'respecting human rights'.

In the approach characterised by morality and ethics, the search for ethical practice is the driver for professional activity. Legal rules are set alongside ethical rules, in pursuit of the exercise of a professional morality in any given situation. The question becomes that of determining the 'right' thing to do in moral terms. If there is no clear answer (as will often be the case in practice), the skill lies in determining the relative merits of different options, balancing the competing imperatives and dilemmas of practice, using ethical principles as guides in this task. Within this approach, law may at times be framed as antithetical to social work values, requiring hostile action to impose solutions that may challenge professional values. However, it is also possible to identify areas of convergence between values in social work practice and the legal rules (Preston-Shoot, *et al.*, 2001).

In the approach characterised by an emphasis on human rights, service users are the drivers of professional activity, from a starting point that social work's core function is to promote social justice and human rights (IASSW, 2001). Knowledge of the law might be much more broadly construed, to include not only the duties and powers that direct social work intervention itself but also the frameworks for challenging inequality and injustice, securing resources and building collective capacity. Skills prioritised are those of consultation, working in partnership, advocacy. The key question becomes that of how power might be balanced more equitably in any given situation.

The components of this triangular model are not mutually exclusive – no one point on the triangle is 'right' whilst others are 'wrong' ways to proceed. Practitioners engaged in promoting rights need to know the technical aspects of the law they use to do this. Law has a key role in regulating the use of power, and technical knowledge of administrative law is important in any professional decision-making process. Moral/ethical codes are inherently bound up with rights, or with notions of their curtailment. Legal duties must be accurately weighed in the balance with moral ones. Rational/technical practice without structural awareness, whilst 'correct' in an administrative sense, will restrict social work to individualised interventions rather than collective agendas.

Where to go from here?

First, there needs to be a stronger articulation, debate and dialogue about what it is we want law to achieve, and therefore about the relationship between law and practice. The debate needs to move beyond the assumptions identified earlier, which obscure the complexities of the relationship, to tackle the core questions of how society should respond to welfare needs and rights. Such an approach addresses the question of why the map is needed in the first place – What is the purpose of the journey? What is the sought destination?

The dialogue and debate needs to involve as wide a stakeholder network as possible, and certainly to include practitioners, professional associations and service users. Whilst different groups will not always agree, there are constructive alliances that can develop to give clear messages to politicians. Those drawing the maps need intelligence from those working on the ground, and from those whose needs and rights are to be addressed through legally informed practice.

Second, drawing upon the model outlined in Figure 17.1, the legal framework must allow for flexibility in the framing of 'problems', to give practitioners scope to respond in ways that are not constrained by individual models of intervention, but can address collective concerns also. Practitioners must have knowledge of such mandates, where they do exist. For example, in the UK, the Race Relations (Amendment) Act 2000 requires public authorities to work towards the elimination of unlawful discrimination and to promote equality of opportunity and good race relations. They must not discriminate, directly or indirectly, in the performance of their duties.

The approach to law, at both practice and policy levels, needs to move beyond the 'rational/technical' model, certainly to recognise the moral/ethical dimension of managing its relationship with the legal mandates, and ultimately to embrace a more rights-based approach. This is not to downplay the importance of a soundly constructed technical framework, and practitioners' knowledge of it – this would be dangerous, a little like setting out on a major expedition but leaving one of the maps in the cupboard at home. Nevertheless, in developing law that is fit for purpose, knowledge from other sources provides a range of filters or lenses that may be used by policy makers and practitioners to subject the legal framework to critical appraisal.

Equally, legal knowledge also must be mediated through values and skills. Values will lead and determine what legal mandates are drawn upon, and how the law is applied. Practitioners need a clear rationale, grounded in professional ethics, for how, when and why the legal framework is used, drawing on maps other than legal ones in order to illuminate and understand the territory they occupy. Relevant skills are those of reading and interpreting maps, using them as frameworks to assist in identifying landmarks on the ground and choosing routes across the territory. Important too are skills in navigating without them, when travelling off-map, or when navigational tools fail.

Third, it is important to build social workers' confidence in the legal arena, and to encourage them to see law as a positive tool. Service users comment that practitioners are ill-at-ease in legal systems, not confident of their place (Braye and Preston-Shoot, 2005). They wish to see lawyers and social workers as allies in the endeavour of securing rights and justice, not as adversaries. This has implications for the kinds of knowledge that practitioners need. It means a focus on aspects of law that empower or promote rights as well as upon those that coerce and constrain. Anti-discrimination legislation, human rights law, housing and employment provision are arguably as important to social work practice as the aspects of law that allow compulsory admission to psychiatric hospital, or removal of a child at risk. A more balanced focus would enable practitioners to work alongside both service users and lawyers to secure goals that are important to service users.

Lastly, as well as improving the maps, it is important to work too on the territory, improving the practice environment, building bridges and supportive structures to assist safe passage through some of the more challenging terrain. This means developing practice structures that connect social workers and lawyers, teachers, healthcare workers. It means engaging in legally informed debate in agencies, working to remove some of the constraints that are experienced by professionals working in corporatised welfare. It means creating structures for service users as stakeholders to articulate clearly their needs and rights in relation to the goals of professional practice. Without attention to the practice environment for legal and ethical practice, the role of law in welfare reform will be compromised, however robust the legal framework.

Notes

1 *R on the application of SSG v Liverpool CC and Secretary of State for the Department of Health and LS (Interested Party)* [2002] 5 CCLR 639.
2 *J.T. v United Kingdom* [2000] 1 FLR 909.
3 *Re F (Adult Patient)* [2000] 3 CCLR 210; *A v A Health Authority* [2002] 5 CCLR 165.
4 *R v Staffordshire CC, ex parte Farley* [1997] Current Law Year Book, 1678.
5 Investigation into Complaint No. 96/C/4315 against Liverpool CC [1999] 2 CCLR 128.
6 For example, in the UK the legal map provided by the Children Act 1989 and related court judgements gives an understanding of what kind of presentation might cause a child to be categorised as a 'child in need' (section 17) or 'at risk of significant harm' (section 47).

References

Alexander, R. (2003) *Understanding Legal Concepts that Influence Social Welfare Policy and Practice*, Pacific Grove, CA: Thomas Brooks Cole.
Beckford Report (1985) *A Child in Trust*, Wembley: London Borough of Brent.
Braye, S. and Preston-Shoot, M. (2005) 'Practice survey', in S. Braye and M. Preston-Shoot, with L.A. Cull, R. Johns, J. Roche (eds) *Knowledge Review. Teaching, Learning and Assessment of Law in Social Work Education*, London: SCIE (Social Care Institute for Excellence).
Brophy, J. and Smart, C. (eds) (1985) *Women-in-law: Explorations in Law, Family and Sexuality*, London: Routledge & Kegan Paul.
Butler-Sloss, E. (1988) *Report of the Inquiry into Child Abuse in Cleveland*, London: HMSO.
Carlisle Report (1987) *A Child in Mind*, London: London Borough of Greenwich.

Charlesworth, S., Turner, J.N. and Foreman, L. (2000) *Disrupted Families: The Law*, Sydney: Federation Press.

Cockburn, C. (1991) *In the Way of Women: Men's Resistance to Sex Equality in Organisations*, London: Macmillan.

Department of Health (DH) (1990) *Community Care in the Next Decade and Beyond: Policy Guidance*, London: HMSO.

—— (1991) *Care Management and Assessment: A Practitioner's Guide*, London: HMSO.

—— (2000) *Framework for the Assessment of Children in Need and Their Families*, London: Stationery Office.

—— (2002) *Fair Access to Care Services. Practice Guidance*, London: DH.

Humphries, B. (2004) 'An unacceptable role for social work: Implementing immigration policy', *British Journal of Social Work*, 34: 93–107.

IASSW (2001) *International Definition of Social Work*, Copenhagen: International Association of Schools of Social Work and International Federation of Social Workers.

Jankovic, J. and Green, R. (1981) 'Teaching legal principles to social workers', *Journal of Education for Social Work*, 17 (13): 28–35.

Kennedy, R. with Richards, J. (2004) *Integrating Human Service Law and Practice*, Melbourne: Oxford University Press.

King, M. and Trowell, J. (1992) *Children's Welfare and the Law: The Limits of Legal Intervention*, London: Sage.

Laming, Lord (2003) *The Victoria Climbié Inquiry, Report of an Inquiry by Lord Laming*, London: HMSO.

Madden, R. and Wayne, R. (2003) 'Social work and the laws: A therapeutic jurisprudence perspective', *Social Work*, 48 (3): 338–47.

Mafile'o, T. (2004) *A Tongan Model of Social Work: Weaving Diversity in the Context of Globalisation*, Paper given at the IFSW/IASSW Global Social Work Congress, Adelaide, October.

Preston-Shoot, M. (2000) 'What if? Using the laws to uphold practice values and standards', *Practice*, 12 (4): 49–63.

Preston-Shoot, M. and Vernon, S. (2002) 'From mapping to travelling: Negotiating the complex and confusing terrain of youth justice', *Youth and Policy*, 77: 47–65.

Preston-Shoot, M., Roberts, G. and Vernon, S. (2001) 'Value in social work law: Strained relations or sustaining relationships?', *Journal of Social Welfare and Family Law*, 23 (1): 1–22.

Reder, P., Duncan, S., Gray, M. (1993) *Beyond Blame: Child Abuse Tragedies Revisited, London:* Routledge.

Schön, D. (1983) *The Reflective Practitioner*, London: Temple Smith.

Further reading

Braye, S. and Preston-Shoot, M. (2006) *Teaching, Learning and Assessment of Law in Social Work Education: Resource Guide*, London: SCIE (Social Care Institute for Excellence).

—— (2009) *Practising Social Work Law*, 3rd edition, Basingstoke: Palgrave Macmillan.

—— (2009) 'Social work and the law', in R. Adams, L. Dominelli and M. Payne (eds) *Themes Issues and Critical Debates*, 3rd edition, Basingstoke: Palgrave Macmillan.

Dalrymple, J. and Burke, B. (2006) *Anti-oppressive Practice: Social Care and the Law, Maidenhead: Open University Press.*

Preston-Shoot, M. (2001) 'A triumph of hope over experience? On modernising accountability in social services: The case of complaints procedures in community care', *Social Policy and Administration*, 35 (6): 701–15.

—— (2008) 'Things must only get better', *Professional Social Work*, March: 14–15.

Stevenson, O. (1988) 'Law and social work education: A commentary on the "Law report"', *Issues in Social Work Education*, 8 (1): 37–45.

18 What are values?

Chris Beckett and Andrew Maynard

This chapter should be read alongside Chapter 19, because values and ethics go hand-in-hand in social work policy and practice, where values refer to what people consider to be 'good', while ethics is concerned with what people consider to be 'right' (Dubois and Miley 1996: 122). In their exploration of values, Beckett and Maynard invite readers to locate themselves in the discussion and, in doing so, they say a little about where they are 'speaking from', that is, as social work academics who are white and black, atheist and Christian, British and Caribbean in family of origin. This reminds us that we need to constantly be aware of the impact of our own biography and structural position on our beliefs and values. We also need to remember that the values we hold dear are located in a specific historical and cultural context (see also Connolly and Harms 2008).

From *Values and Ethics in Social Work: An Introduction*, London: Sage (2005): 5–23.

What do we mean by values?

The word 'value' is used in a number of ways which, at first sight, do not seem to have a huge amount in common. It is used in a financial way, as in 'gold has a higher value than lead', or in a personal way, as in 'I value your company.' Or we speak of values in a cultural sense as in 'Islamic values', 'liberal values' or middle-class values'. We also speak of 'value systems'.

Although 'the value of gold' and 'value systems' are very different kinds of idea there is nevertheless a common ground of meaning. It lies, we suggest, in the notion of preference or choice. When we say to someone 'I value your company', we are really saying that their company is important to us, and that we would choose their company over other things. If an expert on jewellery values your gold ring at £200, he is saying that given the choice between the ring and a sum of money, you should not choose the money unless it is £200 or more.

Similarly, when we speak about the 'value system' of a particular culture we are referring to the things that culture gives a high priority or importance to when making choices. In a liberal democracy, for instance, a high value is given to personal freedom. ('Everyone has the right to liberty,' says the European Convention on Human Rights.) In other societies personal freedom may be seen as less important than other things, such as observance of religious rules, or family loyalty, or social cohesion. We cannot say that one set of values is 'better' than another in any objective sense. We can only note that different cultures use different sets of criteria to make choices, presumably as a result of different circumstances and different traditions.

Values as a guide to action

If all the meanings of the word 'value' relate, as we have suggested, to the idea of choice, they also relate to ideas about what we *ought* to do.

. . . it would be impossible to make choices without values. A purely factual analysis of any given situation can only ever tell us what might be the consequences of different courses of action. But simply knowing the consequences will not help us to choose unless we have some means of determining which set of consequences is preferable. And that is not a factual question but a matter of values.

Values and value systems

We have referred to the term 'value system' but not yet defined it. How does the meaning of 'value system' relate to the meaning of 'value'? Roakeach suggested that what distinguishes a 'value system' is organisation and durability:

> A *value* is an enduring belief that a specific mode of conduct or end-state of existence is personally or socially preferable to an opposite or converse mode of conduct or end-state of existence. A *value system* is an enduring organization of beliefs concerning preferable modes of conduct or end-states of existence along a continuum of relative importance. (1973: 5)

Thus, at any given moment of time we value different things, and this may vary according to our mood or circumstances, but most of us also subscribe to a set of values which is not quite so changeable and which we may be able to define: 'I am a Muslim', 'I am a socialist', 'I am a feminist', 'I believe everyone has the right to . . .', 'I believe a parent ought to . . .'

For most of us, beliefs of these kinds are an important cornerstone of our existence, acting as a filter which defines the things we accept or reject. Value systems inform our actions, they are part of the 'emotional mobilisation' (Day, 1989, cited in Dubois and Miley, 1996: 121) that makes us jump one way as opposed to another. They shape the way we think, the judgements we make, the perceptions we hold about people, and the companions we choose to spend our time with.

Values and social work

. . . when we move from our private life to our professional life, the concept of 'values' takes on an additional dimension. Value questions don't go away when we put on our professional 'hat' – far from it – but they cease to be purely personal.

All professions have to grapple with complex issues involving values, but social work in particular, because of its socially determined nature and its focus on human interactions, constantly involves judgements in which competing values have to be weighed up. At a number of different levels, social workers are provided with frameworks within which to make these decisions:

The level of legislation and policy

Various principles are enshrined in the framework of laws, policies, government guidelines and agency rules within which social work operates. These principles are based, implicitly or explicitly, on certain values. The principles enshrined in legislation are not necessarily in harmony with one another. They can and do conflict. Nor are they necessarily in harmony with other aspects of government decision-making. For instance, the legislation may enshrine one principle, but government policy may make that principle impossible to achieve in practice.

In addition to the framework provided by the law, individual agencies have their own laid-down policies and procedures, their mission statements and guidelines. In the case of statutory agencies these will be based on the agency's legal responsibilities and the policy guidance issued by central government. In the case of non-statutory agencies, these will be generated by the agency itself. Some values will be explicitly stated; others will be implied by what is said.

The level of agency priorities

If someone said 'I really value your opinion' but then never let you get a word in without interrupting or contradicting you, you might question the accuracy of what they said. What people say and what they do are not necessarily the same. Whether looking at yourself, or at an individual, or an organisation – or indeed a whole society – it is necessary to look behind words and stated intentions to get an idea of the values that really guide actions.

If you want to understand an agency's values therefore, it is important to look at its priorities *in practice* as well as its stated intentions. Consider, for instance, an agency that stated that it was committed to working *preventatively* or *proactively*. If you looked at the way it responded to referrals and found out that referrals were only ever followed up if they were dire emergencies, you would have to conclude that in fact working preventatively was not a priority for that agency, whatever it might say, or whatever its staff might like to think.

So part of the values framework within which a social worker operates is their agency's priorities and its expectations about the ways things should be dealt with. These may or may not be reflected in the agency's public statements about its values.

The level of professional ethics and professional values

Another way in which values are, so to speak, enshrined are in guidelines on professional ethics, drawn up to try and establish certain standards of conduct. Doctors, lawyers and accountants all have their codes of professional ethics, as do social workers. Underlying these formal codes typically lie certain values which are seen as being core to that profession.

These ethical guidelines, and the professional values that lie behind them, set a different kind of framework of expectations around professionals which is distinct from those created by legislation, policies and agency priorities. The job of a doctor is different in different settings – a heart surgeon and a GP have very different tasks to perform – and yet certain ethical principles, and a certain professional ethos, are supposed to be common to all doctors. The same is true of social work. And it can happen that professional values come into conflict with the values inherent in legislation, or policy, or agency guidelines.

Personal values

A professional social worker – or any other professional – cannot only be guided by her personal values, but she cannot simply disregard her own personal values either. Personal values, after all, lie behind the decision to go into social work rather than into some other occupation. Many people who go into social work are motivated by a belief that it is important to do something for those who are excluded or disadvantaged by society at large. Some are motivated by religious beliefs or political convictions. Your own personal values will also inevitably influence how you do your job and the decisions and choices that you make. For this reason it is important to be as aware as possible of what those values are and where they come from.

Societal values

Although we are all unique, the values we hold are much less individual than we would perhaps like to think. They are shaped in large part by the society around us and by the particular subsection of society in which we find ourselves: our age group, our gender, our ethnic community, our geographical community, our occupational group, our class . . . and so on.

   We do not notice this all the time because we tend to assume that the values we share with the others around us are just 'common sense'. It is really only when we compare the kinds of assumptions we make now with those made at other times, or that are made now in other places or in other sections of society, that we realise that many of the values that we take for granted are not inevitable, but are the result of a particular and local consensus. The following is a random selection of examples of ways in which societal values can be seen to have changed over time:

- *Sexual behaviour*. In Britain, there has been a huge shift in the last fifty years in what is regarded as acceptable sexual behaviour. Premarital sex is accepted as the norm. Homosexuality has shifted from being a criminal offence to being something which MPs and cabinet ministers openly declare. This shift has not occurred in all societies, however.
- *Corporal punishment*. Fifty years ago caning and other forms of corporal punishment were seen as normal and acceptable in schools and at home. Birching was a sentence available to the courts. Now, in several countries, even smacking with the hand is illegal, although there are still countries where flogging is a normal punishment under the law.
- *Attitudes to childhood*. Historically, and in more traditional societies today, an emphasis is placed on the duties and obligations of children towards their parents. 'Honour thy father and mother,' for instance, is one of the Ten Commandments in the Old Testament. In contemporary Britain, the obligations and duties are seen mainly as flowing in the other direction, as is evidenced by the principle enshrined in Section (1) of the 1989 Children Act that 'the child's welfare should be the paramount consideration'.

You will be able to think of many other examples of areas in which the accepted wisdom of society at large about what is 'right' or 'appropriate' or 'normal' has radically changed in very recent times, and examples too of radical differences in attitude between contemporary societies and cultures: ideas about the roles of men and women, for instance, or attitudes to old people or people who are mentally ill.

Societal values are instilled in us by a socialisation process that begins, for most of us, with the messages we receive from our parents about what is important in life but is then built upon by many other influences: schooling, the peer group and, most importantly in modern culture, by the mass media, which constantly, both explicitly and implicitly, offer us sets of values to absorb.

But even though our personal values may be shaped in large part by the values of the society around us – or the values of the part of society to which we belong – this does not mean that there is no room for conflict. It is inevitable, not only in personal contexts but in professional ones, that we will find ourselves disagreeing with other people about value questions. And it is equally inevitable that even widely held values, with which few people would disagree, will frequently *come into conflict with one another*.

It is in the nature of social work that it is prone to finding itself in difficult places where deeply held societal values collide. And because this involves making compromises in which one principle is partly sacrificed for another, this can often result in social workers seeming, in the eyes of others, to trample on one or other of those deeply held values. For instance on the one hand, because it is a strongly and widely held belief that family life is sacrosanct and private, social workers intervening in families can easily be seen as interfering and oppressive, transgressing against a deep taboo. On the

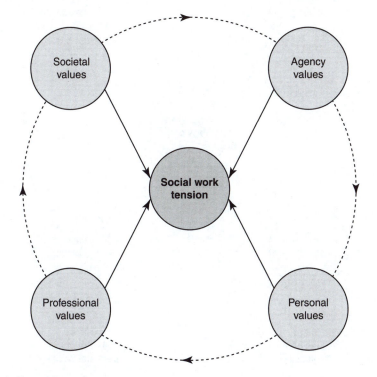

Figure 18.1 Competing values.

other hand, since it is also a strongly and widely held belief that childhood is precious and that children should be protected from harm, the failure of social workers to intervene in families to protect children may be greeted with horror and *also* be seen as transgressive.

Because these societal values exist not only outside of us but also inside, social workers need to be prepared not only for the condemnation of others, but also for powerful feelings of guilt, even if they are clear in their own minds that they have taken the best possible course of action in the circumstances.

Values in tension

Social workers are called upon to perform many complex tasks that involve difficult human interactions and in some instances involve overruling what would normally be regarded as an individual's rights (for instance: compulsory detention under mental health legislation, separation of children and parents under childcare legislation or

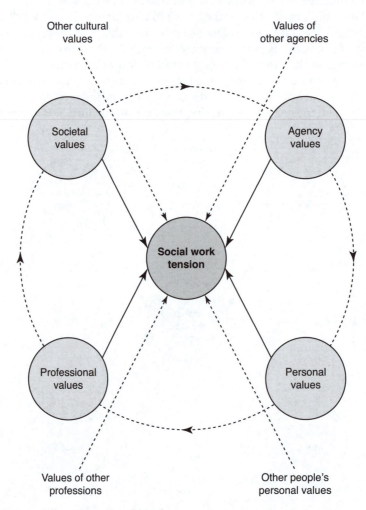

Figure 18.2 Competing values: the wider picture.

the enforcement of court orders on young offenders under youth justice legislation). In trying to come to the right decision about how to respond in any given situation the social worker struggles not only with her own personal feelings, the limitations of her own skill and knowledge, and the constraints imposed by the real world of limited options, she also struggles with a plethora of competing values – societal values, personal values, professional values and the prevailing values of her agency (see Figure 18.1).

This struggle may be experienced as conflict *within* the individual between different and competing personal values and/or internalised societal values but the struggle may also take the form of disagreements with others. It may involve disagreement with colleagues about how to proceed. It may entail disagreements with service users. It may involve struggles with managers or other agencies. There are endless arenas, internal and external, within which value conflicts are played out. Figure 18.2 attempts to illustrate these wider complexities.

References

Connolly, M. and Harms, L. (eds) (2008) *Social Work: Contexts and Practice*, 2nd edition, Oxford University Press: Australia and New Zealand.

Day, P. (1989) *A New History of Social Welfare*, Englewood Cliffs, NJ: Prentice Hall.

Dubois, B. and Miley, K. (1996) *Social Work: An Empowering Profession*, Harlow: Allyn & Bacon.

Roakeach, M. (1973) *The Nature of Human Values*, New York: Free Press.

Further reading

Banks, S. (2006) *Ethics and Values in Social Work*, 3rd revised edition, Basingstoke: Palgrave Macmillan.

Barnes, M. (2006) *Caring and Social Justice*, Basingstoke: Palgrave Macmillan.

Furness, S. and Gilligan, P. (2010) *Religion, Belief and Social Work: Making a Difference*, Bristol: Policy Press.

Horne, M. (1999) *Values in Social Work*, 2nd edition, Aldershot: Ashgate Arena.

Shardlow, S.M. (2009) 'Values, ethics and social work', in R. Adams, L. Dominelli and M. Payne (eds) *Social Work: Themes, Issues and Critical Debates*, 3rd edition, Basingstoke: Palgrave Macmillan, 37–48.

Thompson, N. (1992) *Existentialism and Social Work*, Aldershot: Avebury.

—— (2006) *Anti-discriminatory Practice*, 4th edition, Basingstoke: Palgrave Macmillan.

19 An ethical perspective on social work

Richard Hugman

Richard Hugman is an influential social work academic, now based in Australia, who formerly practised as a social worker in the UK. He has been writing about social work ethics and the social work profession for many years, and is currently advising Unicef on the development of professional social work in Vietnam. This extract connects well with the previous and following chapters by treating professional ethics as both important and situated, historically, socially and culturally.

From M. Davies (ed.) *The Blackwell Companion to Social Work*, 3rd edition, Oxford: Blackwell (2008): 442–8.

Ethics is the branch of philosophy that considers the formation and operation of moral values. In other words, it is the explicit deliberation about what is good or bad and what is right or wrong. Social work attends to core aspects of our society, often focusing on people who are excluded, marginalized, disadvantaged or who lack access to the resources needed to resolve their own problems. Such people include children and their parents, people with disabilities, older people, people with mental health difficulties, people struggling with poverty and lack of access to social infrastructure such as reasonable housing, and so on. These are areas of our lives about which we all tend to hold strong and sometimes conflicting values. So how could ethics not always be at the forefront of our thinking about social work?

The main reason why interest in social work ethics can be said to have grown *again* is that in the 1950s and 1960s the influence of an individualist perspective on ethics tended to predominate. With the development in the 1970s of a greater awareness of the social structural, and hence political, roots of the problems which the service users of social work faced in their lives, questions of ethics (seen as the 'correct actions of individual practitioners') became supplanted by concerns with the politics of practice (for example, Bailey and Brake, 1975; Galper, 1975). The more recent 'return' to ethics as a focus of attention is coterminous with the rise of neo-liberalism in the political sphere that, among other things, has sought to delegitimize the overt political actions of professions. Social work, perhaps more than some other occupations, has responded by looking again at the ethical basis of its values, because ethics is something that cannot be said to be beyond the concern of professions.

A separation of ethics and politics would have made no sense to the early moral philosophers whose work continues to be foundational, either in the Western tradition of Socrates and Plato (around 400 BCE), or in the Eastern tradition of Confucius (around 500 BCE). For all these ancient thinkers ethics and politics were not separate but inherently bound together. Questions about the good person and the good society are two sides of the same coin. For example, we might imagine them asking how social workers who are unjust in their personal relationships can work effectively for social justice, or how just social workers cannot be concerned about social injustices around them. Thus ethics cannot be confined to questions of personal responsibility. Yet at the same time we must be concerned with personal responsibility – professionals exercise considerable power with respect to service users through their knowledge and skills and their access to resources. Failing to take account of this reality does not make it go away. Without a conscious engagement with ethics social workers are poorly equipped to deal with such responsibilities and to act accountably to service users or, indeed, to address issues of injustice, exclusion or disadvantage.

Ethical principles and core approaches

The ethics of social work is, in many ways, actually very similar to that of other caring professions. That is, whether or not social workers may consider themselves to have unique values, the formal statements of ethical principles of the profession are often either identical or very close to those of medicine, nursing, occupational therapy, physiotherapy, school teaching and so on (Hugman, 2005). This is because all such statements are derived from the same stock of concepts in moral philosophy and the wider values of the societies in which these professions have developed. Furthermore, although the formal ethical statements or codes of social workers in various countries differ from each other in detail (Banks, 2006), almost all of them share core characteristics. This is because the professionalization of social work globally has tended to follow a similar pattern, which reflects the emergence of contemporary professionalism as an aspect of modernized, industrialized, urbanized society.

There are two philosophical concepts in particular that underpin almost all social work ethics (and the ethics of other caring professions). The first of these is deontology'. This term is derived from the Greek word 'deon', meaning 'duty'. It refers to ways of understanding what is good and what is right by considering what duties each person has towards other people and the world around them. For example, it may be argued that all human beings should be treated with respect, simply because they are human beings and therefore are all moral entities. So in these terms 'telling a lie' is morally wrong because it treats another person as less than fully human irrespective of the consequences of telling the truth. (The origins of deontology understood in this way is usually attributed to the work of Emmanuel Kant [1724–1804].)

In contrast to deontology, professional ethics in social work also embodies the principles of 'teleology'. This term also comes from a Greek word 'telos' meaning 'the end' and it is the approach that considers something to be good or right at looking at what follows from it. Thus some writers also refer to it as 'consequentialism'. So, for example, whether it is good or right to tell a lie will depend on what are the ends of doing so: the classic example is that of using a lie to protect someone from serious physical harm. Teleology often appears in social work ethics in the form of 'utilitarianism', which is a particular form of the approach. 'Utility' in this sense refers to the way in which something contributes to the greatest possible well-being for the greatest possible number of people. (The origins of utilitarianism are usually seen in the work of Jeremy Bentham [1748–1832] and J. S. Mill [1806–73].)

As these two approaches are inherently in conflict with each other, but both influence professional practice, they have tended to be moderated by taking core principles from them and combining these in a way that downplays their differences. This third approach is sometimes referred to as 'principlism' and is most highly developed in bio-medical and health ethics (Beauchamp and Childress, 2001). The principles that appear in this approach are: respect for people; beneficence (seeking to do good); non-maleficence (seeking not to do harm); justice. As Beauchamp and Childress themselves, among others, have acknowledged, the bringing together of principles from different approaches still leaves it to professions and their individual members to make sense of how these ideas are constituted in practice and how to develop a shared sense of what is good and what is right.

Ethics, professionalism and accountability

As I have already stated, the importance of ethics in a profession such as social work is that all professionals exercise power in relation to the users of their services. While the experience of a junior member of a profession may not always be experienced as 'powerful', the impact of all practice on service users can be said to be powerful in that it has the capacity to affect human lives in profound ways. Indeed, if it does not we perhaps should ask what is the purpose of undertaking such work.

Power does not have to be overt or equated with force. It can take the form of influence or persuasion, for example. The power of a therapist or counsellor would often take such forms, as would the pronouncements of a community development worker. Because of the expertise that professionals are seen to have, their words 'carry weight' and this is often the most effective sort of power in contemporary society.

The sense of responsibility on which professional ethics is based comes from recognizing power while at the same time holding values that emphasize the moral (including the political) standing of service users as equal to that of professionals. The ethical documents of professions thus serve as guidance, which is sometimes quite firm, about the 'good' in practice. Moreover, they also constitute a declaration to the wider society, including service users, about what can be expected of the 'good' practitioner. On these two grounds, taken together, codes of ethics and similar statements can provide an explicit vehicle for accountability (Banks, 2004). In a society such as the USA the implications of a code of ethics may even be seen as contractual, forming the basis by which service users can seek legal redress for actions that breach the terms of a code (Reamer, 2001). In many other countries codes of ethics provide a mechanism for redress that falls short of litigation but in which a professional body may hold practitioners to account for failures to conform to the terms of a code.

Codes of ethics

In the contemporary globalized world it is difficult to think of a profession that does not have a code of ethics. These are the formal statements that represent the values of the professional community. Some national associations, such as those in Australia and in the UK, state that the core values are: human dignity and worth; social justice; service to humanity; integrity; competence (Australian Association of Social Workers

[AASW], 2002, p. 8; British Association of Social Workers [BASW], 2002, p. 2). To these, the national association in the USA adds 'the importance of human relationships' (National Association of Social Workers [NASW], 1999, p. 1).

In addition, codes usually – but not always – contain quite detailed guidance or instruction on how values and principles are to be interpreted in specific aspects of practice (Banks, 2006). For example, in the Australian Association of Social Workers *Code of Ethics (1999)*, each clause in the section on 'ethical practice' begins with or includes the phrase 'social workers will . . .' (AASW, 2002, pp. 11–21). Similar phrasing is used in the codes of the British Association of Social Workers (2002), the New Zealand/ Aotearoa Association of Social Workers (1993) and the National Association of Social Workers (1999).

In some states of the USA and in some provinces of Canada someone who is held to have breached professional ethics may have their registration or licence removed. More recently registration has been introduced in the UK and in New Zealand giving ethics similar importance. In Australia, as yet, the sanction remains that of exclusion from the professional association.

The problem for individual practitioners is that many statements in codes of ethics may at times be open to interpretation, despite the guidance provided for individual application. Although an injunction to 'protect client's records' may be relatively easy to apply, a statement such as 'social workers will acknowledge the significance of culture in their practice' requires a greater degree of interpretation, while the injunction to 'provide a competent and humane service to clients, mindful of fulfilling their duty of care and observing the principles of natural justice' necessitates a sophisticated grasp of ethical concepts by a practitioner.

The IFSW/IASSW joint statement on ethical principles

In 2004 the International Federation of Social Workers (IFSW) and the International Association of Schools of Social Work (IASSW) approved a joint statement on ethical principles in social work that replaces previous ethical documents of the two bodies (IFSW/IASSW, 2004). As the global peak organizations for social work, this statement serves as the basis for national social work associations around the world in the formation of their codes or statements of ethics. The IFSW/IASSW document is not intended to form a blue-print, but rather to act as a guide and as a starting point.

Compared with the previous 'codes' of the two bodies, the 2004 *Statement of Principles* is simplified. It discusses in detail, but briefly, just two core values which are asserted as being core to professional social work: human rights and human dignity, and social justice. These values (which roughly map onto the twin approaches of deontology and teleology) are a reflection of the United Nations and related documents that are cited as the point of reference for social work internationally (such as the UN Declaration on Human Rights). This list is considerably shorter than those of the national associations cited above. Moreover, the implications of the values, and the broad principles that are derived from them, are spelled out succinctly. Human rights and dignity are seen in terms of self-determination, participation, treating each person as a whole and focusing on people's strengths. Social justice is considered to include challenging discrimination, recognizing diversity, seeking equity, challenging unjust policies and working in solidarity (IFSW/IASSW, 2004).

The other point of interest about the IFSW/IASSW *Statement of Principles* is that the document is quite specifically not intended to be a 'code'. This task is left to national associations (who are required to have a code of ethics as part of the conditions of membership of IFSW, for example) (IFSW/IASSW, 2004). This approach recognizes that although there are some core values and principles in social work, such as human rights and social justice, it is appropriate that variations between countries are reflected in specific codes of ethics, for example embodying cultural differences. Nonetheless, the *Statement of Principles* does contain a brief list of short prescriptions of 'good social work', such as not using social work skills to support torture or terrorism, where these were seen to be helpful to defend the core values (personal communication). The point remains that this list is neither exhaustive nor is it enforceable at the local or individual levels of practice by either international organization.

The challenge of 'different' ethics in diverse societies

Although I have indicated that there are some similarities between the ancient ethical traditions of Eastern and Western societies, in the centuries since Confucius and Socrates a greater divergence has opened up. The dominant approaches in professional ethics that have been described, namely deontology, teleology and principlism, are Western. They reflect the impact of scientific thought and what is called 'modernization'. Thus the values expressed in the United Nations documents to which the IFSW/IASSW ethical statement refers, with their foundational principles of human rights and social justice, have been criticized as inherently Western in their outlook. In particular, the concept of 'rights' that exists in Eastern approaches to ethics is somewhat different to that of the West, especially in so far as Eastern ethics tends to prioritize the harmony of the family and the community over the interests of individuals (Wong, 2004). Similar observations may be made about the core values of indigeneous societies, such as Aboriginal Australians or Native Americans, and about post-colonial communities such as traditional Muslim communities in Western countries. Thus some critics have argued that professional ethics as presented by the IFSW and IASSW are not international, but represent an imposition of values from one cultural perspective onto all others (Azmi, 1997).

It is also the case that the approaches of deontology, teleology and principlism do not represent all the possibilities in Western ethical thought. Recent ideas have included the 'ethics of care' (in which the nurturing of caring relationships is a primary value), ethics grounded in the intelligent use of emotions (in which 'compassion' is a primary value) or 'postmodern ethics' (in which, I would argue, an appeal to the Socratic idea of virtue is a very strong element) (Hugman, 2005). However, as Banks (2006) argues, although these approaches provide many useful ideas that can inform how principles may be operationalized in specific situations, they do not provide a firm foundation for the ethics of *a profession*. That is, where membership of an occupation is the one common factor between all social workers (who may be from many different cultures, both men and women, with different identities and experiences) it is insufficient to rely on each individual person applying their own values. Service users should be able to expect something in common between practitioners, so that they can rely on knowing that social workers should protect the privacy of service users, should not exploit service users (for example, sexually or financially) and so on, rather than having to negotiate each of the aspects that are covered by a code of ethics.

Perhaps, then, the solution to diversity is to regard ethical statements, at both the national and international level, as living traditions in the manner of an on-going conversation (Hugman, 2005). At any specific time there will be a written statement on ethics, probably in the form of a code, which applies to the professional community. But this is open to continual debate and reconsideration. The task for each social worker is to be prepared to take part in the conversation and to ensure that the ethical tradition of social work remains alive and continues to grow.

References

Australian Association of Social Workers (AASW) (2002) *Code of Ethics (1999)*, 2nd edition, Canberra: AASW.

Azmi, S. (1997) 'Professionalism and social diversity', in R. Hugman, M. Peelo and K. Soothill (eds) *Concepts of Care*, London: Edward Arnold.

Bailey, R. and Brake, M. (eds) (1975) *Radical Social Work*, London: Edward Arnold.

Banks, S. (2004) *Ethics, Accountability and the Social Professions*, Basingstoke: Palgrave.

—— (2006) *Ethics and Values in Social Work*, 3rd edition, Basingstoke: Palgrave Macmillan.

Beauchamp, T.L. and Childress, J.F. (2001) *Principles of Biomedical Ethics*, 5th edition, Oxford: Oxford University Press.

British Association of Social Workers (BASW) (2002) *Code of Ethics for Social Work*, Birmingham: BASW.

Galper, J. (1975) *The Politics of Social Services*, Englewood Cliffs, NJ: Prentice-Hall.

Hugman, R. (2005) *New Approaches in Ethics for the Caring Professions*, Basingstoke: Palgrave.

International Federation of Social Workers/International Association of Schools of Social Work (IFSW/IASSW) (2004) *Ethics in Social Work: A Statement of Principles*, Berne: IFSW (available at www.ifsw.org, accessed on 16 June 2010).

National Association of Social Workers (NASW) (1999) *Code of Ethics of the National Association of Social Workers*, Washington, DC: NASW.

New Zealand/Aotearoa Association of Social Workers (NZASW) (1993) *Code of Ethics*, Dunedin: NZASW.

Reamer, F.R. (2001) *Ethics Education in Social Work*, Alexandria, VA: NASW.

Wong, D.B. (2004) 'Rights and community in Confucianism', in K.-L. Shun and D.B. Wong (eds) *Confucian Ethics*, Cambridge: Cambridge University Press.

Further reading

Banks, S. and Gallagher, A. (2009) *Ethics in Professional Life: Virtues for Health and Social Care*, Basingstoke: Palgrave Macmillan.

Clark, C.L. (2000) *Social Work Ethics: Politics, Principles and Practice*, Basingstoke: Macmillan

GSCC (General Social Care Council) (2004) *Code of Practice for Social Care Workers* and *Code of Practice for Employers of Social Care Workers*, London: GSCC.

Hugman, R. and Smith, D. (eds) (1995) *Ethical Issues in Social Work*, London: Routledge.

McBeath, G. and Webb, S. (2002) 'Virtue, ethics and social work: Being lucky, realistic and not doing one's duty', *British Journal of Social Work*, 32: 1015–36.

Shardlow, S.M. (2009) 'Values, ethics and social work', in R. Adams, L. Dominelli and M. Payne (eds) *Social Work: Themes, Issues and Critical Debates*, 3rd edition, Basingstoke: Palgrave Macmillan, 37–48.

20 Expanding the philosophical base of social work

Mekada Graham

I have chosen Mekada Graham to end this section on knowledge and values because her writing adds further confirmation to the idea that knowledge and values are always partial and unfinished; moreover, knowledge is, as Foucault (1976) argues, created through power. Graham is a black British social work academic now working in the United States. She argues that until recent years, social work knowledge and values have been built on largely white, Eurocentric ways of thinking, just as feminists have argued that social sciences knowledge has been built on the assumption of men as 'the norm' and women as 'other' (see Harding 1991). Julie Fish (2006) makes a similar point in relation to the implicit heterosexism in social work. In the following extract, Graham offers an African-centred worldview which challenges and unsettles conventional perspectives (see also Linda Tuhiwai Smith on researching indigenous peoples).

From *Social Work and African-centred Worldviews,* Birmingham: Venture Press (2001): 63–74.

African-centred worldviews have emerged as an important cultural foundation source in the study of black people, their lived experiences, social practices, survival, well-being and understanding of the world. The articulation of these worldviews suggests that European and African worldviews have validity only under limiting conditions. However, this standpoint does not imply that only the philosophical traits of a particular worldview characterise people in that ethnic group; rather, this perspective implies that set of philosophical traits of a particular worldview is dominant.

African-centred discourse

African-centred worldviews rest upon the notion of a distinctive African philosophy that embraces various schools of thought which are derived from classical African civilisations as the baseline for conceptions of human beings and the universe. Africa is viewed as the source of historical beginnings, templates of culture, belief systems, philosophies, values and knowledge of the world which all inform African cultural identities.

African-centred social thought has emerged as a critical, deconstructive and reconstructive project that challenges the definitive characterisation of what it is to be human within the context of Enlightenment philosophies. Moreover, this enterprise seeks to organise, study and analyse cultural data in the cultures and philosophies of African people under the umbrella of African philosophy. African-centred endeavours contend that there exists an emotional, cultural, intellectual and psychological connection between all African people wherever they are located. This project seeks to validate the experiences of African peoples as well as critique the exclusion and marginalisation of African knowledge systems from educational and mainstream scholarship. This intellectual exercise began with a decolonised study of Africa from African-centred perspectives. This concept of decolonisation refers to breaking with the ways in which the African human condition is defined and shaped by the dominant context and asserting an understanding of social realities informed by local experiences (hooks, 1984). This trend in African philosophy has its roots in Pan-African social thought and the civil rights movement in the USA it also spans the Caribbean, Europe, Africa and other areas of the diaspora in seeking to free African and African-descended peoples from racialised domination. In this context, the decolonisation of Africa and the Caribbean and the reclamation of indigenous cultures have strongly influenced this discourse.

There are various strands that have shaped and defined African-centred social thought and these include African socialism. Consciencism, scientific socialism and African humanism. These strands draw upon eminent black scholars and activists over the past 200 years who have been instrumental in defining an African-centred intellectual school of thought. Black scholars – notably Ani, Asante, Akbar, Nobles, Hillard, Diop, Obenga, T'Shaka, Blyden, Clarke and Karenga – have been engaged in the process of reclaiming ancient African philosophical systems to interpret a distinctive African school of thought. This project proposes that these ideals can assist in shaping futures for African peoples throughout the world. It is claimed that 'any meaningful and authentic study of peoples of African descent must begin and proceed with Africa as the centre, not periphery' (Abarry, 1990:123).

Liberation philosophies

There have been various definitions and expressions of African-centred social thought. However, they all share a concern to present an alternative way of knowing the world. This intellectual exercise seeks to bring people of African descent from the margins of European social thought to the centre of postmodern history.

According to Asante (1990) the African-centred intellectual idea is distinguished by five characteristics:

- an intense interest in psychological location as determined by symbols, motifs, rituals and signs
- a commitment to finding the subject place of Africans in any social, political, economic or religious phenomenon with implications for questions of sex, gender and class
- a defence of African cultural elements as historically valid in the context of art, music and literature
- a celebration of 'centredness' and agency and a commitment to lexical refinement that eliminates pejoratives about Africans and other people
- a powerful imperative from historical sources to revise the collective text of African people

Asante (1980:5) suggests an African cultural system in which all African people participate, 'although it is modified according to specific histories and nations'. The grounding of African-centred thought is located in *Njia*, 'the collective expression of the Afrocentric worldview based in the historical experience of African people'. Thus, dispensing with the legacy of European Enlightenment representations of Africans in intellectual thought gives rise to new criticism that assists in 'a cultural reconstruction that incorporates the African perspective as a part of an entire human transformation' (1980:6). In this way, African people are given subject place with agency in the study of African phenomena. According to Asante (1980:7), one of the important aspects of this project is the reclamation of the African origins of ancient Egypt (Kemet) and the Nile Valley civilisations. Within this context, classical African civilisations can be 'points of reference for an African perspective in much the same way as Greece and Rome are in the European world'.

Asante (1980:34) maintains that furnished with this new information which will expand human perspectives on knowledge transcultural analysis will become possible. Therefore, armed with this new information and emanating innovative methodologies, 'Africology will transform community and social sciences, as well as arts and humanities and assist in constructing a new, perhaps more engaging way to analyse and synthesise reality'.

African-centred theories propose that this is the most effective way of studying and understanding African people and their communities. This approach suggests an orientation in approaching and interpreting data. Thus African-centred theory may be viewed as mapping the boundaries and contours of this disciplinary field.

African-centred worldviews begin with a holistic conception of the human condition which spans the cosmological (an aspect of philosophy that considers the nature and structure of the universe), ontological (the essence of all things), and axiological (an area of philosophy that considers the nature of values and value preferences in a culture).

African-centred philosophy is a holistic system based upon values and ways of living which are reinforced through rituals, music, dance, story-telling, proverbs, metaphors and the promoting of family; rites of passage, naming ceremonies, child-rearing, birth, death, elderhood and values of governance. The principles and values that underpin the African-centred worldview are:

- the interconnectedness of all things
- the spiritual nature of human beings
- collective/individual identity and the collective/inclusive nature of family structure
- oneness of mind, body and spirit
- the value of interpersonal relationships

African-centred worldviews

The interconnectedness of all things

Within the cosmological perspective of the African-centred worldviews, all elements of the universe – people, animals and inanimate objects – are viewed as interconnected. Since they are dependent upon each other, they are, in essence, considered as one. Human reality is unified and we divide unity into parts only because of the limitations of our present knowledge. Asante (1990) expresses unification through a statement credited to the Zulu peoples: 'I am river, I am mountain, I am tree, I am love, I am emotion, I am beauty. I am lake, I am cloud, I am sun, I am sky, I am mind, I am one with one.'

For Akbar (1976:176), the unity of 'the African cosmos is like a spider web; its least element cannot be touched without making the whole vibrate. Everything is connected, interdependent.' These relationships provide individuals with a sense of purpose and connection with families and community. This is because the self 'cannot be complete if it remains enclosed, but it has to seek out the other if it is to become actualised . . . a person can only be a human when other people are there to complete his or her humaness. The individual cannot be human alone' (Holdstock, 2000:105). Moreover, the maintenance of harmonious social relationships supports the development of positive self-esteem and social competence. Social problems and human dysfunction arise when people become alienated and disconnected from their interdependent human relationships.

The interconnectedness of all things sees no separation between the material and the spiritual 'reality is at one and inseparably spiritual and material' (Myers, 1988:24) as all reality (universe) begins from a single principle. Human beings are perceived as an integral part of nature, and living in harmony with the environment helps them to become one with all reality. The concept of oneness relates to those not yet born and those who have died: all human beings are linked spiritually across time and space. As Schiele (1994:18) declares, 'the focus on interconnectedness recognises that people are spiritual (i.e., nonmaterial) beings who are connected with each other through the spirit of the Creator'. The spiritual aspect of human beings transcends the sphere of time and space.

The interconnectedness of human beings spiritually is translated socially, so that the human being is never an isolated individual but always the person in the community. The community defines the person, as Mbiti (1970:141) explains: 'I am because we are; and because we are, therefore I am.' Holdstock (2000:105) captures the essence of this concept when he uses the Zulu expression, '*umuntu ngumuntu ngabantu*', which means that a person is a person through other persons. Self-knowledge is rooted in 'being centred in one's self, one's own experience, one's history' (Verharen, 1995:65). To become aware of the cultural self is an important process that connects a person spiritually to others within a culture. It is the universal network of energies that generates sustenance for individuals and communities and, in so doing, self-knowledge within the context of one's cultural base and connection with others provides the basis for transformation, spiritual development and wellbeing.

The spiritual nature of human beings

Spirituality forms the cornerstone of African-centred worldviews and is the essence of human beings. Spirituality has been defined as 'that invisible substance that connects all human beings to each other and to a creator' (Schiele, 1994:18). The spiritual essence of human beings requires a shift in thinking towards valuing human beings above the social and economic status which has been assigned to them. For example, who you are, your personhood, comes about through your relationship with the community. As Karenga (1997) proposes, personhood evolves through the process of becoming and this negates the idea that personhood is achieved simply by existence. The process of being is marked by successive stages of integration or incorporation into the community. Life is a series of passages: a process whereby a person is accorded the challenge togrow, change and develop to attain moral, intellectual and social virtues within the context of community.

Collective / individual identity and collective / inclusive nature of the twinlineal family structure

The individual cannot be understood separately from other people (Myers, 1988). The collective nature of identity is expressed in the African proverb 'I am because we are and because we are therefore I am' (Mbiti, 1970:141). These philosophical assumptions transmit to the psyche a sense of belonging to the collective and of being part of the whole. This is because mutuality and individuality are inextricably linked in the concept of self. The individual's moral growth and development facilitates the growth of others (Holdstock, 2000).

From these assumptions of collective identity follows the emphasis upon human similarities or commonalities rather than upon individual differences. The collective nature of human beings entails collective responsibility for what happens to individuals. 'Whatever happens to the individual happens to the whole group and whatever happens to the whole group happens to the individual' (Mbiti, 1970:141). The collective identity of human beings links the conception of the family to its structures and functioning. Twinlineal is a term used for black families, referring to the fact that African family lineages come from both the mother and father rather than *only* the mother or father as in matrilineal and patrilineal family systems. The family structure also includes members who are not biologically related and an extensive network of cousins (T'Shaka, 1995). This has immediate implications for social work: 'social workers have found themselves utterly confused when they have attempted to list, define or describe black families utilising the guidelines which have grown from their own experiences' (Akbar, 1976:180).

The notion of half-siblings prevalent within social work theory and practice, for example, is incomprehensible; it does not exist within an African-centred worldview.

The underlying precept of 'half-sibling' becomes a value-based supposition within social work practice that is manifested where contact arrangements with 'half-siblings' may be viewed as less important than those with 'full siblings'. In my experience, and that of many other professionals working in the field of child-care, neither these concepts nor these assumptions reflect the realities of black children. Thus the ethnocentric worldview constructs a 'universalism' of social work practice and imposes a value system and construct which may compromise the psychological wellbeing of black children.

For the same reason, the therapeutic tool of the ecomap does not capture the realities of some black families or of the network of cousins and other family members beyond the 'extended family'. This more complex picture, of families which include members who are not biologically related, is reflected in developing African-centred designs for social work practice where there is an emphasis on being part of a group, spiritually as well as physically, as an essential ingredient of identity. The failure of the social work profession to comprehend this critical proposition is one of the reasons why black professionals and the black community were so vociferously opposed to the one-way traffic of transracial placements. The children were considered a loss to the whole community, not just physically but as a loss felt spiritually by the collective – the whole community – worldwide.

African-centred worldviews regard children as the collective responsibility of communities. The African proverb, 'It takes a village to raise a child', expresses the view that child-rearing is a collective responsibility, rather than a concern for individual nuclear families. Children are highly valued in general, as 'of the community', and they therefore cannot be deemed illegitimate (Suda, 1997).

Oneness of mind, body and spirit and the value of interpersonal relationships

There is no division between mind, body and spirit in African-centred paradigms. They are each given equal value and are believed to be interrelated (Mbiti, 1970). The development and knowledge of self, mind, body and spirit are the halmark of human objectives to seek divinity through *Maat* (truth, justice, righteousness, harmony, balance, order, propriety, compassion and reciprocity) within the self and through reaching a state of optimal health (Chissell, 1994). To promote personhood, optimal health requires optimal emotional health, physical health, intellectual health and spiritual health. These principles underlie the need to achieve harmony with the forces of life. King (1994:20) outlines the process of achieving a harmonious way of living. He suggests the combination of co-operating with natural forces that influence events and experiences while at the same time 'taking responsibility for one's life by consciously choosing and negotiating the direction and paths one will follow'.

African-centred worldviews include the concept of balance. The task of all living things is to maintain balance in the face of adverse external forces. When this inner peace is compromised, the psychological, social and physical wellbeing of a person is threatened.

Using these values and principles as a guide, Karenga (1993) has developed a theory of cultural and social change. The Kwaida theory proposes that examples of alienation, degradation, self-hatred and dysfunction within black communities may be directly related to a misplaced consciousness. Karenga (1993) contends that this is symptomatic of a cultural crisis that faces communities in European/Western contexts where marginalisation and institutional racism are an integral part of societies. The philosophy of Kwaida is expressed as an orientation towards corrective action that includes the reconstruction of cultural values on the basis of a critical reading of African cultural antecedents. Thus Kwaida is a prescriptive theory of cultural and social change located in seven basic areas of cultural and social life. These correctives are advanced in the areas of religion, history, social, economic and political organisations, creativity and ethos (Karenga, 1993).

The core of the Kwaida theory advances seven principles, the *Nguzo Saba*, to provide a guide to cultural and social change and the organisation of black life. These include *Umoja* (unity), *Kujichagulia* (self-determination), *Ujima* (collective work and responsibility), *Ujamaa* (co-operative economics), *Nia* (purpose), *Kuumba* (creativity) and *Imani* (faith).

References

Abarry, A. (1990) 'Afrocentricity: Introduction', *Journal of Black Studies*, 21: 123–5.
Akbar, N. (1976) 'Rhythmic patterns in African personality', L. King, V. Dion, V. and W. Nobles

(eds) *African Philosophy: Assumptions and Paradigms for Research on Black People*, Los Angeles, CA: Fanon Research Development Center.

Asante, M. (1980) 'International/intercultural relations', in M. Asante and A. Vandi (eds) *Contemporary Black Thought: Alternative Analyses in Social and Behavioural Science*, Beverley Hills, CA: Sage.

—— (1990) *Kemet, Afrocentricity and Knowledge*, Trenton, NJ: Africa World Press.

Chissell, J.T. (1994) *Pyramids of Power! An Ancient African-centred Approach to Optimal Health*, Baltimore, MD: Positive Perceptions.

Fish, J. (2006) *Heterosexism in Health and Social Care*, Basingstoke: Palgrave Macmillan.

Foucault, M. (1976) *The History of Sexuality Volume 1*, New York: Random House.

Harding, S. (1991) *Whose Science? Whose Knowledge? Thinking from Women's Lives*, Milton Keynes: Open University Press.

Holdstock, T. (2000) *Re-examining Psychology: Critical Perspectives and African Insights*, London: Routledge.

hooks, b. (1984) *Feminist Theory: From Margin to Center*, Boston, MA: South End Press.

Karenga, M. (1993) *Introduction to Black Studies*, 2nd edition, Los Angeles, CA: University of Sankore Press.

—— (1997) *Kwanzaa: A Celebration of Family, Community and Culture*, Los Angeles, CA: University of Sankore Press.

King, A. (1994) 'An Africocentric cultural awareness program for incarcerated African-American males', *Journal of Multicultural Social Work*, 3 (4): 17–28.

Mbiti, J. S. (1970) *African Religions and Philosophy*, Garden City, NY: Anchor Books.

Myers, L. (1988) *Understanding an Afrocentric World View: Introduction to Optimal Psychology*, Dubuque, IA: Kendall/Hunt.

Schiele, J. (1994) 'Afrocentricity as an alternative worldview for equality', *Journal of Progressive Human Services*, 5 (1): 5–25.

Smith, L.T. (1999) *Decolonizing Methodologie: Research and Indigenous Peoples*, London: Zed Books and University of Otago Press..

Suda, C. (1997) 'Street children in Nairobi and the African cultural ideology of kin-based support system: Change and challenge', *Child Abuse Review*, 6 (3): 199–217.

T'Shaka, O. (1995) *Return to the African Mother Principle of Male and Female Equality*, Volume 1, Oakland, CA: Pan Afrikan.

Verharen, C. (1995) 'Afrocentrism and acentricim: A marriage of science and philosophy', *Journal of Black Studies*, 26 (1): 62–76.

Further reading

Dominelli, L. (2002) *Anti-oppressive Social Work Theory and Practice*, Basingstoke: Palgrave Macmillan.

—— (2008) *Anti-racist Social Work*, 3rd edition, Basingstoke: Palgrave Macmillan.

Graham, M. (2007) *Black Issues in Social Work and Social Care*, Bristol: Policy Press.

Graham, M.J. (1999) 'The African-centred worldview: Developing a paradigm for social work', *British Journal of Social Work*, 29 (2): 251–67.

Holloway, J.S. and Keppel, B. (eds) (2007) *Black Scholars on the Line: Race, Social Science, and American Thought in the Twentieth Century*, Notre Dame, IN: University of Notre Dame Press.

Nziri, V. (2009) *Social Care with African Families*, London: Routledge.

Obama, B. (2008) *Dreams from My Father: A Story of Race and Inheritance*, Edinburgh: Canongate.

Part III

Skills and practice in social work

Commentary 3

It has been challenging to find a way through the material which might be included in this section of the reader. As already discussed, social work makes use of a range of skills, models and methods which are built on different theoretical approaches drawn from psychology, social psychology, sociology, philosophy, education, the law, etc. These are discussed in a number of social work texts, including Coulshed and Orme (2006), Lishman (2007), Nash *et al.* (2005), Sheldon and Macdonald (2009), Trevithick (2005) and Watson and West (2006). At the same time, social work practice takes place in a wide range of settings which include fieldwork, day-care, residential and community work; health, education and (in Scotland) criminal justice services; in the statutory, voluntary and private sectors (see Adams *et al.* 2009; Cree and Myers 2008; Davies 2008; Wilson *et al.* 2008). It will never be possible to cover all the skills and practice with which social work engages in this section. Furthermore, it is arguable whether skills and practice can ever be learned from reading about them. As demonstrated consistently over many years, learning is only ever fully integrated when it is applied in practice (Kolb 1984; Boud and Miller 1996; Gould and Taylor 1996). As Kolb explains:

> . . . learning, and therefore knowing, requires both a grasp of figurative representation of experience and some transformation of that experience . . . the creation of knowledge and meaning, occurs though the active extension and grounding of ideas *and* experiences in the external world and through internal reflection about the attributes of these experiences and ideas.
>
> (Kolb 1984: 42, 52)

Nevertheless, I believe that it is possible to present a number of skills, methods and models which are likely to be useful in most social work settings. All the approaches which I have selected value the individual, whilst also seeing that person in the context of their biography, their family, community and society. They also all bear witness to an underlying commitment to anti-oppressive values and social justice.

To begin at the beginning. Social workers work with people who are in need of help of one kind or another, whether they are individuals, members of families or groups. To be able to do this, they must first be able to communicate and engage with people, hence to draw on communication skills (Chapter 21). They must then be able, with the service user/users, to work out what the nature of the problem is:

that is, to carry out an assessment and then to evaluate their intervention to see whether or not it worked, and what more (if anything) needs to be done (discussed in Chapter 22). At this point, they will have to be able to see the individual and their problem in context, and an ecological or systems approach will be useful here (Chapter 23). Sometimes people experience a number of issues all at the same time, and a problem-solving approach like crisis intervention may enable the worker and service user to see a way forward (Chapter 24). They must also remember that individuals are more than the sum of their problems, or, in other words, that everyone has resources (individual, family and community) that can and should be built on; a strengths approach may facilitate this (Chapter 25). Professionals are not the only people with answers, as an exploration of advocacy (Chapter 26) illustrates. Moreover, social work practitioners frequently work alongside others (professionals and lay people) in the context of current practice (Chapter 27). But, to repeat, social work is not only about individuals and families. Social workers must recognise that what may benefit people most is action at a community level, not an individual level, and in this respect, Chapters 28 and 29 offer useful suggestions. Chapter 30 ends the book where we began, with an acknowledgement that we are living and working in uncertain times, and that, because of this, our practice must remain open, flexible and, above all, critically reflective.

Key questions

1   Can good social work practice be taught and, if so, how?
2   Pick a model or method from this section. What is it about it that speaks to you most and why?
3   What do we need to do to ensure that anti-oppressive practice and social justice remain at the heart of the social work agenda?

References

Adams, R., Dominelli, L. and Payne, M. (eds) (2009) *Social Work: Themes Issues and Critical Debates*, 3rd edition, Basingstoke, Palgrave Macmillan.

Boud, D. and Miller, N. (1996) *Working with Experience: Animating Learning*, London: Routledge.

Coulshed, V. and Orme, J. (2006) *Social Work Practice*, 4th edition, Basingstoke: Palgrave Macmillan.

Cree, V.E. and Myers, S. (2008) *Social Work: Making a Difference*, Bristol: Policy Press/ BASW.

Davies, M. (ed.) (2008) *Blackwell Companion to Social Work*, 3rd edition, Oxford, Blackwell.

Gould, N. and Taylor, I. (1996) *Reflective Learning for Social Work*, Aldershot: Arena.

Kolb, D.A. (1984) 'A comparative study of professional education in social work and engineering', in D.A. Kolb (ed.) *Experiential Learning*, New York: Prentice Hall.

Lishman, J. (ed.) (2007) *Handbook for Practice Learning in Social Work and Social Care*, London: Jessica Kingsley.

Nash, M., Munford, R. and O'Donoghue, K. (2005) *Social Work Theories in Action*, London: Jessica Kingsley.

Sheldon, B. and Macdonald, G. (2009) *A Textbook of Social Work*, London: Routledge.

Trevithick, P. (2005) *Social Work Skills: A Practice Handbook*, 2nd edition, Maidenhead: Open University Press.

Watson, D. and West, J. (2006) *Social Work Process and Practice: Approaches, Knowledge and Skills*, Basingstoke: Palgrave Macmillan.

Wilson, K., Ruch, G., Lymbery, M. and Cooper, A. (2008) *Social Work: An Introduction to Contemporary Practice*, Harlow: Essex Pearson Education.

Further reading

Teater, B. (2010) *An Introduction to Applying Social Work Theories and Methods*, Buckingham: Open University Press.

21 The communication skills of therapeutic dialogue

Gerard Egan

The starting point for all social work practice is to be able to engage with people and genuinely hear what they are saying. This demands an ability to communicate both verbally and non-verbally and a capacity to build relationships, or to have what Neil Thompson calls 'people skills'. Of course, communication is never divorced from the setting and context within which it takes place. This means that a home visit to someone who has asked for social work help is likely to be very different in tone and substance to a meeting in an office with someone who is an 'involuntary client' (Trotter 1999). There may also be differences according to culture and ethnicity (Dominelli 2008; Graham 2001; Robinson 2007). In spite of this, there are basic guidelines which may be helpful whatever the setting or context, and Gerard Egan's book, *The Skilled Helper*, now in its ninth edition, is as good an introduction to the subject as any, and one which is widely used by a range of social work authors; readers are encouraged to get hold of the book, not just this heavily edited extract. Egan is Emeritus Professor of Psychology and Organizational Studies at Loyola University of Chicago.

From *The Skilled Helper: A Problem-Management and Opportunity-Development Approach to Helping*, 9th edition, Belmont, CA: Brooks/Cole (2010): 131–50.

I. VISIBLY TUNING IN: THE IMPORTANCE OF EMPATHIC PRESENCE

Helping and other deep interpersonal transactions demand a certain robustness or intensity of presence. Visibly tuning in to others contributes to this presence. It is an expression of empathy that tells clients that you are with them, and it puts you in a position to listen carefully to their concerns. Your attention can be manifested in both physical and psychological ways. Because nonverbal behavior can play an important part in empathic communication, let's start by briefly exploring nonverbal behavior as a channel of communication.

Nonverbal behavior as a channel of communication

The face and body are extremely communicative. We know from experience that even when people are together in silence, the atmosphere can be filled with messages. Sometimes clients' facial expressions, bodily motions, voice quality, and physiological responses communicate more than their words do. The following factors, on the part of both helpers and clients, play an important role in the therapeutic dialogue:

- bodily behavior, such as posture, body movements, and gestures
- eye behavior, such as eye contact, staring, and eye movement
- facial expressions, such as smiles, frowns, raised eyebrows, and twisted lips
- voice-related behavior, such as tone of voice, pitch, volume, intensity, inflection, spacing of words, emphasis, pauses, silences, and fluency
- observable autonomic physiological responses, such as quickened breathing, blushing, paleness, and pupil dialation
- physical characteristics, such as fitness, height, weight, and complexion
- space, that is, how close or far a person chooses to be during a conversation
- general appearance, such as grooming and dress

People constantly 'speak' to one another through their nonverbal behavior. Effective helpers learn this 'language' and how to use it effectively in their interactions with their clients. They also learn how to 'read' relevant messages embedded in the nonverbal behavior of their clients.

Helpers' nonverbal behavior

Before you begin interpreting the nonverbal behavior of your clients, take a look at yourself. You speak to your clients through all the nonverbal categories outlined above. At times your nonverbal behavior is as important as, or even more important than, your words. Your nonverbal behavior influences clients for better or for worse. Clients read cues in your nonverbal behavior that indicate the quality of your presence to them. Attentive presence can invite or encourage them to trust you, open up, and explore the significant dimensions of their problem situations. Half-hearted presence can promote distrust and lead to clients' reluctance to reveal themselves to you. Part of listening, then, is being sensitive to clients' reactions to your nonverbal behavior.

SOLER: Guidelines for visibly tuning in to clients

There are certain key nonverbal skills you can use to visibly tune in to clients. These skills can be summarized in the acronym SOLER. Because communication skills are particularly sensitive to cultural differences, care should be taken in adapting what follows to different cultures. What follows, however, is only a framework.

S: Face the client Squarely   That is, adopt a posture that indicates involvement. In North American culture, facing another person squarely is often considered a basic posture of involvement. It usually says, 'I'm here with you; I'm available to you.' Turning your body away from another person while you talk to him or her can lessen your degree of contact with that person. Even when people are seated in a circle, they usually try in some way to turn toward the individuals to whom they are speaking. The word squarely here should not be taken too literally. 'Squarely' is not a military term. The point is that your bodily orientation should convey the message that you are involved with the client. If, for any reason, facing the person squarely is too threatening, then an angled position may be more helpful. The point is not inches and angles but the quality of your presence. Your body sends out messages whether you like it or not. Make them congruent with what you are trying to do.

O: Adopt an Open posture   Crossed arms and crossed legs can be signs of lessened involvement with or availability to others. An open posture can be a sign that you're open to the client and to what he or she has to say. In North American culture, an open posture is generally seen as a nondefensive posture. Again, the word 'open' can be taken literally or metaphorically. If your legs are crossed, this does not mean that you are not involved with the client. But it is important to ask yourself, 'To what degree does my present posture communicate openness and availability to the client?' If you are empathic and open-minded, let your posture mirror what is in your heart.

L: Remember that it is possible at times to Lean toward the other   Watch two people in a restaurant who are intimately engaged in conversation. Very often they are both leaning forward over the table as a natural sign of their involvement. The main thing is to remember that the upper part of your body is on a hinge. It can move toward a person and back away. In North American culture, a slight inclination toward a person is often seen as saying, 'I'm with you, I'm interested in you and in what you have to say.' Leaning back (the severest form of which is a slouch) can be a way of saying, 'I'm not entirely with you' or 'I'm bored.' Leaning too far forward, however, or doing so too soon, may frighten a client. It can be seen as a way of placing a demand on the other for some kind of closeness or intimacy. In a wider sense, the word 'lean' can refer to a kind of bodily flexibility or responsiveness that enhances your communication with a client. Bodily flexibility can mirror mental flexibility.

E: Maintain good Eye contact   In North American culture, fairly steady eye contact is not unnatural for people deep in conversation. It is not the same as staring. Again, watch two people deep in conversation. You may be amazed at the amount of direct eye contact. Maintaining good eye contact with a client is another way of saying, 'I'm with you; I'm interested; I want to hear what you have to say.' Obviously, this principle is not violated if you occasionally look away. Indeed, you have to if you don't want to stare. But if you catch yourself looking away frequently, your behavior may give you a hint about some kind of reluctance to be with this person or to get involved with him or her, or it may say something about your own discomfort. In other cultures, however, too much eye contact, especially with someone in a position of authority, is out of order. I have learned much about the cultural meaning of eye contact from my Asian students and clients.

R: Try to be relatively Relaxed or natural in these behaviors   Being relaxed means two things. First, it means not fidgeting nervously or engaging in distracting facial expressions. The client may wonder what's making you nervous. Second, it means becoming comfortable with using your body as a vehicle of personal contact and expression. Your being natural in the use of these skills helps put the client at ease.

II. ACTIVE LISTENING: THE FOUNDATION OF UNDERSTANDING

Visibly tuning in to clients is not, of course, an end in itself. We tune in both mentally and visibly in order to listen to what clients have to say – their stories, complaints, points of view, intentions, proposals, decisions, and everything else. Listening carefully to a client's concerns seems to be a concept so simple to grasp and so easy to do that one may wonder why it is given such explicit treatment here. Nonetheless, it is amazing how often people fail to listen to one another. Full listening means listening actively, listening accurately, and listening for meaning. Listening is not merely a skill. It is a rich metaphor for the helping relationship itself – indeed, for all relationships.

Forms of poor listening

Effective listening is not a state of mind, like being happy or relaxed. It's not something that just happens. It's an activity. In other words, effective listening requires work. Let's first take a look at the opposite of active listening. All of us have been, at one time or another, both perpetrators and victims of the following forms of inactive or inadequate listening.

- nonlistening
- partial listening
- tape-recorder listening

Empathic listening: listening to clients' stories and their search for solutions

The opposite of inactive or inadequate listening is empathic listening, listening driven by the value of empathy. Empathic listening centers on the kind of attending, observing, and listening – the kind of 'being with' – needed to develop an understanding of clients and their worlds. Although it might be metaphysically impossible to actually get inside the world of another person and experience the world as he or she does, it is possible to approximate this.

Empathic participation in the world of another person obviously admits of degrees. As a helper, you must be able to enter clients' worlds deeply enough to understand their struggles with problem situations or their search for opportunities with enough depth to make your participation in problem management and opportunity development valid and substantial. If your help is based on an incorrect or invalid understanding of the client, then your helping may lead him or her astray. If your understanding is valid but superficial, then you might miss the central issues of the client's life.

Focused listening: experiences, thoughts, behaviors, and affect

In many ways helping is a talking game. Therefore, the kind and quality of talk are both crucial. Listening at its best is both focused and unbiased. Two forms of focus are offered here. First, the problem-management helping model itself, because it is not theory- or school-focused, helps counselors organize what they are hearing without prejudice. Problem-management and opportunity-development dialogue is at the heart of helping. Helpers listen intently to clients' stories to help them search for solutions.

Listening for strengths, opportunities, and resources

If you listen only for problems, you will end up talking mainly about problems. And you will shortchange your clients. Every client has something going for him or her. Your job is to spot clients' resources and help them invest these resources in managing problem situations and opportunities. If it is true that people generally use only a fraction of their potential (Maslow, 1968), then there is much to be tapped.

One section of the positive psychology movement focuses on strengths, especially strengths that clients have but fail to use as they struggle with problem situations (Aspinwall and Staudinger, 2003; Peterson and Seligman, 2004). Just the list of the strengths examined in a book on positive psychological assessment, edited by Lopez and Snyder (2003), gives the reader a lift – hope, optimism, self-efficacy, problem-solving, internal locus of control, creativity, wisdom, courage, positive emotions, self-esteem, love, emotional intelligence, forgiveness, humor, gratitude, faith, morality, coping, and well-being. Though we might long for a world in which striving for these virtues was a priority, listening for hints of any or all of these capabilities in our clients is a first step.

Putting it all together: listening to the client's integrated narrative

When clients talk about their concerns, they mix all forms of discourse – thoughts, stories, experiences, emotions, actions, evolving decisions, points of view, proposed actions, strengths, resources – together. This is the client's narrative.

Narrative therapy focuses on clients' understanding of their stories and how their experiences, thoughts, emotions, and actions fit into the context of the story. This approach can help clients do three things: put untold aspects of the client's past into the life narrative, emotionally enter and reauthor their own stories, and/or construct new meanings in old stories or find new meaning in stories that emerge during therapy.

While listening is important, there is no need to go overboard on listening. Remember that you are a human being listening to a human being, not a vacuum cleaner indiscriminately sweeping up every scrap of information. Effective dialogic listening helps both you and your client discover the kind of meaning needed to move forward in managing problem situations and spotting and developing life-enhancing opportunities.

Understand clients through context

People are more than the sum of their verbal and nonverbal messages. Listening, in its deepest sense, means listening to clients themselves as influenced by the contexts in which they 'live, move, and have their being.' As mentioned earlier, it is important to interpret a client's nonverbal behavior in the context of the entire helping session. It is also essential to help clients understand their stories, points of view, and messages and the emotions that permeate them through the wider context of their lives. Tiedens and Leach (2004), in their edited book *The Social Life of Emotions*, develop the theme that emotions cannot be understood independently of the social relationships and groups in which they occur. All the things that make people different – culture, personality, personal style, ethnicity, key life experiences, education, travel, economic status, and other forms of diversity – provide the context for the client's problems and unused opportunities. Key elements of this context become part of the client's story, whether they are mentioned directly or not. Effective helpers listen through this wider context without being overwhelmed by the details of it.

References

Aspinwall, L.G. and Staudinger, U.M. (eds) (2003) *A Psychology of Human Strengths: Fundamental Questions and Future Directions for a Positive Psychology*, Washington, DC: American Psychological Association.

Dominelli, L. (2008) *Anti-racist Social Work*, 3rd edition, Basingstoke: Palgrave Macmillan.

Graham, M. (2001) *Social Work and African-centred Worldviews*, Birmingham: Venture Press.

Lopez, S.J. and Snyder, C.R. (2003) *Positive Psychological Assessment: A Handbook of Models and Measures*, Washington, DC: American Psychological Association.

Maslow, A.H. (1968) *Toward a Psychology of Being*, 2nd edition, New York: Van Nostrand Reinhold.

Peterson, C. and Seligman, M.E.P. (2004) *Character Strengths and Virtues: A Classification Handbook*, New York: Oxford University Press.

Robinson, L. (2007) *Cross-cultural Child Development for Social Workers*, Basingstoke: Palgrave Macmillan.

Tiedens, L.Z. and Leach, C.W. (2004) *The Social Life of Emotions*, New York: Cambridge University Press.

Trotter, C. (1999) *Working with Involuntary Clients: A Guide to Practice*, London: Sage.

Further reading

Brown, C. and Augusta-Scott, T. (2006) *Narrative Therapy: Making Meaning, Making Lives*, Thousand Oaks, CA: Sage.

Kadushin, A. (1997) *The Social Work Interview: A Guide for Human Service Professionals*, 4th edition, New York: Columbia University Press.

Koprowska, J. (2007) 'Communication skills in social work', in M. Lymbery and K. Postle (eds) *Social Work. A Companion to Learning*, London: Sage, 123–33.

McLeod, J. (2007) *Counselling Skill*, Maidenhead: Open University Press.

Mearns, D. and Thorne, B. (2007) *Person-centred Counselling in Action*, 3rd edition, London: Sage.

Moss, B. (2007) *Communication Skills for Health and Social Care*, London: Sage.

Rogers, C.R. (1980) *A Way of Being*, Boston, MA: Houghton Mifflin.

—— (2003) *Client-centred Therapy: Its current practice, implications and theory*, Revised edition, London: Constable.

Thompson, N. (2009) *People Skills*, 3rd edition, Basingstoke: Palgrave Macmillan.

—— (2003) *Communication and Language: A Handbook of Theory and Practice*, Basingstoke: Macmillan.

White, M. and Epston, D. (1990) *Narrative Means to Therapeutic Ends*, London: W.W. Norton & Company.

22 Assessment, monitoring and evaluation

Brian Sheldon and Geraldine Macdonald

In their review of approaches to assessment, Crisp *et al.* (2005) assert that there is no single understanding and theory about assessment in social work. This is hardly surprising, given that assessment takes place in so many different ways and for so many different reasons. Increasingly, assessment in social work is equated with assessment of risk (Cree and Wallace 2009). The nature of an assessment will be determined by whether it is being conducted by a sole practitioner or by one who is part of a multi-disciplinary or inter-agency team (see Barrett *et al.* 2005; Morris 2008). And assessments may be either 'needs' or 'resources' led. Although the language of current policy statements is always couched in terms which suggest that service users should have choices about the services which support them (referred to as 'personalisation' or a 'person-centred approach'), the reality is that agencies have to take resources into account when assessing what packages of care might be made available to an individual (Petch 2008). The selected extract by Brian Sheldon and Geraldine Macdonald, social work academics in England and Northern Ireland, provides a good overview of things to be considered in making an assessment and evaluating practice of any kind.

From *A Textbook of Social Work*, London: Routledge (2009): 95–111.

General points

We are taking these three stages together, conscious of the convention that chapters on evaluation usually come at the end of books. But what may be claimed at the end stage is dependent upon the quality of the original assessment, the goals arising from it, and the measures against which progress has been monitored. Working the other way, the accuracy of assessments can only be judged against measures of progress and, ultimately, by the outcomes which result. Otherwise, as computer programmers say, 'garbage in, garbage out'. There are some other general points to make about assessments and why they can be problematic:

1   First, we should be sure that there is one. Obvious as this point might seem, inquiry after inquiry in both the childcare and mental health fields have found, instead, case notes which amount to little more than collections of factual data intermingled with more speculative material, giving the impression that these comments were put there more for storage purposes than as the considered basis for a plan.

The lack of a comprehensive assessment and consequent care and protection plan was a feature in the death of Victoria Climbié (see Laming, 2003) and many others. That this issue should keep arising has stretched public and political patience to breaking-point. Even allowing for the deceptive power of hindsight, as Lord Laming remarked: 'this is not exactly rocket science'.

2   Increasingly the approach to assessment has been to standardize assessment and planning into 'tick-box', 'write-in' forms with too little regard for questions of validity and reliability. This may secure the gathering of information across a range of domains, but does not, in and of itself, secure an assessment, which entails the critical appraisal of the information gathered.

The clients of social workers, given increasingly high eligibility thresholds, will usually be in a state of imminent crisis, and disinclined to sit down and run through an account of the long and winding road which led them to our door – or we to theirs. Nevertheless, as consumers ourselves, say, of the health service, we expect to receive a medical assessment prior to intervention except in the most dramatic of circumstances. When we don't get one, as in the case of 'reflex prescribing' by GPs, we feel uneasy. In social work we have allowed 'something must be done' pressures from the media, from employers and from clients themselves to distract us from a technically necessary activity. This is vital for ourselves if we are to do our jobs properly and necessary for our clients who usually have hopes about receiving effective aid – or at least of convincing us that they have no case to answer. In our experience, where the need to put together a 'map' of problems over a decent period of time (covering likely causes and effects, and usually involving more than 'the' identified client or intended beneficiary) is explained, then time and patience can usually be found. After all, most of the complaints against Social Services departments refer not to the *longueurs* of contact but to frustrations about short, glancing consultations resulting in clients being endlessly referred elsewhere.

3   Social histories entail establishing an overview of major categories of past events, mapping and exploring current relationships and so on, so that current events may be viewed within the context of a person's life. Social histories have fallen out of fashion of late, probably because they are time-consuming, and because in previous decades there never seemed to be *quite* enough information on which to proceed. So, a few years ago, we flipped to very quick 'appraisals', largely of risk (to the department as much as to clients themselves). These provide a limited picture of how problems have built up and therefore little information on potential leverage points.

4   There is a beguiling idea, long in circulation, that 'assessment is an ongoing process'. Well yes, it is, but it cannot be never-ending. The reality is that it is very easy to postpone an assessment in the face of urgent or neglected problems with statutory implications. But then we know of many cases where once 'first aid' measures have been taken the other, slower burning aspects of cases are neglected, only to recur later in more threatening forms. The authors therefore advocate a definite 'diagnostic' phrase to work, focusing on the *aetiology* of problems by getting clients to 'rewind' the 'video-tapes' of their lives and take stock.

5   However, this word 'problems' seems to give some social workers and academics semantic indigestion. Therefore they tend to coat the word with euphemisms such as 'unmet needs'. Strangely though, clients who come our way, either directly or via research projects, usually see themselves as drowning in *problems*. Recognizing this

does not entail denial of people's strengths. A good assessment will identify, affirm and capitalize on these.

6   . . . we do not take the view that subjectivity can be completely eliminated from assessments; or that given a detailed enough protocol, the case notes should contain only objectively verifiable 'facts'. However, given that we know we have these semi-automatic cognitive tendencies, does it not behove us to take precautions when the welfare of others is at stake? For example, remembering is an active, socially constructed process, bearing little resemblance to any camera or taperecorder-like activity. What we remember about ourselves and others and what we forget is strongly influenced by psychological factors: . . .

Stages in assessment (see Figure 22.1)

Referral and early engagement

The ideal shape for any assessment procedure is, metaphorically, that of the funnel or tun dish: wide open to start with and then tapering off.

People come forward for help, or are impelled forward, in complex ways. Therefore the *route to referral* is the natural starting point for assessment. Clients may have been to several agencies before receiving what they regard as useful assistance or none. Some will feel that they have already told their stories, and may be reluctant to go through the whole process again.

Previous contacts can also result in a 'shaping' process, whereby clients are persuaded that their difficulties are of a certain kind, with certain origins, and with certain preferred solutions in prospect. There is also a large literature in social psychology on the subliminal power of initial impressions and of reputation which, it appears, can

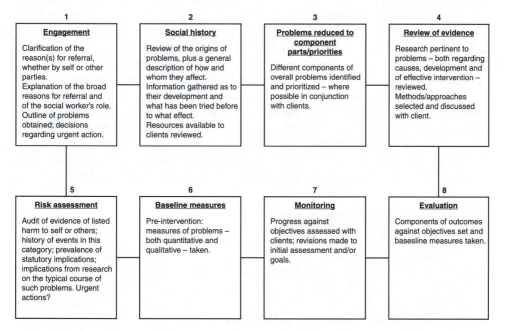

Figure 22.1 Stages in assessment.

be more powerful influences than the *content* of what is said or done (see Cohen, 1964; Zimbardo, 2000).

Another aspect of pre-assessment experience is the way in which clients are received when they seek help. Rooms give messages. They may be welcoming and homely, or impersonal and threatening.

Social histories

Patterns of unfolding interaction and their consequences for individuals and members of the family as a whole are the stuff of a good family assessment (and may also be important when working with individuals).

Staff should take notes during the conduct of an assessment because, as we have seen, memory is fallible; because clients' stories are full of dates, times and sequences which can easily get jumbled up, and because it is natural for listeners unconsciously to add in material to a narrative to round it off and make it 'coherent'. Yet sometimes it is the very 'incoherency' of accounts which make for the most interesting starting points. But also, imagine being interviewed by a financial adviser about your pension prospects with him or her nodding sympathetically throughout, but never writing anything down.

Current family relationships and circumstances

This part of the social history is also concerned with qualitative issues (i.e. how relationships between family members have developed over time and what patterns of typical interaction have added to or subtracted from their problems), but it is mainly concerned with their current impact (i.e. given certain situations, frustrations or dissatisfaction, which persons would typically intervene, how, and why? Who would not, and why?). This focus on contemporary manifestations recognizes that although most problems have historical roots, they have their main force in the here and now.

Well-functioning families exhibit a number of characteristics which render them resilient: (1) they provide opportunities for the expression of ideas and feelings in the expectation of being listened to; (2) no big family secrets exist which everyone pretends not to know; (3) there is a valuing of the different responsibilities and attributes of others; (4) there are rules that are flexible, explained, reinforced, but also *enforced* when necessary; (5) there are positive expectations of growth and change; (6) good role models are available and discipline relies on these rather than on ever more detailed instructions; (7) love is shown and love returned, and 'second chances' are given. Writing this list is easy; creating and sustaining these principles in adverse circumstances is hard.

Financial, material and housing circumstances

Few referrals come to us which are not a mixture of material and psycho-social problems. Clients are often under heavy financial pressure due to chronically low income, debt, insecure and/or unsuitable housing and so on. Material problems of this kind add to the emotional burdens of families and, in turn, relationship problems can distract from sensible approaches to them. Clients (perhaps all of us at one time or another) are therefore often caught up in vicious circles; often hiding away from financial problems, rather than approaching them constructively and incrementally. Similarly, many clients do not claim all the financial benefits due to them. This is a particular problem with older people who, for historical reasons, associate means-tested benefits with remnants of the Poor Law.

Officialdom does little other than generally to encourage claimants, but then sends them complex forms to fill in. The current pension credit scheme, for example, can add substantially to the income of older people, but one-third of those entitled to it fail to claim. A good basic grasp of the social security system (maze) is thus essential knowledge for social workers (see Dowling, 1998).

Health

Close attention to any physical or mental health problem is essential, as these conditions can strongly affect social functioning even when they are not the main people is ill-health or worries about its prospect. These emotional factors can, in turn, lead to self-neglect, poor nutrition, self-imposed social isolation, and to a worsening of the very physical health problems which started the cycle.

Education

If the family one is working with has children of school age then, whether they present with problems or unexplained shortfalls in performance or not, it is wise to enquire about their educational experiences since it is rare that this sphere does not affect the others. Bullying, for example, can have substantial effects on family life and often children disguise the fact that it is taking place. The child suicide, child depression and deliberate self-harm statistics hide thousands of such experiences.

Sometimes, however, influences on family life are less dramatic, as when children are just 'not doing well', find some subjects difficult, feel a failure, and so reject school and start truanting. Blunt consequences fall heavily on parents these days given new attendance legislation, and this is particularly the case where they have problems of their own. These may not look like high-profile problems but they have manifold consequences.

Reducing problems to their component parts

'What exactly is it that is threatening, worrying, or troublesome?' should be an early question. 'Where and how often do these events occur; what do clients do themselves to ameliorate them, and with what results?' should be the next one. Problems usually have cognitive, emotional and behavioural components.

Another approach is to look at how and where problems begin and at what feeds them, since recurring difficulties often have identifiable 'triggers', are maintained by the reactions they get (e.g. '*You can stay out all night for me, it's your life*' ('good, you said it')), but sometimes these early precursors may yield to diversionary action.

Beginning with a list of problems is sensible. If clients have trouble helping to make one, for example, by saying '*everything*', then little thought experiments such as 'Imagine that it is a year from now and you are much happier, (1) what would have to have gone from your life, and (2) what would have to have come into it?' Or, 'If someone was able to record on CCTV everything that happened in your house/at work/at school on a typical day, what would they see/not see?' Or, 'If in six months things have improved for you, what would we see and hear that is different?' Sometimes single difficulties are central and give rise to satellite 'problems'.

We have seen a number of children who have spent long periods in care present with sharply different problems, showing, for example, aggression, self-centredness and serious risk-taking behaviour. Such children have learned to distrust the motives of others; they *expect* adults to let them down; they have few secure, counteractive relationships, and so they decide to look after themselves in whatever way seems safe at the time. As W.H. Auden (1994) observed, '*Those to whom evil is done, do evil in return.*' The 'evil' does not have to be intentional, by the way.

Whatever the direction of casual probabilities, it is sensible to start off by offering help with 'here-and-now' problems, and then to move backwards.

Risk assessment

Once the social worker has achieved an overview of current problems and has developed some ideas about their aetiology, it behoves her or him to undertake an assessment of any potentially serious risks posed. Given the high eligibility for service thresholds now in operation, most cases which come our way are likely to warrant this. We have to highlight this issue somewhere in the assessment sequence, but in reality it pervades all the stages under discussion, hence the vertical lines in Figure 22.1.

Over the past few years a host of risk assessment instruments, national standards frameworks and departmental guidelines have been developed. However much comfort we allow ourselves to feel regarding these attempts, there are some provisos to enter about them.

1   We inhabit an organizational and political culture which sees risks as virtually always foreseeable by someone; which sees the (as it turns out) mistaken priority accorded to certain *other* allegedly risky cases (where nothing has yet happened) over the one where something did, as evidence of culpable misjudgement. In this fraught atmosphere we have – at a conceptual level – a difficulty in separating out risk that is *estimatable probabilities* from 'anyone's guess' *uncertainties*.

   The tangible result of this confusion, and of the developing 'blame culture', is professional defensiveness, covert self-protection, and 'going-through-the-motions' behaviour by staff (ask any social worker in private). Take this example from the inquiry into the death of Kimberly Carlisle (London Borough of Greenwich 1987):

   > I walked with the family to the door of the building and watched as they walked across the road to where their old ear was parked. I still have a clear mental picture of the way they each walked across the road and got into the car, parents holding children by the hand, children leaping around in the car as they got in, laughing, shouting and playing happily with each other. It was almost an archetype of a happy family scene.

   The inquiry chairman's response was to observe that 'Far from being reassured, [the social worker] should have been alive to the risk of being manipulated. Plainly he had been deceived' (p. 112). Plainly? Certainly, with hindsight, we know that that family was not a 'happy family', though even with hindsight we do not know that 'manipulation' and 'deception' were present in that scene – even dysfunctional families can have happy moments. And the implicit criticism is sustainable only with the benefit of hindsight; the invited counterfactual (removal on the basis of this 'happy scene') is not plausible.

Where such wishful standards of professional prescience exist, the outcome is unlikely to be that social workers will be more careful; rather it will encourage them speculatively to record *absolutely everything*. Too much information, not properly sifted, not looked into sceptically, is a greater enemy of good assessment than too little.

2   Many of the risk assessment schedules in use, which are intended to guide staff towards greater objectivity and consistency, are the products of a retrospective identification of factors present in cases where death or serious harm has occurred. Only recently have such guidelines been subjected to validity and reliability testing. Validity raises the question as to whether an instrument actually measures what it purports to measure or just collateral factors. Reliability raises the questions as to whether two or more different people or one and the same person would, at different times, come close in their views as the result of using a given schedule (for a sober, evidence-based debate on such matters see Macdonald and Macdonald, 1999a).

3   There is another problem, this time regarding allegedly measurable uncertainties. Supposing we had a risk assessment schedule with an 84 per cent reliability level who would decline to use it? But we are usually dealing with very large numbers of people who fall within a given orbit: millions of children, thousands of mentally ill people and so on, and we know very little about the base rates of 'suspicious' collateral circumstances in these populations.

The problem, then, with all but *massively* accurate screening instruments (we have none, nor does psychiatry, nor does education), is that when applied to large populations they yield discomfiting numbers of false positives (not really a risk at all) and false negatives (not a risk on paper but one in actuality). Therefore the risk of harm through hyper-vigilant good intentions should be as much to the forefront of our thinking as the risk of harm through lack of watchfulness.

4   The next point concerns *types* of suspected harm – because risk is not a unitary phenomenon. Some bad events seem to come out of nowhere. Then there are slowly developing risks where problems and provocations steadily mount and it is difficult for staff to appreciate the significance of the pattern. Then there is the occupational hazard of inurement to risks. Desensitization to squalid living conditions and threats to the development of children have featured in many inquiry reports and we need to guard against confusing weary acceptance of what seems chronic with non-judgemental 'acceptance'.

5   All the caveats discussed in this section aside, some risks *are* foreseeable.

It is thus important to distinguish between the general watchfulness that most social workers adopt when working in risky areas and formal risk assessments undertaken at a particular point in time and designed to answer specific questions about the likelihood of harm. The former approach is an integral part of our responsibility to recognize, for example, children in need of protection, or older people at risk of falling. The latter entails using a formalized approach designed to improve the quality of decision-making by providing a clear framework for the collection, organization and interpretation of information.

Given all these compromising factors, what then is the most secure way of approaching risk assessment?

1   First, get to know the risks associated with the problems you are dealing with, and their base rates.
2   Piece together the chronology of events, including contacts with other agencies, and collect information from all relevant parties.
3   Be explicit and transparent. Make it clear *what* information you have gathered, why you have gathered it, and what you think its significance is. Say what story you think it tells, estimate what it says about the likelihood of the risks you are concerned with, and over what time period. Spell out the things you think might contain the risk, including those services and supports that other agencies or other people can introduce.
4   Monitor the impact of particular forms of intervention and consider the length of time it is taking to bring about a given level of change. Is this in line with, or at odds with, the interventions literature for this approach? The latter point is particularly important when the risks one is dealing with are cumulative.
5   As new information comes to light, reassess – preferably with a supervisor – your estimates of likely danger. Even though we can rarely estimate the absolute probability of something bad happening, we can, and should, be able to make a stab at estimates of relative probability. For reasons of self-protection too, 'show your working out' regarding changing risk levels and anchor decisions in events as much as in conversations. *Invite* your supervisor to alert you to any logical 'jumps' or *non sequiturs* in your assessments. This process of active review is perhaps one of the most important aspects of risk assessment.

However, what is too little realized is that not taking a considered risk can be the most hazardous option of all. 'Frozen watchfulness' is a condition that not only affects abused children, but whole organizations.

Setting intermediate and longer term objectives

In social work, intermediate and longer term objectives, and qualitative and quantitative factors tend to get mixed up together. This is partly due to the complexity of the cases with which we deal, but it also results from inadequate training in these matters, and from a stubborn occupational attachment to the heart-warmingly all-encompassing. Therefore, it is wise to address the question 'How shall we know, and be able to show others that we have achieved this?' That is, how shall we know, over and above our subjective feelings, that something worthwhile has happened? Positive views from clients should by no means be neglected, but one should also expect to see tangible behavioural or circumstantial change to give these statements credibility.

It is our experience that most clients value interim feedback on progress, both with tasks that they have agreed to pursue themselves and in respect of those undertaken on their behalf. Here are the necessary steps:

1   Introduce early on the idea of the need to monitor key events, whether of a positive type (which it is hoped will increase), or of a problematic type (which it is hoped will decrease), or both.
2   Negotiate with clients as to what measures would best represent progress, and try politely to squeeze out vagueness of expression by asking for examples.

3 Introduce the idea of record-keeping regarding both hoped for qualitative and quantitative changes. Diaries are useful.
4 Standardized instruments (see Fischer and Corcoran, 1994) may be used to assess change on a before-and-after basis.
5 Work with clients to produce estimates of the likely duration of attempts to change something. We know from the literature on task-centred casework that this can have motivating effects. If the work is likely to be lengthy it can help 'pace' clients and immunize them against disappointment.
6 Do not be afraid to redefine goals and objectives, or to try out new approaches to problems; just restart the monitoring scheme each time.
7 Give positive feedback to clients on any progress made. Many live lives where there is little encouragement available, only inspection.

Evaluation

We have four recommendations to make:

1 Do one. Most case records contain nothing worthy of the name. In place of evaluations we tend to get summaries at the end.
2 Evaluation should be given a *much* higher profile on qualifying courses and in-service training than it currently has.
3 We need *baseline information* before proceeding, and we regard the routine absence of this information from Social Services' records as a serious fault.
4 Single case designs have been around for years, and relevant books and articles are full of practice examples of their use (see Sheldon, 1983, 1995).

The strictures discussed above apply to projects as well as cases.

Conclusions

We have tried to set down what we think are the characteristics of a good assessment, and make no apology for it being an 'ideal type'. That is we know well that organizational factors, crises, shortage of time, uncooperative clients and changing caseload priorities will probably hinder the completion of stages in any neat order. The point is that if the social worker has a structure in her or his head, or better still in his or her notebook, then they will know that some information is still missing, and can pursue it if the opportunity arises.

References

Barrett, G., Sellman, D. and Thomas, J. (2005) *Interprofessional Working in Health and Social Care: Professional Perspectives,* Basingstoke: Palgrave Macmillan.
Cohen, A.R. (1964) *Attitude Change and Social Influence*, New York: Basic Books.
Cree, V.E. and Wallace, S.J. (2009) 'Risk and Protection', in R. Adams, M. Payne and L. Dominelli (eds) *Practising Social Work in a Complex World*, 2nd edition, Basingstoke: Palgrave Macmillan, 42–56.
Crisp, B., Green Lister, P. Anderson, M.R. and Orme, J. (2005) *Learning and Teaching in Social Work Education: Textbooks and Frameworks on Assessment*, London: Social Care Institute for Excellence (SCIE).

Dowling, M. (1998) *Poverty*, Birmingham: Venture Press.

Fischer, J. and Corcoran, K. (1994) *Measures for Clinical Practice, Volume 1*, London: Free Press.

Laming, Lord (2003) *The Victoria Climbié Inquiry, Report of an Inquiry by Lord Laming*, London: HMSO.

London Borough of Greenwich (1987) *A child in Mind: Report of the Commission of Inquiry into the circumstances surrounding the death of Kimberley Carlisle*, London: London Borough of Greenwich.

Macdonald, G.M. and Macdonald, K.I. (1999) 'Perceptions of risk', in Parsloe, P. (ed.) (1999) *Risk Assessment in Social Care and Social Work*, London: Jessica Kingsley.

Morris, K. (ed.) (2008) *Social Work and Multi-agency Working: Making a Difference*, Bristol: Policy Press.

Petch, A. (2008) 'Social work with adult service users', in M. Davies (ed.) *The Blackwell Companion to Social Work*, 3rd edition, Oxford: Blackwell, 236–50.

Sheldon, B. (1983) 'The use of single case experimental designs in the evaluation of social work', *British Journal of Social Work*, 13 (1): 477–500.

—— (1995) *Cognitive Behavioural Therapy: Research, Practice and Philosophy*, London: Routledge.

Zimbardo, P.G. (2000) *Psychology and Life*, 13th edition, New York: HarperCollins.

Further reading

Frost, N. (2009) 'Evaluating practice', in R. Adams, L. Dominelli and M. Payne (eds) *Practising Social Work in a Complex World*, 2nd edition, Basingstoke: Palgrave Macmillan, 296–307.

Kemshall, H. and Pritchard, J. (eds) (1996) *Good Practice in Risk Assessment and Risk Management*, London: Jessica Kingsley.

McIvor, G. (2007) 'Assessment in criminal justice', in J. Lishman (ed.) *Handbook for Practice Learning in Social Work and Social Care*, London: Jessica Kingsley.

Milner, J. and O'Byrne, P. (2009) *Assessment in Social Work*, 3rd edition, Basingstoke: Palgrave Macmillan.

Parker, J. and Bradley, G. (2007) *Social Work Practice: Assessment, Planning, Intervention and Review*, 2nd edition, Exeter: Learning Matters.

Shaw, I. and Shaw, A. (1997) 'Keeping social work honest: Evaluating as profession and practice', *British Journal of Social Work*, 27: 847–69.

Walker, S. and Beckett, C. (2004) *Social Work Assessment and Intervention*, London: Russell House.

23 The ecological systems metaphor in Australasia

Keiran O'Donogue and Jane Maidment

This chapter moves beyond engagement and assessment to the first of the chapters which examine intervention with service users. Given the prominence I have already placed on seeing individuals in context, this chapter will consider the usefulness of ecological and systems theories to social work practice. Although these approaches have distinct histories and backgrounds, they also have much in common, as our extract will demonstrate (see also Barber 2002). An ecological approach seeks to understand the centrality of the person in their environment (see Bronfenbrenner 1979) while a systems perspective such as that developed by Pincus and Minahan proposes that four systems must be addressed in social work practice: 'the change agent system' (the practitioner and their colleagues and agency); 'the client system' (the service user and their networks); 'the target system' (the 'people who need to be changed to accomplish the goals of the change agent'); and 'the action system' ('the change agent and the people he works with and through to accomplish his goals and influence the target system') (1973: 63). In this extract, Keiran O'Donogue and Jane Maidment, both social work academics in New Zealand, discuss the pros and cons of using an ecological system approach in practice in Australasia.

From M. Nash, R. Munford and K. O'Donogue (eds) *Social Work Theories in Action*, London: Jessica Kingsley (2005): 39–45.

Key ecological systems concepts

Ecological concepts

Ecology is described as concerned with the interrelationship and adaptation of organisms with each other and with their surroundings, be they organic or inorganic (Mattaini and Meyer 2002; Ungar 2002). Central to this interrelationship and adaptation is the concept of *level of fit*, which concerns the degree of balance and reciprocity between the person's needs, capacities and aspirations and the resources and expectations accessible and available in their environment (Gitterman 1996a). According to Gitterman (1996b), when the degree of balance and reciprocity between these two aspects is positive, the *level of fit* achieves the condition of *adaptedness*, in which the exchanges or interactions between them is likely to facilitate the actualization of both human and environmental development. However, when the personal and environmental exchanges are not positive they are described as *dysfunctional* and have the potential to inhibit, frustrate, damage and oppress both human and environmental potential (Gitterman 1996b). When people perceive an imbalance between the demands of their environment and their ability to mobilize resources to manage such demands, the result is stress. According to Gitterman (1996b, p.391), stress can only be relieved by improving: a) the level of person and environment fit through change in the person's perception or behaviour, or b) the environment's response to the person, or c) the quality of exchanges between both person and environment.

The second key ecological concept is that of the *environment*. The environment is a multidimensional entity, which contains physical, social and cultural aspects (Germain 1979; Kemp *et al.* 1997). It contains dynamic and interactive features that are mediated through place, time and space, as well as human beings' perceptions, structures, relationships and meaning-making activities. According to Kemp *et al.* (1997, p.85), the levels of the environment include the following:

- the perceived environment, that is, the environment as constructed in individual and collective systems of meaning and belief
- the physical environment, both natural and built
- the social/interactional environment, comprised largely of human relationships at various levels of intimacy, and including family, group and neighbourhood networks and collectivities
- the institutional and organizational environment
- the cultural and socio-political environment.

The ecological concepts of *habitat* and *niche* are important terms for understanding the impact of the environment on people. A person's habitat is the location where a person is found and will involve all of the levels of the environment described above, but particularized to their locale. A person's niche, on the other hand, involves the person's place and status within the habitat. According to Rapp (1998), a niche can be either entrapping or enabling. An entrapping niche is one in which people are marginalized, with minimal available resources or support and little prospect of social mobility and/or belonging. An enabling niche is the opposite of an entrapping niche and is one that provides resources and support that enable social mobility, social belonging and social connectivity (Rapp 1998).

Systems concepts

As mentioned above, the systems concepts of reciprocal influence, circular causality, structure and unpredictability will be briefly outlined in this section. The first concept, reciprocal influence, refers to the idea that all parts of a system share an influence upon each other. A fairly common example of reciprocal influence comes to our attention when people leave a system. The second concept is circular causality, which sees an effect or outcome influencing its own cause (Ridley 2003). This differs from linear causality in which an effect or outcome is caused by something specific.

Structure is our third key concept and involves the system's patterns of organization, which guide and maintain its functioning. Within each system there are subsystems, and every individual system is also part of a bigger system or suprasystem (Agass and Preston-Shoot 1990). Individual systems and subsystems are differentiated by *boundaries*, non-physical dividers that separate one system from another. Boundaries vary in type and in the amount of information they receive and transmit. Generally, problems occur in systems when the boundaries are either too open or too closed and the structure is either too rigid or too flexible (Rothery 2001). *Unpredictability* is our fourth key systems theory concept and this is based upon the circular and recipro-cal nature of systems in which everything effects everything else in a system. The terms *equifinality* and *multifinality* describe the nature of this unpredictability well. Equifinality means that similar or the same ends are achieved from different starting points, whereas multifinality means that similar or the same starting points result in multiple and differing outcomes. What these terms and the concept of unpredictability reveal is that the system's response to the social worker's intervention influences the outcome, and because of the complex nature of systems and (human persons) they do not act predictably (Rothery 2001).

The ecomap

The ecomap, developed by Hartman (1978), is the most commonly used and longstand-ing visual tool used by social workers to find their way through the complexity of person and environment information. It is a diagrammatic illustration of where the client locates him- or herself in relation to the surrounding systems, and shows the nature of those relationships using a legend of symbols denoting differing types of connections between the systems. Drawing an ecomap can be a useful way for the practitioner and client together to gain an appreciation of where the major stressors and supports exist in the client's life. It is possible to condense a great range of complex information succinctly in diagrammatic form. In this way, developing an ecomap can be used as part of the assessment process, to be referred back to over time, reviewed, and used as a means for evaluating ongoing relationships, social supports, stressors, and changes in the level of fit between the client and their environment. Once clients have become accustomed to illustrating relationships using ecomaps, it is not uncommon for them to invent their own signs, images and symbols to describe these, which serves further to personalize and enrich the depth of information conveyed in these diagrams. Figure 23.1 shows an eco-map for the brief case study outlined below.

> Matt (19) comes to the community mental health team for assessment, having been referred by his GP. In the referral letter, the GP notes that Matt has just recently returned to live with his parents after breaking up with his girlfriend, Sue (17). Together, Matt and Sue have a daughter, Zoe, who is just a few months old.

Near the end of the first discussion with Matt, the practitioner begins to draw an ecomap of people and institutions that currently impact on Matt's life (see Figure 23.1).

In the centre of the ecomap is a small genogram of Matt's immediate family. Both of Matt's parents, Carl and Joan, work in paid employment. Carl enjoys his work and does not see himself retiring for some time. Joan works 'on call' at a hospital canteen, work she has done for a long time. She does not particularly enjoy the job, but continues to help 'save for retirement'. Joan's mother, Ida, has moderate dementia, and although she still lives at home, needs a lot of input from Joan and community services. Both Joan and Carl have a strong work ethic and are displeased that Matt has just lost his job due to a prank at work that compromised health and safety regulations. Matt has broken up with his partner, Sue, during the last month. He has a poor relationship with Sue's

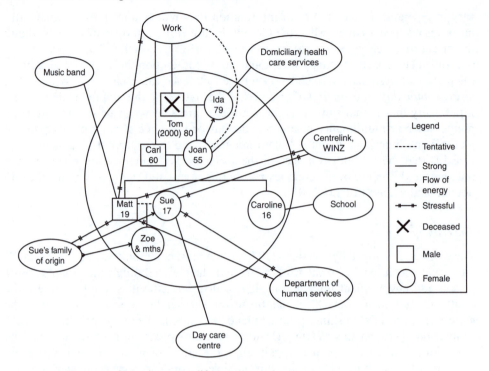

Figure 23.1 Ecomap of Matt's current life.

parents, and now has infrequent contact with his daughter, Zoe. Both Matt and Sue have had conflicted contact with Centrelink (Work and Income [WINZ] or Social Security Department), with disputes over benefit eligibility. They have also had some difficult contact with the Department of Human Services (Department of Child, Youth and Family or Department of Child Protective Services) when a neighbour reported a dispute at their flat shortly after the birth of Zoe. During this contact, the worker from the Department organized for Zoe to attend day care a couple of times a week. Sue has now established some good links with the staff at the centre.

From the discussion and development of the ecomap with Matt it becomes clear that his only really supportive and positive relationships at the moment are connected with the band he plays in on Friday and Saturday nights. He feels his parents favour his sister, whom he describes as 'goody two-shoes' and who excels at school work. He misses Sue and Zoe, has a sense of failure about losing his job, is angry with his father for 'going on' about work, and has little to do with his mother who is juggling the care of Ida (her mother) with her own part-time work. The ecomap provides Matt and the social worker with some clues about where to begin with intervention.

Critique of ecological systems approach

The following section provides a critique of an ecological systems approach context-ualized within an Aotearoa/New Zealand and Australian locale. This critique will pay particular attention to a range of defining features that greatly influence the person-in-environment transactions, some of which these two countries share, and others that are unique to each country.

Mixed perceptions of an ecosystemic paradigm

One of the major strengths of using an ecological systems perspective to understand client issues is that it incorporates an analysis of both formal and informal networks around the client, including relationships with individuals, groups, family, community and the environment as a whole. In this way, it is a perspective that can help the worker and client gain an appreciation of the multiple factors that contribute to, or inhibit client wellbeing. The examination of boundaries between the client system and others enables a fluid interpretation in terms of what constitutes healthy relationships and boundary setting within differing cultural contexts.

On a more contentious note, the degree to which an ecological systems approach does or does not acknowledge the notions of power, oppression and marginalization is the subject of enduring debate (Ungar 2002; Greif 2003). Since both Australia and New Zealand share a history punctuated by indigenous dispossession and alienation from the land, compromised indigenous human rights, and poor statistics for wellbeing amongst indigenous populations, questions of authority and self-determination are important. Early users of systems theory focused on the notions of relationship, 'goodness of fit' and successful *adaptation* of the individual within the environment (Ungar 2002). These early interpretations of systems and an ecological perspective have been criticised for being dominated by a narrow focus on psycho-social imperatives. However, more recent applications of these ideas have emphasized the integral connectedness between client spirituality and notions of wellbeing, acknowledging economic and political determinants (Anglem and Maidment 2004). In this way, emerging models of practice derived from an ecological systems analysis overtly recognize the unique and differing cultural interpretations of how the person-in-environment transactions might justifiably occur.

Further evidence of this evolving politicization of ecological systems analysis can be found in literature in which the notion of 'environment' is redefined in ways that explicitly acknowledge the social, political and economic determinants of powerlessness in individual daily living arrangements and institutional structures (Chung and Pardeck 1997). Thus, while the perspective can be interpreted as being apolitical, in that it does not specifically promote a particular ideological position to address structural change, it includes a framework that can be used to identify where change processes at micro, meso and macro levels of intervention need to occur.

For indigenous populations in both countries the relationship with the natural environment is powerfully linked to questions of personal identity, spiritual strength and ongoing survival (Hunter 2000; Patterson 1999; Ruwhiu 2001). An ecological systems understanding of functioning, which integrates environmental perspectives, is therefore particularly relevant for work with these populations. Nevertheless, it is an approach that has also been criticized as being hard to test empirically, and overly inclusive (Payne 1997; Wakefield 1996a, 1996b). Both of these 'limitations', however, come from a non-indigenous position. This position privileges positivist inquiry, fails to acknowledge the importance of broad kinship networks, and overlooks the integral relationship indigenous populations have with the land and other natural habitats such as flora, fauna and the waterways.

The ecological systems framework has been further criticized for providing no guidance to practitioners in terms of suggesting what methods to use, or when and how to intervene with the client-system (Mancoske, cited in Payne 1998; Wakefield 1996a). This is a fair criticism, as it is not a prescriptive model of practice, and as such does not provide a concise 'recipe' for client intervention in the way that task-centred social work or brief solution-focused therapy does so well. Nevertheless, it is a perspective that can be used by practitioners and clients to analyze and understand the complex network of relationships and systems that influence the client's world. In this way, the framework provides the means to trace and map the major sources of client tension and support, using visual cues such as the ecomap. This process promotes joint client and worker understanding of the issues at hand, and assists with the engagement and rapport building so necessary in the initial stages of contact.

One of the more unique features of an ecological systems perspective is that it can illustrate and take account of the non linear passage of time and interactions between different parts of the system in a way that other perspectives do not. This is particularly important in relation to working with indigenous communities, where temporal considerations cannot be limited to a linear understanding based on the notion of cause and effect. In the *Dreaming*, 'from any particular point in time, the past may be the future and the future may be the present. Time does not extend back through a series of pasts' (Hume 2003, p.38).

As outlined above, an ecological systems approach to working with clients has both its strengths and weaknesses. In selecting what theoretical principles to use to guide practice, the important considerations for the worker must centre on how the client might best be able to move forward in a positive direction, the nature of the presenting issues, and what framework might address these in the most constructive way. An ecological systems analysis can be used on its own, or in conjunction with other perspectives to inform this process.

References

Agass, D. and Preston-Shoot, M. (1990) 'Defining the theory: A systems Approach', in D. Agass and M. Preston-Shoot (eds) *Making Sense of Social Work*, London: Macmillan.

Anglem, J. and Maidment, J. (2004) 'Introduction to assessment', in J. Maidment and R. Egan (eds) *Practice Skills in Social Work and Welfare*, Sydney: Allen & Unwin.

Bronfenbrenner, U. (1979) *The Ecology of Human Development Experiments by Nature and Design*, Cambridge, MA: Harvard University Press.

Chung, W.S. and Pardeck, J.T. (1997) 'Treating powerless minorities though an ecosystem approach', *Adolescence*, 32 (127): 625–34.

Germain, C. (1979) 'Introduction: Ecology and social work', in C. Germain (ed.) *Social Work Practice: People and Environments*, New York: Columbia University Press.

Gitterman, A. (1996a) 'Ecological perspective: Response to Jerry Wakefield', *Social Service Review*, 70 (3): 472–6.

—— (1996b) 'Life model theory and social work treatment', in F. Turner (ed.) *Social Work Treatment*, 4th edition, New York: Free Press.

Greif, G. (2003) 'In response to Michael Ungar's "A deeper, more social, ecological social work practice" debate with authors', *Social Service Review*, 77 (2): 306–11.

Hartman, A. (1978) 'Diagrammatic assessment of family relationships', *Social Casework*, 59: 465–76.

Hume, L. (2003) *Ancestral Power: The Dreaming, Consciousness and Aboriginal Australians*, Melbourne: Melbourne University Press.

Hunter, B. (2000) 'Looking after country – the ACF indigenous program takes shape', *Habitat Australia*, 28: 4, 23.

Kemp, S., Whittaker, J. and Tracy, E. (1997) *Person–Environment Practice: The Social Ecology of Interpersonal Helping*, New York: Adeline de Gruyter.

Mancoske, R. (1981) 'Sociological perspectives on the ecological model', *Journal of Sociology and Social Welfare*, 8 (4): 710–32 cited in Payne, M. (1998) *Modern Social Work Theory*, 3rd edition, Basingstoke: Palgrave Macmillan: pp 158–9.

Mattaini, M. and Meyer, C. (2002) 'The ecosystems perspective: Implications for practice', in M. Mattaini, C. Lowery and C. Meyer (eds) *The Foundations of Social Work Practice*, 3rd edition, Washington, DC: NASW Press.

Patterson, J. (1999) 'Respecting nature: The Maori way', *The Ecologist*, 29 (1); 33–9.

Payne, M. (1997) *Modern Social Work Theory*, 2nd edition, Basingstoke: Macmillan.

Pincus, A. and Minahan, A. (1973) *Social Work Practice: Model and Method*, Itasca, IL: F.E. Peacock.

Rapp, C. (1998) *The Strengths Model: Case Management with People Suffering from Severe and Persistent Mental Illness*, New York: Oxford University Press.

Ridley, M. (2003) *Nature Via Nurture: Genes, Experience and What Makes Us Human*, London: Fourth Estate.

Rothery, M. (2001) 'Ecological systems theory', in P. Lehmann and N. Coady (eds) *Theoretical Perspectives for Direct Social Work Practice: A Generalist–Eclectic Approach*, New York: Springer Publishing.

Ruwhiu, L. (2001) 'Bicultural issues in Aotearoa/New Zealand', in M. Connolly (ed.) *New Zealand Social Work*, Auckland: Oxford University Press.

Ungar, M. (2002) 'A deeper, more social, ecological social work practice', *Social Service Review*, 76 (3): 480–97.

Wakefield, J. (1996a) 'Does social work need the eco-systems perspective? Part 1. Is the perspective clinically useful?', *Social Service Review*, 70 (1): 1–32.

—— (1996b) 'Does social work need the eco-systems perspective? Part 2. Does the perspective save social work from incoherence?', *Social Service Review*, 70 (2): 182–213.

Further reading

Barber, J. G. (2002) *Social Work with Addictions*, 2nd edition, Basingstoke: Palgrave Macmillan.

Bilson, A. and Ross, S. (1999) *Social Work Management and Practice: Systems Principles*, 2nd edition, London: Jessica Kingsley.

Jack, G. (1997) 'An ecological approach to social work with children and families', *Child and Family Social Work*, 2 (1): 109–20.

—— (2000) 'Ecological influences on parenting and child development', *British Journal of Social Work*, 30 (6): 703–20.

Pardeck, J.T. (1996) *Social Work Practice: An Ecological Approach*, Westport, CT: Greenwood Publishing.

Payne, M. (2005) *Modern Social Work Theory*, 3rd edition, Basingstoke: Palgrave Macmillan.

Reynolds, M. and Holwell, S. (eds) *Systems Approaches to Managing Change: A Practical Guide*, New York: Springer.

24 Bridging the past and present to the future of crisis intervention and crisis management

Albert R. Roberts

Social workers work with people who are in crisis all the time; people whose normal coping mechanisms have broken down, and they are, quite literally, at the end of their tether. Crisis intervention theory and practice offer a helpful way of responding to people in crisis, and Albert Roberts, Professor in Criminal Justice and Social Work at Rutgers, the State University of New Jersey in Pitscataway, is one of the best authorities on this subject in the world. In locating this extract, it is important to acknowledge that crisis intervention, like task-centred practice (see Reid and Epstein 1972; Doel 2002), is a problem-solving approach, drawing on the early work of Helen Perlman (1957). It also shares with a task-centred approach the idea that it is most helpful to work with people who are in trouble in a short-term, focused way, instead of offering longer term support (as shown in research including a classic study by Mayer and Timms published in 1970). More recently, these ideas have been developed further in solution focused brief therapy (SFBT) where the focus shifts to understanding solutions, not problems (Ansbacher and Ansbacher 1998; Cree and Myers 2008). In the selected extract, Albert Roberts describes the historical beginnings of crisis intervention theory, and offers a useful model for practice now and in the future.

From *Crisis Intervention Handbook: Assessment, Treatment and Research*, Oxford: Oxford University Press, (2005): 11–21.

Crisis reactions and crisis intervention

A *crisis* can be defined as a period of psychological disequilibrium, experienced as a result of a hazardous event or situation that constitutes a significant problem that cannot be remedied by using familiar coping strategies. A crisis occurs when a person faces an obstacle to important life goals that generally seems insurmountable through the use of customary habits and coping patterns. The goal of crisis intervention is to resolve the most pressing problem within a 1- to 12-week period using focused and directed interventions aimed at helping the client develop new adaptive coping methods.

Crisis reaction refers to the acute stage, which usually occurs soon after the hazardous event (e.g., sexual assault, battering, suicide attempt). During this phase, the person's acute reaction may take various forms, including helplessness, confusion, anxiety, shock, disbelief, and anger. Low self-esteem and serious depression are often produced by the crisis state. The person in crisis may appear to be incoherent, disorganized, agitated, and volatile or calm, subdued, withdrawn, and apathetic. It is during this period that the individual is often most willing to seek help, and crisis intervention is usually more effective at this time (Golan, 1978).

Crisis intervention can provide a challenge, an opportunity, and a turning point within the individual's life. According to Roberts and Dziegielewski (1995), crisis clinicians have been encouraged to examine psychological and situational crises in terms of 'both danger and opportunity' (p. 16). The aftermath of a crisis episode can result in either a highly positive or a highly negative change. Immediate and structured crisis intervention guided by Roberts's seven-stage model facilitates crisis resolution, cognitive mastery, and personal growth, rather than psychological harm.

A divorce, a robbery, a broken engagement, being the victim of a domestic assault, and being the close relative of a person killed in an automobile accident or a plane crash are all highly stressful occurrences that can result in an active crisis state. The persons involved may exhibit denial, intense anxiety, and confusion; they may express anger and fear, or grief and loss, but they can all survive. Crisis intervention can reduce immediate danger and fear, as well as provide support, hope, and alternative ways of coping and growing.

Persons in acute crisis have had similar reactions to traumatic events, from initial feelings of disruption and disorganization to the eventual read-justment of the self. During the impact phase, survivors of victimization and other crisis-producing events often feel numb, disoriented, shattered, fearful, vulnerable, helpless, and lonely. The survivors may seek help, consolation, and advice from friends or professionals within several hours or days after the traumatic or stressful life event.

Helping a person in crisis – whether it be in the aftermath of a violent crime, a suicide attempt, a drug overdose, a life-threatening illness, a natural disaster, a divorce, a broken romance, or an automobile crash – requires exceptional sensitivity, active listening skills, and empathy on the part of the crisis intervenor. If a hotline worker, crisis counselor, social worker, or psychologist is able to establish rapport with the person in crisis soon after the acute crisis episode, many hours of later treatment may be averted.

Defining a crisis and crisis concepts

Crisis may be viewed in various ways, but most definitions emphasize that it can be a turning point in a person's life. According to Bard and Ellison (1974), crisis is 'a subjective reaction to a stressful life experience, one so affecting the stability of the individual that the ability to cope or function may be seriously compromised' (p. 68).

It has been established that a crisis can develop when an event, or a series of events, takes place in a person's life and the result is a hazardous situation. However, it is important to note that the crisis is not the situation itself (e.g., being victimized); rather, it is the person's *perception of and response to* the situation (Parad, 1971, p. 197).

The most important precipitant of a crisis is a stressful or hazardous event. But two other conditions are also necessary to have a crisis state: (a) the individual's perception that the stressful event will lead to considerable upset and/or disruption; and (b) the individual's inability to resolve the disruption by previously used coping methods . . .

Crisis intervention refers to a therapist entering into the life situation of an individual or family to alleviate the impact of a crisis to help mobilize the resources of those directly affected (Parad, 1965).

In conceptualizing crisis theory, Parad and Caplan (1960) examine the fact that 'crises have a peak or sudden turning point'; as the individual reaches this peak, tension increases and stimulates the mobilization of previously hidden strengths and capacities. They urge timely intervention to help individuals cope successfully with a crisis situation. Caplan (1961) states that 'a relatively minor force, acting for a relatively short time, can switch the balance to one side or another, to the side of mental health or the side of mental ill health' (p. 293).

There is a general consensus among clinical social workers, counselors, psychologists, and emergency services workers that the following characterize a person in crisis:

1   Perceiving a precipitating event as being meaningful and threatening
2   Appearing unable to modify or lessen the impact of stressful events with traditional coping methods
3   Experiencing increased fear, tension, and/or confusion
4   Exhibiting a high level of subjective discomfort
5   Proceeding rapidly to an active state of crisis – a state of disequilibrium

Basic tenets of crisis theory

As mentioned earlier, a crisis state is a temporary upset, accompanied by some confusion and disorganization, and characterized by a person's inability to cope with a specific situation through the use of traditional problem-solving methods. According to Naomi Golan (1978), the heart of crisis theory and practice rests in a series of basic statements:

> Crisis situations can occur episodically during "the normal life span of individuals, families, groups, communities and nation." They are often initiated by a hazardous event. This may be a catastrophic event or a series of successive stressful blows which rapidly build up a cumulative effect. (p. 8)

> The impact of the hazardous event disturbs the individual's homeostatic balance and puts him in a vulnerable state. (p. 8)

> If the problem continues and cannot be resolved, avoided, or redefined, tension rises to a peak, and a precipitating factor can bring about a turning point, during which self-righting devices no longer operate and the individual enters a state of a disequilibrium . . . (an) active crisis. (p. 8)

Duration of the crisis

Persons cannot remain indefinitely in a state of psychological turmoil and survive. Caplan (1964) noted, and other clinical supervisors have concurred, that in a typical crisis state equilibrium will be restored in 4 to 6 weeks. However, the designation of 4 to 6 weeks has been confusing. Several authors note that crisis resolution can take from several weeks to several months. To clarify the confusion concerning this period, it is useful to explain the difference between restoring equilibrium and crisis resolution.

Disequilibrium, which is characterized by confusing emotions, somatic complaints, and erratic behavior, is reduced considerably within the first 6 weeks of crisis intervention. The severe emotional discomfort experienced by the person in crisis propels him or her toward action that will result in reducing the subjective discomfort. *Thus, equilibrium is restored*, and the disorganization is time limited.

Viney (1976) aptly describes *crisis resolution* as restoration of equilibrium, as well as cognitive mastery of the situation and the development of new coping methods. Fairchild (1986) refers to crisis resolution as an adaptive consequence of a crisis in which the person grows from the crisis experience through the discovery of new coping skills and resources to employ in the future. In this handbook, crisis intervention is viewed as the process of working through the crisis event so that the person is assisted in exploring the traumatic experience and his or her reaction to it. Emphasis is also placed on helping the individual do the following:

- Make behavioral changes and interpersonal adjustments.
- Mobilize internal and external resources and supports.
- Reduce unpleasant or disturbing affects related to the crisis.
- Integrate the event and its aftermath into the individual's other life experiences and markers.

The goal of effective crisis resolution is to remove vulnerabilities from the individual's past and bolster him or her with an increased repertoire of new coping skills to serve as a buffer against similar stressful situations in the future.

Historical development

As far back as 400 B.C., physicians have stressed the significance of crisis as a hazardous life event. Hippocrates himself defined a crisis as a sudden state that gravely endangers life. But the development of a cohesive theory of crisis and approaches to crisis management had to await the twentieth century. The movement to help people in crisis began in 1906 with the establishment of the first suicide prevention center, the National Save-a-Life League in New York City. However, contemporary crisis intervention theory and practice were not formally elaborated until the 1940s, primarily by Erich Lindemann and Gerald Caplan.

Lindemann and his associates at Massachusetts General Hospital introduced the concepts of crisis intervention and time-limited treatment in 1943 in the aftermath of Boston's worst nightclub fire, at the Coconut Grove, in which 493 people perished. Lindemann (1944) and colleagues based the crisis theory they developed on their observations of the acute and delayed reactions of survivors and grief-stricken relatives of victims. Their clinical work focused on the psychological symptoms of the survivors and on preventing unresolved grief among relatives of the persons who had died. They found that many individuals experiencing acute grief often had five related reactions:

1   Somatic distress
2   Preoccupation with the image of the deceased
3   Guilt
4   Hostile reactions
5   Loss of patterns of conduct

Furthermore, Lindemann and colleagues concluded that the duration of a grief reaction appears to be dependent on the success with which the bereaved person does his or her mourning and 'grief work.' In general, this grief work involves achieving emancipation from the deceased, readjusting to the changes in the environment from which the loved one is missing, and developing new relationships. We learned from Lindemann that people need to be encouraged to permit themselves to have a period of mourning and eventual acceptance of the loss and adjustment to life without the parent, child, spouse, or sibling. If the normal process of grieving is delayed, negative outcomes of crises will develop. Lindemann's work was soon adapted to interventions with World War II veterans suffering from 'combat neurosis' and bereaved family members.

Gerald Caplan, who was affiliated with Massachusetts General Hospital and the Harvard School of Public Health, expanded Lindemann's pioneering work in the 1940s and 1950s. Caplan studied various developmental crisis reactions, as in premature births, infancy, childhood, and adolescence, and accidental crises such as illness and death. He was the first psychiatrist to relate the concept of homeostasis to crisis intervention and to describe the stages of a crisis. According to Caplan (1961), a crisis is an upset of a steady state in which the individual encounters an obstacle (usually an obstacle to significant life goals) that cannot be overcome through traditional problem-solving activities. For each individual, a reasonably constant balance or steady state exists between affective and cognitive experience. When this homeostatic balance or stability in psychological functioning is threatened by physiological, psychological, or social forces, the individual engages in problem-solving methods designed to restore the balance. However, in a crisis situation, the person in distress faces a problem that seems to have no solution. Thus homeostatic balance is disrupted, or an upset of a steady state ensues.

Caplan (1964) explains this concept further by stating that the problem is one in which the individual faces 'stimuli which signal danger to a fundamental need satisfaction ... and the circumstances are such that habitual problem-solving methods are unsuccessful within the time span of past expectations of success' (p. 39).

Caplan also described four stages of a crisis reaction. The first stage is the initial rise of tension that comes from the emotionally hazardous crisis-precipitating event. The second stage is characterized by an increased level of tension and disruption to daily living because the individual is unable to resolve the crisis quickly. As the person attempts and fails to resolve the crisis through emergency problem-solving mechanisms, tension increases to such an intense level that the individual may go into a depression. The person going through the final stage of Caplan's model may experience either a mental collapse or a breakdown, or may partly resolve the crisis by using new coping methods. J. S. Tyhurst (1957) studied transition states – migration, retirement, civilian disaster, and so on – in the lives of persons experiencing sudden changes. Based on his field studies on individual patterns of responses to community disaster, Tyhurst identified three overlapping phases, each with its own manifestations of stress and attempts at reducing it:

1   A period of impact
2   A period of recoil
3   A postraumatic period of recovery

Tyhurst recommended stage-specific intervention. He concluded that persons in transitional crisis states should not be removed from their life situation, and that intervention should focus on bolstering the network of relationships.

In addition to building on the pioneering work of Lindemann and Caplan, Lydia Rapoport was one of the first practitioners to write about the linkage of modalities such as ego psychology, learning theory, and traditional social casework (Rapoport, 1967). In Rapoport's first article on crisis theory (1962), she defined a crisis as 'an upset of a steady state' (p. 212) that places the individual in a hazardous condition. She pointed out that a crisis situation results in a problem that can be perceived as a threat, a loss, or a challenge. She then stated that there are usually three interrelated factors that create a state of crisis:

1 A hazardous event
2 A threat to life goals
3 An inability to respond with adequate coping mechanisms

In their early works, Lindemann and Caplan briefly mentioned that a hazardous event produces a crisis, but it was Rapoport (1967) who most thoroughly described the nature of this crisis-precipitating event. She clearly conceptualized the content of crisis intervention practice, particularly the initial or study phase (assessment). She began by pointing out that in order to help persons in crisis, the client must have rapid access to the crisis worker. She stated: 'A little help, rationally directed and purposefully focused at a strategic time, is more effective than more extensive help given at a period of less emotional accessibility' (Rapoport, 1967, p. 38).

This point was echoed by Naomi Golan (1978), who concluded that during the state of active crisis, when usual coping methods have proved inadequate and the individual and his or her family are suffering from pain and discomfort, a person is frequently more amenable to suggestions and change. Clearly, intensive, brief, appropriately focused treatment when the client is motivated can produce more effective change than long-term treatment when motivation and emotional accessibility are lacking.

Rapoport (1967) asserted that during the initial interview, the first task of the practitioner is to develop a preliminary diagnosis of the presenting problem. It is most critical during this first interview that the crisis therapist convey a sense of hope and optimism to the client concerning successful crisis resolution. Rapoport suggested that this sense of hope and enthusiasm can be properly conveyed to the client when the interview focuses on mutual exploration and problem solving, along with clearly delineated goals and tasks. The underlying message is that client and therapist will be working together to resolve the crisis.

Crisis intervention models and strategies

In order to become an effective crisis intervenor, it is important to gauge the stages and completeness of the intervention. The following seven-stage paradigm should be viewed as a guide, not as a rigid process, since with some clients stages may overlap.

Roberts's (1991) seven-stage model of crisis intervention (Figure 24.1) has been utilized for helping persons in acute psychological crisis, acute situational crises, and acute stress disorders. The seven stages are as follows:

1 Plan and conduct a thorough assessment (including lethality, dangerousness to self or others, and immediate psychosocial needs).

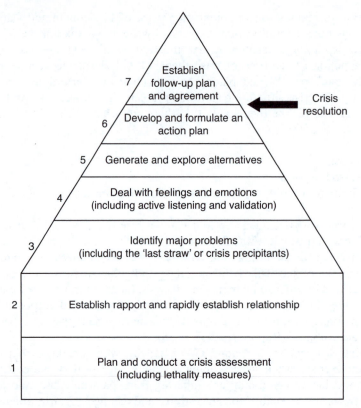

Figure 24.1 Roberts's seven-stage crisis intervention model.

2   Make psychological contact, establish rapport, and rapidly establish the relation-
    ship (conveying genuine respect for the client, acceptance, reassurance, and a
    nonjudgmental attitude).
3   Examine the dimensions of the problem in order to define it (including the last
    straw or precipitating event).
4   Encourage an exploration of feelings and emotions.
5   Generate, explore, and assess past coping attempts.
6   Restore cognitive functioning through implementation of action plan.
7   Follow up and leave the door open for booster sessions 3 and/or 6 months later.

References

Ansbacher, H.L. and Ansbacher, R.R. (eds) (1998) *Individual Psychology of Alfred Adler:
    A Systematic Presentation in Selections from his Writings*, New York: HarperCollins.
Bard, M. and Ellison, K. (1974) 'Crisis intervention and investigation of forcible rape', *The Police
    Chief*, 41 (May): 68–73.
Caplan, G. (1961) *An Approach to Community Mental Health*, New York: Grune & Stratton.
—— (1964) *Principles of Preventive Psychiatry*, New York: Basic Books.
Cree, V.E. and Myers, S. (2008) *Social Work: Making a Difference*, Bristol: Policy Press/BASW.
Doel, M. (2002) 'Task centred work', in R. Adams, L. Dominelli and M. Payne (eds) *Social
    Work: Themes Issues and Critical Debates*, Basingstoke: Palgrave.

Fairchild, T.N. (1986) *Crisis Intervention Strategies for School-based Helpers*, Springfield, IL: Charles C. Thomas.

Golan, N. (1978) *Treatment in Crisis Situations*, New York: Free Press.

Lindemann, E. (1944) 'Symptomatology and management of acute grief', *American Journal of Psychiatry*, 101: 141–48.

Mayer, J. and Timms, N. (1970) *The Client Speaks*, London: Routledge & Kegan Paul.

Parad, H.J. (ed.) (1965) *Crisis Intervention: Selected Readings*, New York: Family Service Association of America.

—— (1971) 'Crisis intervention', in R. Morris (ed.) *Encyclopedia of Social Work Vol 1*, New York: National Association of Social Workers, 196–202.

Parad, H.J. and Caplan, G. (1960) 'A framework for studying families in crisis', *Social Work*, 5 (3): 3–15.

Perlman, H.H. (1957) *Social Casework: A Problem Solving Process*, Chicago, IL: University of Chicago Press.

Rapoport, L. (1962) 'The state of crisis: some theoretical considerations', *Social Service Review*, 36: 211–17.

—— (1967) 'Crisis-oriented short-term casework', *Social Service Review*, 41: 31–43.

Reid, W.J. and Epstein, L. (1972) *Task Centred Casework*, New York: Columbia University Press.

Roberts, A.R. (1991) 'Conceptualizing crisis theory and the crisis intervention model', in A.R. Roberts (ed.), *Contemporary Perspectives on Crisis Intervention and Prevention*, Englewood Cliffs, NJ: Prentice Hall, 3–17.

Roberts, A.R. and Dziegielewski, S.F. (1995) 'Foundation skills and applications of crisis intervention and cognitive therapy', in A.R. Roberts (ed.) *Crisis Intervention and Time-limited Cognitive Treatment*, Thousand Oaks, CA: Sage, 3–27.

Tyhurst, J.S. (1957) 'The role of transition states – including disasters – in mental illness', in *Symposium on Preventive and Social Psychiatry*, Washington, DC: Water Reed Army Institute of Research, 1–23.

Viney, L.L. (1976) 'The concept of crisis: A tool for clinical psychologists', *Bulletin of the British Psychological Society*, 29: 387–95.

Further reading

Doel, M. and Marsh, P. (2005) *The Task-centred Book*, London: Routledge.

James, R.K. and Gilliland, B.E. (2001) *Crisis Intervention Strategies*, 4th edition, Belmont, CA: Wadsworth.

Kanel, K. (2003) *A Guide to Crisis Intervention*, 2nd edition, Pacific Grove, CA: Brooks/Cole.

Myer, R.A. (2001) *Assessment for Crisis Intervention: A Triage Assessment Model*, Belmont, CA: Brooks/Cole.

O'Hagan, K. (1986) *Crisis Intervention in Social Services*, Basingstoke: Macmillan.

—— (1991) 'Crisis intervention in social work', in J. Lishman (ed.) *A Handbook of Theory for Practice Teachers in Social Work*, London: Jessica Kingsley.

Payne, M. (2005) *Modern Social Work Theory*, 3rd edition, Basingstoke: Palgrave Macmillan.

Reid, W.J. and Shyne, A.W. (1969) *Brief and Extended Casework*, New York: Columbia University Press.

25 Power in the people

Dennis Saleebey

Since the first edition of this book was published in 1992, strengths-based approaches have made a major contribution to developing a social work practice which is empowering and values-led, as demonstrated in settings as diverse as children and families, mental health, criminal justice and community social work across the world. Strengths-based approaches, as the title suggests, focus on identifying the strengths which service users have in themselves, their families, their wider lives and communities, and building from these. The notion of 'resilience', central to research findings on children at risk, has resonance with this approach (see Masten *et al.* 1990; Smith and Carslon 1997), as do solution-focused approaches (highlighted in the previous chapter) and cognitive behavioural approaches (see Sheldon 1995; Sheldon and Macdonald 2009). Strengths-based approaches see the relationship between the social worker and the service user as fundamental to motivating change (see Nash *et al.* 2005), a message taken forward in the review of social work in Scotland (Scottish Executive 2006) and also reflected in earlier research by Prochaska and diClemente (1984) on helping people with addictions problems. The extract is taken from the fourth edition of the groundbreaking book by Dennis Saleebey who is based at the University of Kansas in the US.

From *The Strengths Perspective in Social Work Practice*, 4th edition, Boston, MA: Pearson Education (2006): 7–22.

THE STRENGTHS PERSPECTIVE: PHILOSOPHY, CONCEPTS, AND PRINCIPLES

I want to discuss two major philosophical principles as a way of staking out the claims of the strengths perspective, but in the context of the sometimes numbing and usually complex realities of daily life.

Liberation and empowerment: heroism and hope

Liberation is founded on the idea of possibility: the opportunities for choice, commitment, and action whether pursued in relative tranquility or in grievous circumstance. We have fabulous powers and potentials. Some are muted, unrealized, and immanent. Others glimmer brilliantly about us. All around are people and policies, circumstances and conventions, contingencies and conceptions that may nurture and emancipate these powers or that may crush and degrade them. Somewhere within, and we may call it by different names, lies the longing for the heroic: to transcend circumstances, to develop one's own powers, to face adversity down, to stand up and be counted. All too often social institutions, oppressors, other people, some even with good intentions, tamp out this yearning or distort it so that it serves the interests and purposes of others. Nonetheless, however muted, this precious craving abides. It is incumbent on the healer, the humane leader, the shaman, the teacher, and, yes, the social worker to find ways for this penchant for the possible and unimaginable to survive and find expression in life-affirming ways. Of course, things go more smoothly if people simply play their roles, pay their taxes, and stifle their opinions. Liberation exerts tremendous pressure on the repressive inclinations of institutions and individuals. Collectively, liberation unleashes human energy and spirit, critical thinking, the questioning of authority, challenges to the conventional wisdom, and new ways of being and doing. But liberation may also be modest and unassuming. We may try out new behaviors, forge new relationships, or make a new commitment. Hope and the belief in the possible is central to liberation. Before his death, the great pedagogue of liberation, Paulo Freire, wrote in his last book, *Pedagogy of Hope* (1996), that he had previously underestimated the power of hope.

I would go so far as to say that the central dynamic of the strengths perspective is precisely the rousing of hope, of tapping into the visions and the promise of that individual, family, or community. Circumstances, bad luck, unfortunate decisions, the harshness of life lived on the edge of need and vulnerability, of course, may smother these. Nonetheless, it is the flicker of possibility that can ignite the fire of hope.

The heroism of everyday life is all around us. People carrying on in the midst of mind-searing stress; people coming to the fore when the needs around them require someone to act and to act out of the ordinary; people whose moral imagination allows them to see, even in distant and unfamiliar places, the utter humanity of those who suffer (Glover, 2000). 9/11 is an instructive example. Fire and police personnel, rescue teams, the people who risked their lives and faced serious harm in helping to clear away the hellish debris (Langewiesche, 2003), social workers who met with survivors and witnesses to help ease the psychological and interpersonal wreckage of the trauma; people trapped in the inferno, facing certain death, who called their loved ones to tell them goodbye and to express their love: many of these pushed the boundaries of the heroic outward and upward. Clearly, the destruction wrought on that day was a deliberate, heinous, and murderous crime. But even on the other side, given their point of view, the terrorists thought themselves to be heroic.

Alienation and oppression: anxiety and evil

The circumstances around us will not let us deny the existence of harsh and tyrannical institutions, relationships, circumstances, and regimes. Bigotry, hatred, war, slaughter, repression, and, more quietly but no less devastating, setting people aside, treating them as the despised other, and acting as though they are not fully human, are all daily reminders of the existence of evil, brutality, and despotism.

. . . from the ashes of destruction, mayhem, and oppression may emerge the human spirit, the capacity for the heroic. So we can never dismiss the possibility of redemption, resurrection, and regeneration.

We have seen that the preoccupation with problems and pathologies, while producing an impressive lode of technical and theoretical writing, may be less fruitful when it comes to actually helping clients grow, develop, change directions, realize their visions, or revise their personal meanings and narratives. What follows is a brief glossary of terms supporting an orientation to strengths as well as a statement of the principles of practice central to a strengths perspective. These are meant to give you a vital sense of what a frame of mind devoted to the strengths of individuals and groups requires.

THE LEXICON OF STRENGTHS

'We can act,' wrote William James (1902) in reflecting upon Immanuel Kant's notions about conceptions, 'as *if* there were a God; feel as *if* we were free; consider nature as *if* she were full of special designs; lay plans as *if* we were to be immortal; and we find then that these words **do** [emphasis added] make a genuine difference in our moral life' (p. 55). Language and words have power. They can elevate and inspire or demoralize and destroy. If words are a part of the nutriment that feeds one's sense of self, then we are compelled to examine our dictionary of helping to see what our words portend for clients. Any approach to practice speaks a language that, in the end, may have a pronounced effect on the way that clients think of themselves and how they act. Not only that, our professional diction has a profound effect on the way that *we* regard clients, their world, and their troubles. In the strengths approach to practice, some words are essential and direct us to an appreciation of the assets of individuals, families, and communities.

A simple device for framing and remembering the essentials of the strengths perspective can be found in Figure 25.1.

These words capture, I think, the core values of the strengths lexicon. The central dynamic of strength discovery and articulation lies in hope and possibility; the vision of a better future or quality of life.

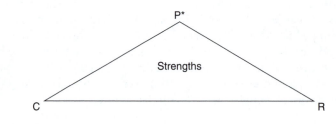

Where C stands for:

Competence, capacities, courage

And P symbolizes:

Promise, possibility, positive expectations

And R signifies:

Resilience, reserves, resources

Figure 25.1

*Thanks to my daughter Meghan for suggesting this.

Plasticity (and the placebo effect). It is a miracle of the brain that it 'never loses the power to transform itself on the basis of experience and that the transformation can occur over short intervals. . . . your brain is different today than it was yesterday' (Restak, 2003, p. 8). It was once thought that after adolescence the brain is pretty much structural monolith, hardly changing. But now, thanks to sophisticated imaging techniques, it is clear that the brain, in ways minute and substantial, continually undergoes change. We have a marvelous capacity to alter, extend, and reshape behavior, feeling, and cognition. Of course, much of what happens here is beyond our conscious recognition.

The placebo effect has been long noted (even before modern medicine although it was not called that). Whatever else this means, it does, I think, bespeak the power of hope, positive expectations, and belief in the healing ministration. It seems odd that we would not have made more of the placebo effect (even if it is only a short-term one).

Empowerment. Although rapidly becoming hackneyed, empowerment indicates the intent to, and the processes of, assisting individuals, groups, families, and communities to discover and expend the resources and tools within and around them.

To discover the power within people and communities, we must subvert and abjure pejorative labels; provide opportunities for connections to family, institutional, and communal resources; assail the victim mind-set; foreswear paternalism; trust people's intuitions, accounts, perspectives, and energies; and believe in people's dreams. Barbara Levy Simon (1994) builds the concept of empowerment with five necessary ideas: collaborative partnerships with clients and constituents; an emphasis on the expansion of client strengths and capacities; a focus on both the individual or family and the environment; assuming that clients are active subjects and agents; and directing one's energies to the historically disenfranchised and oppressed. The strengths of individuals and communities are renewable and expandable resources. Furthermore, the assets of individuals almost always lie embedded in a community of interest and involvement. Thus, the ideas of community and membership are central to the strengths approach.

Membership. To be without membership is to be alienated, to be at risk for marginalization and oppression. People need to be citizens, responsible and valued members of a community. To sever people from the roots of their 'place' subverts, for all, civic and moral vigor. The strengths orientation proceeds from the recognition that all of those whom we serve are, like ourselves, members of a species, entitled to the dignity, respect, and responsibility that comes with such membership. There is another meaning of membership and that is that people must often band together to make their voices heard, get their needs met, to redress inequities, and to reach their dreams.

Resilience. A growing body of inquiry and practice makes it clear that the rule, not the exception, in human affairs is that people do rebound from serious trouble, that individuals and communities do surmount and overcome serious and troubling adversity.

Resilience is not the cheerful disregard of one's difficult and traumatic life experiences; neither is it the naive discounting of life's pains. It is, rather, the ability to bear up in spite of these ordeals. Damage has been done. Emotional and physical scars bear witness to that. In spite of the wounds, however, for many the trials have been instructive and propitious. Resilience is a process – the continuing growth and articulation of capacities, knowledge, insight, and virtues derived through meeting the demands and challenges of one's world, however chastening.

Healing and wholeness.   Healing implies both wholeness and the inborn facility of the body and the mind to regenerate and resist when faced with disorder, disease, and disruption. Healing also requires a beneficent relationship between the individual and the larger social and physical environment. The natural state of affairs for human beings, evolved over eons of time and at every level of organization from cell to self-image, is the repair of one's mind and body. Just as the resilience literature assures us that individuals have naturally occurring self-righting tendencies, even though they can be compromised (Werner and Smith, 1992), it seems also the case that all human organisms have the inclination for healing. This evolutionary legacy, of course can be compromised by trauma, by environmental toxins, by bodily disorganization, and, not the least, by some of our professional intervention philosophies and systems. But, the bottom line is this: . . . So healing and self-regeneration are intrinsic life support systems, always working and, for most of us, most of the time, on call. Such a reality has dramatic implications, not just for medicine but for all the helping professions. At the least, it challenges the assumption of the disease model that only experts know what is best for their clients and that curing, healing, or transformation comes exclusively from outside sources.

Dialogue and collaboration.   Humans can only come into being through a creative and emergent relationships with others. Without such transactions, there can be no discovery and testing of one's powers, no knowledge, no heightening of one's awareness and internal strengths. In dialogue, we confirm the importance of others and begin to heal the rift between self, other, and institution.

The idea of collaboration has a more specific focus. When we work together with clients we become their agents, their consultants, stakeholders with them in mutually crafted projects. This requires us to be open to negotiation and to appreciate the authenticity of the views and aspirations of those with whom we collaborate. Our voices may have to be quieted so that we can give voice to our clients. Comfortably ensconced in the expert role, sometimes we may have great difficulty assuming such a conjoint posture.

Suspension of disbelief.   It would be hard to exaggerate the extent of disbelief of clients' words and stories in the culture of professionalism. While social work because of its enduring values may fancy itself less culpable in this regard than other professions, a little circumspection is warranted.

Professionals have contained the affirmation of clients in a number of ways:

- by imposing their own theories over the theories and accounts of clients
- by using assessment in an interrogative style designed to ascertain certain diagnostic and largely preemptive hypotheses that, in the end, confirm suspicions about the client
- by engaging in self-protective maneuvers (like skepticism) designed to prevent the ultimate embarrassment for a professional – being fooled by or lied to by a cunning client

The frequent talk about manipulative and resistant clients in many social agencies may stem from the fear of being made the fool. To protect self-esteem, nonnormative life-styles, self-interests, or benefits, clients may have a vested interest in not telling the truth. But we must consider the possibility that avoiding the truth may be a function of the manner in which the professional pursues and/or asserts the truth. The professional's knowledge, information, and perspective are privileged and carry institutional and legal weight. The client's do not.

PRINCIPLES OF THE STRENGTHS PERSPECTIVE

What exactly is a perspective? It is not a theory. Theories seek to explain some phenomena, or at least describe them analytically. It is not a model. Models are meant to represent, logically and graphically, some aspect of the world. A perspective is somewhat harder to define. At the least it is a standpoint, a way of viewing and understanding certain aspects of experience. It is a lens through which we choose to perceive and appreciate. It provides us with a slant on the world, built of words and principles. We have already reviewed some of the words. What follows now are some of the principles.

The principles that follow are the guiding assumptions and regulating understandings of the strengths perspective. They are tentative, still evolving, and subject to revision. They do, however, give a flavor of what practicing from a strengths appreciation involves.

Every individual, group, family, and community has strengths.   While it may be hard at times to invoke, it is essential to remind oneself that the person or family in front of you and the community around you possess assets, resources, wisdom, and knowledge that, at the outset, you probably know nothing about. First *and* foremost, the strengths perspective is about discerning those resources, and respecting them and the potential they may have for reversing misfortune, countering illness, easing pain, and reaching goals. To detect strengths, however, the social work practitioner must be genuinely interested in, and respectful of, clients' stories, narratives, and accounts – the interpretive angles they take on their own experiences. These are important 'theories' that can guide practice. The unearthing of clients' identities and realities does not come only from a ritual litany of troubles, embarrassments, snares, foibles, and barriers. Rather, clients come into view when you assume that they know something, have learned lessons from experience, have hopes, have interests, and can do somethings masterfully. These may be obscured by the stresses of the moment, submerged under the weight of crisis, oppression, or illness but, nonetheless, they abide.

In the end, clients want to know that you actually care about them, that how they fare makes a difference to you, that you will listen to them, that you will respect them no matter what their history, and that you believe that they can build something of value with the resources within and around them. But most of all, clients want to know that you believe they can surmount adversity and begin the climb toward transformation and growth.

Trauma and abuse, illness and struggle may be injurious but they may also be sources of challenge and opportunity.   The Wolins (1997) point out that the 'damage model' of development so prevalent in today's thinking only leads to discouragement, pessimism, and the victim mind-set. It also foretells a continuing future of psychopathology and troubled relationships. Individuals exposed to a variety of abuses, especially in childhood, are thought always to be victims or to be damaged in ways that obscure or override any strengths or possibilities for rebound. In the Wolins' 'challenge model,' children are not seen as merely passive recipients of parental unpredictability, abuse, disappointment, or violence. Rather, children are seen as active and developing individuals who, through these trials, learn skills and develop personal attributes that stand them in good stead in adulthood. Not that they do not suffer. They do. Not that they do not bear scars. They do. But they also may acquire traits and capacities that are preservative and life affirming. There is dignity to be drawn from having prevailed over obstacles to one's growth and maturing. The Wolins (1993) refer to this as 'survivor's pride.' It is a deep-dwelling sense of accomplishment in having met life's challenges and walked away, not without fear, even terror, and certainly not without wounds. Often this pride is buried under embarrassment, confusion, distraction, or self-doubt. But when it exists and is lit, it can ignite the engine of change.

Assume that you do not know the upper limits of the capacity to grow and change and take individual, group, and community aspirations seriously.   Too often, professionals assume that a diagnosis, an assessment, or a profile sets the parameters of possibility for their clients. In our personal lives, looking back, we sometimes marvel at the road we traveled – a road that we, at the outset, might not have even considered taking – and the distance that we have come. For our clients, too often, we cannot imagine the prospect of similar dizzying and unanticipated destinations. The diagnosis or the assessment becomes a verdict and a sentence. Our clients will be better served when we make an overt pact with their promise and possibility. This means that we must hold high our expectations of clients and make allegiance with their hopes, visions, and values.

It is becoming increasingly clear that emotions have a profound effect on wellness and health. When people believe that they can recover, that they have prospects, that their hopes are palpable, their bodies often respond optimally. That does not mean that people do not get sick. It does mean that when people are sick, healers can make an alliance with the body's regenerative powers and augment them with real but nonetheless fortifying and uplifting expectations (Weil, 1995).

We best serve clients by collaborating with them.   The role of expert or professional may not provide the best vantage point from which to appreciate clients' strengths and assets. A helper may best be defined as a collaborator or consultant: an individual clearly presumed, because of specialized education and experience, to know some things and to have some tools at the ready but definitely not the only one in the situation to have relevant, even esoteric, knowledge and understanding.

We make a serious error when we subjugate clients' wisdom and knowledge to official views. There is something liberating, for all parties involved, in connecting to clients' stories and narratives, their hopes and fears, their wherewithal and resources rather than trying to stuff them into the narrow confines of a diagnostic category or treatment protocol. Ultimately a collaborative stance may make us less vulnerable to some of the more political elements of helping: paternalism, victim-blaming (or, more currently, victim-creating), and preemption of client views. It is likewise important to get the stories and views of clients out to those who need to hear them – schools, agencies, employers, local governments, churches, and businesses. This is part of the role of advocacy.

Every environment is full of resources.   In communities that seem to amplify individual and group resilience, there is awareness, recognition, and use of the assets of most members of the community (Kretzmann and McKnight, 1993). Informal systems and associations of individuals, families, and groups, social circuits of peers, and intergenerational mentoring work to assist, support, instruct, and include all members of a community (Schorr, 1997). In inclusive communities, there are many opportunities for involvement, to make contributions to the moral and civic life of the whole; to become, in other words, a citizen in place. No matter how harsh an environment, how it may test the mettle of its inhabitants, it can also be understood as a potentially lush topography of resources and possibilities. In every environment, there are individuals, associations, groups, and institutions who have something to give, something that others may desperately need: knowledge, succor, an actual resource or talent, or simply time and place. Such resources usually exist outside the usual matrix of social and human service agencies. And, for the most part, they are unsolicited and untapped. Melvin Delgado (2000), in his articulation of the capacity-enhancement approach to urban social work practice, describes the five critical assumptions of that approach: '(1) The community has the will and the resources to help itself; (2) it knows what is best for itself; (3) ownership of the strategy rests within, rather than outside, the community; (4) partnerships involving organizations and communities are the preferred route for initiatives; and (5) the use of strengths in one area will translate into strengths in other areas . . . a ripple effect' (p. 28).

Caring, caretaking, and context.   The idea that care is essential to human well-being does not sit well in a society beset by two centuries of rugged individualism. Deborah Stone (2000) says that we have three rights to care. First, all families must be permitted and assisted in caring for their members. Second, all those paid caregivers need to be able give the support and quality care that is commensurate with the highest ideals of care without subverting their own well-being. Finally, a right to care boils down to this: that all people.

   In one sense, social work is about care and caretaking. Ann Weick (2000) makes the case that social caretaking as an activity is the profession's hidden and first) voice; hidden because it is also woman's voice. Caretaking is, in a diffuse sense, also the work of the strengths perspective.

SOME PRELIMINARY THOUGHTS

Finally, the research on the effectiveness of a strengths approach, although very preliminary, suggests that it may be an effective and economical framework for practice or case management (Rapp, 1998). Related research on power of mind/health realization; resilience-based practice; solution-focused therapy; community-building; and the research done on the critical factors in successful therapy provide some associated support for the elements of a strengths perspective that make a difference. Research actually done from the vantage point of a strengths approach includes the views and concerns of the stakeholders (subjects and clients) from the outset. The results of the research are to be used to achieve stated objectives of the stakeholders and/or to aid in the solving of identified problems.

References

Delgado, M. (2000) *Community Social Work Practice in an Urban Context: The Potential of a Capacity-enhancement Perspective*, New York: Oxford University Press.

Freire, P. (1996) *Pedagogy of Hope: Reliving Pedagogy of the Oppressed*, New York: Continuum.

Glover, J. (2000) *Humanity: A Moral History of the Twentieth Century*, New Haven, CT: Yale University Press.

James, W. (1902) *The Varieties of Religious Experience,* New York: Modern Library.

Kretzmann, J.P. and McKnight, J.L. (1993) *Building Communities from the Inside Out: Toward Finding and Mobilizing a Community's Assets*, Evanston, IL: Northwestern University, Center for Urban Affairs and Policy Research.

Langewiesche, W. (2003) *American Ground: Unbuilding the World Trade Center*, New York: North Point Press.

Masten, A.S., Best, K.M. and Garmezy, N. (1990) 'Resilience and development: Contributions from the study of children who overcome adversity', *Development and Psychopathology*, 2: 425–44.

Nash, M., Munford, R. and O'Donogue, K. (eds) (2005) *Social Work Theories in Action*, London: Jessica Kingsley.

Prochaska, J.O. and diClemente, C.C. (1984) *The Transtheoretical Approach: Crossing the Traditional Boundaries of Therapy*, Homewood, IL: Dow Jones-Irwin.

Rapp, C.A. (1998) *The Strengths Model: Case Management with People Suffering from Severe and Persistent Mental Illness*, New York: Oxford University Press.

Restak, R. (2003) *The New Brain: How the Modern Age is Rewiring your Mind*, New York: St Martin's Press.

Schorr, L.B. (1997) *Common Purpose: Rebuilding Families and Neighborhoods to Rebuild America*, New York: Anchor/Doubleday.

Scottish Executive (2006) *Changing Lives*, Edinburgh: The Scottish Executive.

Sheldon, B. (1995) *Cognitive Behavioural Therapy: Research, Practice and Philosophy*, London: Routledge.

Sheldon, B. and Macdonald, G. (2009) *A Textbook of Social Work*, London: Routledge.

Simon, B.L. (1994) *The Empowerment Tradition in Social Work: A History*, New York: Columbia University Press.

Smith, C. and Carlson, B.E. (1997) 'Stress, coping, and resilience in children and youth', *The Social Service Review*, 71 (2): 231–56.

Stone, D. (2000) 'Why we need a care movement', *The Nation*, 270: 13–15.

Weick, A. (2000) 'Hidden voices', *Social Work*, 45: 395–402.

Weil, A. (1995) *Spontaneous Healing*, New York: Knopf.

Werner, E. and Smith, R.S. (1992) *Overcoming the Odds*, Ithaca, NY: Cornell University Press.

Wolin, S.J. and Wolin, S. (1993) *The Resilient Self: How Survivors of Troubled Families Rise Above Adversity*, New York: Villard.

Wolin, S. and Wolin, S.J. (1997) 'Shifting paradigms: Taking a paradoxical approach', *Resiliency in Action*, 2: 23–8.

Further reading

Aspinwall, L.G. and Staudinger, U.M. (eds) (2003) *A Psychology of Human Strengths: Fundamental Questions and Future Directions for a Positive Psychology*, Washington, DC: American Psychological Association.

Healy, K. (2005) *Social Work Theories in Context*, Basingstoke: Palgrave McMillan.

Jack, R. (2005) Strengths-based practice in statutory care and protection work', in M. Nash, R. Munford and K. O'Donogue (eds) (2005) *Social Work Theories in Action*, London: Jessica Kingsley, 174–88.

Lopez, S.J. and Syder, C.R. (2003) *Positive Psychological Assessment: A Handbook of Models and Measures*, Washington, DC: American Psychological Association.

McIvor, G. and Raynor, P. (eds) (2007) *Developments in Social Work with Offenders*, London: Jessica Kingsley.

Munford, R. and Sanders, J. (2005) 'Working with families. Strengths-based approaches', in M. Nash, R. Munford and K. O'Donogue (eds) (2005) *Social Work Theories in Action*, London: Jessica Kingsley, 158–73.

Peterson, C. and Seligman, M.E.P. (2004) *Character Strengths and Virtues: A Classification Handbook*, New York: Oxford University Press.

Thomas, C. and Davis, S. (2005) 'Bicultural strengths-based supervision', in M. Nash, R. Munford and K. O'Donogue, K. (eds) (2005) *Social Work Theories in Action*, London: Jessica Kingsley, 189–204.

26 Disabled people and self-directed support schemes

Simon Prideaux, Alan Roulstone,
Jennifer Harris and Colin Barnes

There has been a revolution in approaches to care over the last 30 years or so, with the closure of long-stay hospitals for people with physical and intellectual (learning) disabilities and mental health problems, and the new emphasis on care in, and by, the community. As self-advocacy movements such as the Disabled People's Movement and People First (to name but two) have grown in strength and influence, so governments have increasingly seen self-directed and sponsored care as the way forward for those in our community who need support. But what part should social work and social workers play in this new world? If, as some analyses suggest, social work in the past was 'part of the problem', how can it now become 'part of the solution'? The following extract, from a journal article by four UK academic researchers, raises these issues in the context of a discussion of work and welfare. We might take the discussion further and ask: where is social work here?

From *Disability & Society*, 24 (5): 557–69 (2009).

Introduction

This article critically explores and contextualises recent shifts towards self-directed support services for disabled people and their families in the UK. It will be agued that these new methods of service delivery have much wider socio-economic implications and promise for the 21st century than have been accounted for to date. Although the focus here is on the UK experience, it is evident that self-directed support systems or 'cash for care' services are increasingly recognised as a positive way forward across much of the post-industrial world (Ratzka 2007; Ungerson 2002; Ungerson and Yeandle 2007). This promise is encapsulated in the new social relations of support at the heart of such schemes. In short, they are social relations that challenge existing notions of the binary distinction between work and welfare. Consequently, this article identifies the altered features of the social relations of self-directed support systems and raises new questions about the meaning of work and conventional assumptions surrounding disabled users using these schemes as welfare dependents. This is borne out by the nature of state funded, user-directed support systems which are akin to running a small business: one which provides important social and economic advantages for all concerned at the local and national level in all advanced capitalist societies.

Background

As in many 'developed' nations, self-directed support systems in the UK are rooted in disabled people's struggle for equality and justice and have been known under various guises, such as 'self-operated care schemes' and 'self-directed care'. Since the mid 1990s these schemes have been delivered via what is widely referred to as direct payments and more recently individual budgets (Barnes and Mercer 2006). Direct payments are cash payments made by local councils and/or the Independent Living Fund to individuals who have been assessed as requiring 'social care services' (Hasler *et al.* 1999). Individual budgets are currently less widely used but extend this idea to include funding from other sources, such as health authorities and employment agencies (Department of Health 2008). Both systems are complex in their delivery arrangements but, nonetheless, have the potential to open up a whole new dimension to work and employment relations for disabled people.

Hitherto the literature has focused mainly on the social benefits of self-directed support for disabled people and their families. Other studies have identified some economic savings from 'cash for care' type schemes. Where applicable, these studies have tended to focus on comparisons between the cost of traditional services with direct payment schemes and have not taken account of the economic and social implications for informal 'carers', relatives and friends (Ungerson 2002; Ungerson and Yeandle 2007). Key features of the social relations of support pertinent to these schemes are rarely identified or discussed, particularly in relation to the knowledge and variety of qualities and skills necessary to organisze, manage and effectively operate self-support systems that achieve a lifestyle compatible with the philosophy of independent living. All of which raise poignant questions about traditional notions of disability, dependence and work.

Therefore, a more fruitful approach would be for future research and policy initiatives to adopt a more thorough and holistic analysis of the less acknowledged socio-economic costs and benefits of self-directed support systems for service users, their families, personal assistants (PAs) and local/national economies. This is essential if we are to recognise the variety of skills that disabled people must acquire when operating user-led services and employing professional 'carers', 'care attendants' or PAs. The skills acquired by PAs when supporting disabled service users in both the home and in the work environment (where the employment of PAs has provided the opportunity for a disabled person to work in the paid labour market) should also be explored. Furthermore, consideration has to go beyond the service users and their PAs to include the role of informal, unpaid 'carers' who may be relieved of their support roles and thus enabled to secure employment in the paid workplace. It must also address the increased employment opportunities for all concerned and, most notably, account for the potential tax revenues that may accrue from such activities both locally and nationally.

In policy terms, it is remarkable that despite notions of 'independent living' underpinning state funded, self-operated support, the 'independence' of disabled people is not freed from the wider policy discourses of welfare dependency. In this respect, it is noteworthy that direct payments and individual budgets continue to emanate primarily from the UK government's Department of Health rather than the Department for Work and Pensions and/or the Department for Business, Enterprise and Regulatory Reform (BERR). This suggests that the wider policy grasp of self-directed support is rooted in outdated administrative and governmental structures. There is an urgent need, therefore, to reconfigure the extent to which user-led support systems like direct payments and individual budgets may transform our understanding of the dependent/ interdependent continuum in terms of disability policy and practice.

As with feminism, we face particular challenges in disability studies in that main-stream constructions of disablement are largely negative, imposed and non-negotiable in policy and political discourse. Historically, disability has been understood as a medical and individual problem. More recently, these interpretations have given way to social model understandings of disability which focus on society's failure to accom-modate the individual needs of disabled people rather than their impairment as the cause of their disadvantage (Barnes *et al.* 2002). This new approach has generated theoretical perspectives clustered around the notion of independent living, which is both a philosophy and a practical solution to the problem of disability. Indeed, the independent living concept:

> refers to all disabled people having the same choice, control and freedom as any other citizen at home, at work and as members of the community. This does not mean disabled people 'doing everything for themselves', but it does mean that any practical assistance required should be under the control of disabled individuals. (Barnes and Mercer 2006, 33)

Giving disabled people control of their support needs is an integral aspect of independent living. Certainly, the recent announcement by the Health Secretary (Department of Health 2007a) to extend user-led support funding to older people for 'home care' bears testament to the perceived success of these systems. To date, the main beneficiaries of these services have been younger disabled people and they are acknowledged in the literature to have had a positive effect on their lives (Department of Health 2007b; Glasby and Littlechild 2002; Woodin 2006). Prima facie evidence suggests that not only has state funded, self-operated provision changed the social relations of support, it has also benefited the economy as, for instance, direct payment users employ others for their 'care'. In turn, the employment of PAs has the additional benefit of providing a number of disabled people with the opportunity to undertake paid work elsewhere should they choose to do so. Again, economic benefits accrue. Interestingly, though, there has been little explicit acknowledgement of the economic benefits that this work has on the UK balance sheet.

Work and welfare: a helpful dichotomy?

When viewed in their entirety the legislation, implications and implementations of state funded, user-controlled support schemes operate under an essential dichotomy. On the one hand, within the guidelines for implementation there appears to be an implicit recognition that the recipient of such provision must become an 'active' employer, whether or not they are represented by their nominees or advocates. On the other hand, entitlement to funding is firmly tied to eligibility for, and receipt of, social support services. This conjures up a contrasting image of 'passivity' that tends to act against the central aims and objectives of user-directed support, which are to promote independent living. Nevertheless, a growing number of disabled people in the UK are becoming employers of PAs (perhaps as many as five or six people over the course of a week). This adds a new dimension to what is meant by 'work' and employment. Even so, such

a dimension is still not sufficiently recognised in policy documents and 'work' literature. Interestingly, utilising direct payment type schemes to employ PAs is not 'paid
employment' in the conventional sense, yet it critically differs from 'unpaid domestic
labour' or 'voluntary work'.

Some social policy writers have expressed concern that the move toward cash
payments offers an example of welfare states 'distancing themselves from how the care
needs are satisfied' (Daly and Lewis 2000, 294) or may actually reinforce the commodification of welfare services (Williams 2001). Others suggest that the employment
of PAs is creating another pool of low paid, often insecure 'personal care' jobs for a
predominantly female workforce (Ungerson 1999). Whilst these might be reasonable
concerns, and the extent to which direct payment packages afford adequate levels of
support and remuneration ought to be queried, they are, without doubt, key questions
that fail to invalidate the support and scope for greater user control. It would be
far more useful if these critics directed their attention to the policies of those who
determine and control the levels of funding available to individual service users, which,
in turn, determines the wage levels of PAs. Moreover, the UK, in common with
most developed societies, has a long tradition of paid domestic service and the transfer
of paid work from the 'care sector' to the 'domestic employment' arena does not
represent the creation of 'new' employment.

In explicitly acknowledging the true economic costs and benefits of self-operated
support systems use our aim is to challenge the traditional, 'welfarist' assumptions
that characterise disabled people using these schemes as 'benefit claimants'. The other
challenge is to place the analytical framework of user-controlled services into a more
appropriate theoretical, economic and policy context. Indeed, a new language of 'social
entrepreneurs' or 'active citizens' should be applied to those disabled people who
employ PAs.

The challenge to social policy

'Welfarist' assumptions based on 'care' and paternalism have been present from the
outset of the welfare state in the UK. Ever since Beveridge set out his five giants of
'squalor', 'disease', 'ignorance', 'idleness' and 'want', welfare policies have been based
upon perceived needs of the time. All were bolstered by fixed assumptions about marriage, gender roles, ability and full employment. All were firmly set in the context of
established moral and national boundaries (Williams 1989). With the onset of 'stagfla-
tion' (a term developed to describe an economy suffering from stagnation and high
inflation) in the 1970s and the rising spectre of high unemployment in the midst of
increasing globalisation these assumptions and the post-war welfare settlement itself
were deemed inappropriate and ineffective. Monetarist policies combined with calls for
welfare rights to be replaced, or at least balanced, by a renewed sense of individual
'responsibility' or 'obligation' came to the forefront of welfare debates in the UK.
Integral to this shift toward 'responsibility' was the belief that there was a growing body
of 'irresponsible' welfare recipients who did not want to work, lived a life of crime and
significantly contributed to increasing rates of illegitimacy and lone parenthood. This
'underclass', which more recently included disabled people (cf. Field 2008, and his
assertions about Incapacity Benefit), was commonly believed to represent a significant
drain on the public 'purse' and in part was seen to contribute to the destabilisation of
the economy.

Such beliefs still persist. So too does the inextricable link between work in the paid labour market and welfare provision. Indeed, New Labour's self-declared ambition to achieve 'nothing less than a change of culture among benefit claimants' (Department for Social Security 1998, ch. 3.2) gives further credence to this viewpoint. As a consequence, policy aims concentrated on 'supply side' policies, such as job search advice, rehabilitation and financial inducements (Roulstone 2000).

It is logical to assume that social inclusion should be about countering the dynamics and multidimensional aspects of social exclusion. Inclusion in these terms would entail the involvement of hitherto excluded individuals or groups in decision-making and political processes about making access to employment and material resources easier and about opening the doors to cultural integration so that neighbourhoods do not become neglected, marginalised and run down. Current policy trends do not, however, take such a wide view of social inclusion. Of late, work in the paid labour market, or at least actively seeking such work, is seen as the only means by which social inclusion can be fully achieved (Levitas 1998; Prideaux 2001, 2005).

Indeed, our current understanding of social inclusion does not incorporate the activities and problems faced by users of self-directed support systems. To counter this, Barnes and Mercer (2005) provided the starting point for a root and branch reform of the way in which the social and economic value of disabled people is constructed. They called for a critical re-evaluation of orthodox sociological theories of work, unemployment and under-employment relating to the exclusion of disabled people from the workplace. It is argued that previous analyses of work and disability have failed to address in sufficient depth or breadth the various social and environmental barriers that confront disabled people. Consequently, it is argued that a reconfiguration of the meaning of work for disabled people (which draws upon and is commensurate with disabled people's perspectives expressed in the philosophy of independent living) and a social model analysis of their oppression is needed. In short, it is imperative that the realities of work are fundamentally reconfigured in a way that completely acknowledges the wider social and economic contributions of disabled people.

Typologies of work

Arguably, state funded, self-operated personal support represents the first step towards a dynamic reconceptualisation of 'work' and provides a new understanding that appropriately reflects the activities and efforts of disabled people to overcome unwarranted and enforced dependence. Taken in this context, such schemes represent a significant shift away from the 'welfarist' paternalism implicit in the individual/medical model of disability towards the social model of disability and its emphasis upon barrier removal and 'user control'.

To reinforce this fledgling reconceptualisation, a more extensive typology of 'work' in its various forms is given below. It is a typology that presents 'work' as a definitional continuum: one where 'work' is defined as purely contractual at one end of the continuum, while at the other it includes the range of ways in which human effort and endeavour are encapsulated more fully. Such reappraisals have profound implications for our understanding of the valued and valorised lives of previously excluded policy categories emanating from the outmoded definition of working and rewarded citizens.

The ensuing list summarises both the traditional ways of thinking about 'work' (largely as work in the paid labour market) and the challenges over time to that rather restrictive interpretation. Nonetheless, this is not to suggest that a linear shift from the 'traditional' model to the 'post-welfarist' model of work has occurred. Indeed, the interpretation of work in the 'majority world' [a term which more accurately reflects the social context in which most of the world's population live as it moves from geographical notions of space, wealth and power (Stone, 1999)] has for some time been very different to those employed in 'advanced' industrial economies. The term 'post-welfarist' is, in current policy terms, more of an aspiration in many policy areas and not without contestation. In the field of self-directed support services, however, provision falls most squarely into a framework that turns established assumptions about 'work' and 'employment' on their head. Here, then, is an introductory typology with which to begin this reconceptualisation.

(1) *Industrial*. Work is largely seen as paid work. Paid work is a series of economic and social exchanges for gain between two or more people. It is work that is socially and economically valorised as 'real' and is motivated by gain and/or survival.
(2) *Progressive*. Work can be understood as paid and unpaid transactions without which social and economic activity, integration and cohesion would be severely restricted. This would include unpaid support and household maintenance, for which both formal and informal transaction may take place.
(3) *Majority world*. Those economic and social exchanges transacted in cash, kind, barter or promissory understanding (or which is socially unacknowledged, such as foraging and scavenging) that form a diverse matrix of formal and informal activity ranging from begging through to paid contractual work. All function as ways of 'making out'.
(4) *Post-welfarist*. Modes of economic and social activity in 'advanced' industrial society that take account of all forms of paid and unpaid activity, including employees, employers, unpaid support and new social and economic arrangements such as direct payment recipients acting as employers, and which questions assumed ideas around welfare dependency and non-working constituencies. This model recognises that recipients of social goods such as monies for social support may be used as the basis for employment of others and more akin in policy terms to running a small business than to assumed ideas about welfare dependency.

Within this framework state funded, self-operated support schemes fit squarely into the post-welfarist typology. This is significant, as it acknowledges that previous discourses and welfare systems construed disabled people as either able to work (paid contractual work) or eligible for support (with all the connotations of 'passivity' that have been attached to this latter aspect over time). A post-welfarist typology begs many questions of existing dichotomies of work/welfare: it is a typology which challenges previously harmful policy binaries that were, and remain, based on traditional notions of work and social valuations (Roulstone and Barnes 2005). Post-welfarist ideas challenge notions of value being attached purely to contractual exchange values. There is, therefore, a need to widen and fully acknowledge the growing diversity of social and economic exchanges that arise from new social relations of support.

Final word

Direct payment type schemes could and should be placed in a more appropriate theoretical, economic and policy context. Quite simply, it is our contention that they represent the first step towards a reconceptualisation of 'work' that will facilitate a new and more pertinent understanding of the activities and efforts undertaken by disabled people. All of which has particular implications for both disabled and non-disabled people across the world, given growing concerns over the future stability of the global economy as a result of the economic recession which began with the near collapse of the international monetary system in 2008 and the ongoing struggle for a more equitable and just society (Barnes and Mercer 2009).

References

Barnes, C. and Mercer. G. (2005) 'Disability, work and welfare: Challenging the social exclusion of disabled people, *Work, Employment and Society*, 19 (5): 527–45.
—— (2006) *Independent Futures: Creating User Led Disability Services in a Disabling Society*, Bristol: Policy Press.
—— (2009) *Exploring Disability*, Cambridge: Polity Press.
Barnes, C., Oliver, M. and Barton, L. (2002) *Disability Studies Today*, Cambridge: Polity Press.
Daly, J. and Lewis, J. (2000) 'The concept of social care and the analysis of contemporary welfare states', *British Journal of Sociology*, 51 (2): 281–98.
Department of Health (2007a) *Frequently Asked Questions on Direct Payments*, London: Department of Health, www.shaw-trust.org.uk/files/frequently_asked_question_on_direct _payments.pdf/(accessed on 25 June 2010).
Department of Health (2007b) *A Guide to Receiving DPs from Your Local Council: A Route to Independent Living*, London: Department of Health Publications.
Department of Health (2008) *Evaluation of the Individual Pilot Programme: Final Report*, London: Department of Health Publications.
Department for Social Security (1998) *New Ambitions for Our Country: A New Contract for Welfare*, Green Paper, Department for Social Security Cm3805, London: Stationery Office.
Field, F. (2008) *A Failure to Destroy Benefit Serfdom*, Frank Field, www.frankfield.com/(accessed on 16 June 2010).
Glasby, J. and Littlechild, R. (2002) *Social Work and DPs*, Bristol: Policy Press.
Hasler, F., Campbell, J. and Garb, G. (1999) *Direct Routes to Independence*, London: Policy Studies Institute.
Levitas, R. (1998) *The Inclusive Society? Social Exclusion and New Labour*, Basingstoke: Macmillan.
Prideaux, S. (2001) 'New Labour, old functionalism: The underlying contradictions of welfare reform in the US and the UK', *Social Policy & Administration*, 35 (1): 85–115.
—— (2005) *Not So New Labour: A Sociological Critique of New Labour's Policy and Practice*, Bristol, UK: Policy Press.
Ratzka, A. (2007) *Independent Living and Direct Payments: A Swedish Perspective*, Paper presented at the Independent Living 2007 Conference, June 5, Dublin, Ireland.
Roulstone, A. (2000) 'Disability, dependency and the new deal for disabled people', *Disability & Society*, 15 (3): 427–45.
Roulstone, A. and Barnes, C. (eds) (2005) *Working Futures? Disabled People, Policy and Social Inclusion*, Bristol: Policy Press.
Stone, E. (ed.) (1999) *Disability and Development: Learning from Action and Research on Disability in the Majority World*, Leeds: Disability Press.

Ungerson, C. (1999) 'PAs and disabled people: An examination of a hybrid form of work and care', *Work, Employment and Society*, 13: 583–600.

—— (2002) 'Care as a commodity', in B. Bytheway, V. Bacigalupo, J. Bornat, J. Johnson and S Spurr (eds) *Understanding Care, Welfare and Community: A Reader*, London: Routledge, 351–61.

Ungerson, C., and Yeandle, S. (eds) (2007) *Cash for Care in Developed Welfare States*, Basingstoke: Palgrave.

Williams, F. (1989) *Social Policy: A Critical Introduction. Issues of Race, Gender and Class*, Cambridge: Polity Press.

—— (2001) 'In and beyond New Labour: Towards a new political ethics of care', *Critical Social Policy*, 21 (4): 467–93.

Woodin, S. (2006) *Social Relations and Disabled People: The Impact of DPs*, PhD thesis, Leeds: University of Leeds.

Further reading

Apis, S. (1997) 'Self-advocacy for people with learning difficulties: Does it have a future?', *Disability & Society*, 12 (4): 647–54.

Barnes, C. (1993) *Making Our Own Choices: Independent Living and Personal Assistance*, Belper: Ryburn Press.

Bateman, N. (2000) *Advocacy Skills for Health and Social Care Professionals*, 2nd edition, London: Jessica Kingsley.

Brandon, D. and Brandon, T. (2001) *Advocacy in Social Work*, Birmingham: Venture Press.

Campbell, J. and Oliver, M. (1996) *Disability Politics: Understanding Our Past, Changing Our Future*, London: Routledge.

Charlton, J.I. (1998) *Nothing about Us Without Us: Disability Oppression and Empowerment*, Berkley, CA: University of California Press.

Gray, B. and Jackson, R. (eds) (2002) *Advocacy and Learning Disability*, London: Jessica Kingsley.

Jackson, R. (2005) 'Does advocacy have a future?', *Journal of Developmental Disabilities*, 12 (1): 19–30.

Oliver, M. and Barnes, C. (1998) *Social Policy and Disabled People: From Exclusion to Inclusion*, London: Longman.

Tufail, J. and Lyon, K. (2007) *Introducing Advocacy: The First Book of Speaking Up – A Plain Text Guide to Advocacy*, London: Jessica Kingsley.

27 Models for interprofessional collaboration

Audrey Leathard

This chapter picks up a theme which has already been touched on in various chapters, that is interprofessional or multi-agency working. As has been already stated, social workers increasingly work with other professional groups and in settings where they are in a professional minority. This inevitably brings tension, value differences and, sometimes, ethical dilemmas. It also, however, brings the possibility of learning from each other and working to provide the best possible support to, and with, service users. The selected extract is set in the context of England and Wales policy and legislation, but the models which Audrey Leathard introduces are applicable anywhere.

From *Interprofessional Collaboration: From Policy to Practice in Health and Social Care*, London: Brunner-Routledge (2003): 94–113.

The additive and multiplicative effects models

Don Rawson (1994) has creatively argued that two distinct versions of the effects of interprofessional work are possible. Under the *additive effects model*, each profession adds its own particular contribution where interprofessional practice is defined as the sum of the professional perspectives. No one group controls the area in total but contributions from each of the professional groups involved must be taken into account and this is best achieved when professions work together. However under the *multiplicative effect model*, combined, integrated efforts can achieve more than is possible simply by adding contributions. Interprofessional work can thus generate new potential and enhance the input of individuals whereby professionals thus working together can produce a magic between groups. The multiplicative effects model thus underpins collaborative potential in the belief that the whole can become greater than the sum of the parts.

Expressed mathematically, the *additive effects model* reflects a lower score, for example: $2 + 2 + 2 + 2 + 2 = 10$, which achieves less than *multiplicative effects*: $2 \times 2 \times 2 \times 2 \times 2 = 32$. The outcome suggests a nice mathematical justification to support interprofessional collaboration.

Models for professionals working together

Collaborative grading

In one of the first studies on *Interprofessional Collaboration in Primary Health Care Organisations*, Gregson *et al.* (1991, 1992) developed indices for the degree of collaboration between district nurses, general practitioners and health visitors in a stratified random sample of 20 district health authorities in England. Table 27.1 displays the outcome: a taxonomy of collaboration adapted from work by Armitage (1983) on joint working in primary health care.

By the early 1990s, the results showed a relatively low level of joint working between doctors and nurses (24 per cent) and an even lower score for doctors and health visitors working together (8 per cent). At the highest level of collaboration – multidisciplinary working – for both groups, the scores were the same and minimal in both cases (3 per cent). Gregson *et al.* (1992) concluded overall that only 27 per cent of general practitioners and district nurses with patients in common and 11 per cent of general practitioners and health visitors 'collaborated'. While valuable in providing a useful grading approach, one problem is to perceive what actually counts as collaboration across the rating elements. The five terms used in the model can be interpreted differently in a span of potential collaboration. However, by the early twenty-first century, if a similar study were to be conducted in the UK, the 'collaborative' elements, however interpreted, would undoubtedly achieve a higher score but the arena has become more complex as other professional groups have increasingly worked in primary health care teams. Further, from 2002, with the development of care trusts between health and social care services, a sixth level could now usefully be introduced under 'integration'.

Models of interprofessional collaboration

In the light of the White Paper *The New NHS* (Secretary of State for Health 1997), the New Labour government outlined a strategy of joint working underpinned by a partnership approach at the front line. In this context, Hudson (1998) pins down collaboration under four different models of joint working (Table 27.2) that span lower to higher levels of collaborative involvement.

At the lower level of collaboration, *communication* can vary from simply giving

Table 27.1 A taxonomy of collaboration

1 No direct communication	Members who never meet, talk or write to each other
2 Formal, brief communication	Members who encounter or correspond but do not interact meaningfully
3 Regular communication and consultation	Members whose encounters or correspondence include the transference of information
4 High level of joint working	Members who act on that information sympathetically, participate in general patterns of joint working; subscribe to the same general objectives as others on a one-to-one basis in the same organisation
5 Multidisciplinary working	Involvement of all workers in a primary health care setting

Source: Gregson *et al.* (1992).

Table 27.2 Models of interprofessional collaboration

• Communication	Interactions are confined to the exchange of information
• Coordination	Individuals remain in separate organisations and locations but develop formal ways of working across boundaries
• Co-location	Members of different professions are physically located alongside each other
• Commissioning	Professionals with a commissioning remit develop a shared approach to the activity

Source: Hudson (1998: 26–7).

information or, with a little more structure, can lead to formal agreements between primary care practices and social services. *Coordination* can cover various forms of shared assessment and joint provision. *Co-location* has generally referred to social services staff based in a general practice from which evaluated arrangements have usually been favourable. However, *commissioning* can include not only the three previous elements, but also a higher level of collaboration where joint commissioning takes place between primary health care practices and social services departments. However, as Hudson (1998: 26–7) points out, what is also needed is a strategy of planning for joint working where health and social care needs are held together. Meanwhile, partnership prospects can be challenged by professional and cultural barriers, different perceptions of costs and benefits, as well as different patterns of employment, accountability and decision-making.

A model for interprofessional consultation

From a background of psychiatry and psychotherapy, Steinberg (1989) sets out to consider the ways and means of how professionals and patients can work together based on the viewpoint that interprofessional consultation is one form of collaborative work. While good consultation is likely to be educational, consultation uniquely provides a joint method of enquiry into the 'fundamental nature of problems and ways of responding to them' (Steinberg 1989: 14). Consultation can therefore provide new approaches to understanding problems and innovative management strategies. Consultation can equally demonstrate where an institution or organisation is failing and where training, staffing or supervision are inadequate. The categories in Table 27.3 reflect the wide arena in which consultative work can operate.

From the model presented, Steinberg (1989: 23) argues that consultation, through the various mechanisms suggested, may be the most appropriate way to bring people together with different skills and experience. Although perceived essentially as a teaching and learning experience based on shared appraisal, the model also points a way forward, more widely, for professionals to work together effectively in practice.

Models for interprofessional practice

In a consideration of how groups of professionals can work together, Don Rawson (1994) has devised a mapping of sets in Figure 27.1.

The model of sets can be applied to various fields of interprofessional practice to elucidate what aspects of the sets are working well and where problems need to

Table 27.3 Categories of consultative work

1 The circumstances under which undertaken	• Single *ad-hoc* consultation: both urgent and non-urgent • Planned consultations: either a series or indefinite
2 The overall aim	• Primarily problem-solving, with training as a secondary benefit • Primarily training, with problem-solving as an additional benefit
3 The focus of the work	• Client-centred; consultee-centred; work-centred
4 The people involved	• Individual • Group: open or closed
5 Continuing reappraisal at a more informal level: circularity in consultation	• What are the facts of the situation? • Who is involved? • What are the feelings? • How does the situation look now?

Source: Modified from Steinberg (1989: 23, 65).

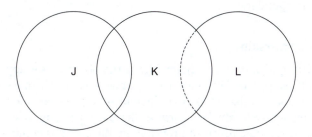

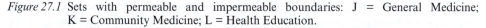

Figure 27.1 Sets with permeable and impermeable boundaries: J = General Medicine; K = Community Medicine; L = Health Education.

Source: Rawson (1994: 43). Reproduced by kind permission of Brunner-Routledge.

be addressed. As Rawson (1994: 43) points out, the intersection of different types of professional work is likely to blur tasks and responsibilities that can lead some professionals involved to try to recreate their own specialisms and work relationships. A further challenge to joint working is the likelihood that different groups in the health and welfare professions may well be at different levels of development in working practices. Levels of expertise, job descriptions and standard operating procedures can well influence who gives way and on what issues.

Nevertheless, as constant changes occur in the structure of the services for health and social care, Figure 27.1 demonstrates the possibility that some boundaries may dissolve (denoted by a dotted line) whereupon professional responsibilities may be transferred, shared or absorbed by one group. As applied hypothetically to Figure 27.1, health education work may become eclipsed by community medicine, which then has the potential to take over or assimilate the field. As boundaries become impermeable, so professionals have to reach an agreement over work sharing and involvement that is mutually acceptable or agree to differ. As Rawson (1994: 44) points out, to survive intact professions, which are overshadowed by more powerful rivals, have to make their professional concerns functionally dissimilar. One alternative model for the professions is to uphold a new common purpose to realign, assimilate or meld the older occupational groupings into an interprofessional engagement and outlook. A more ambitious model is to dissolve boundaries through seamless care which, in theory, is the intention behind the integration of health and social care provision for care trusts in the future.

Agencies, sectors and organisations working together

One crucial factor in the provision of health and social care has been the need to bring various professional groups to work together across agencies and sectors. A selection of models now looks at this angle then considers wider possibilities for organisational joint working. The first model (Figure 27.2) shows an approach with regard to service provision for child health and social services for children in need.

Here is a model that accommodates specific professional input for certain aspects of the health and social services but is a clear arena for joint working. A neat division of responsibilities can be seen but, as the Audit Commission (1994a: 3) has pointed out, the overlap of responsibilities between social services and health authorities requires major adjustments to the way agencies work and relate to each other. However, change can soon shift the boundaries.

Public/private partnerships

A further analytical advantage of Figure 27.3 is the potential for application. As the public and private sector have been increasingly drawn together within specific contexts, one can reset the model (Table 27.4) for a different sphere of evaluation.

The interest for analysis can be to assess the customer and cost effectiveness of ventures across the separate forms of provision in Table 27.4 is comparison with joint working and partnership outcomes as well as the potential for drawing up the advantages and disadvantages of each section. However, the problem in the application of the model in Table 27.4 is the sheer complexity of the issues whether in the public or private sector or with regard to working in partnership.

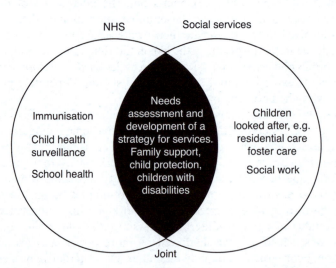

Figure 27.2 Services provided by the NHS and Social Services. Many activities fall within the remit of both NHS and Social Services.

Source: Audit Commission (1994a: 3), Exhibit 2. Reproduced by kind permission of the Audit Commission.

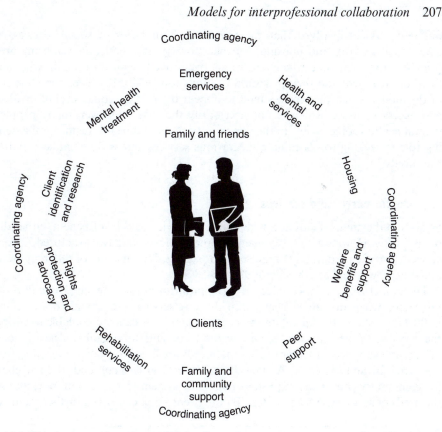

Figure 27.3 The elements of an appropriate service.

Source: Audit Commission (1994b: 17). Adapted from J. Carson and T. Sharma (1994) 'In-patient psychiatric care. What helps? Staff and patient perspectives', *Journal of Mental Health*, 3: 99–104. Reproduced by kind permission of the *Journal of Mental Health* (http://www.tandf.co.uk).

Table 27.4 Public/private partnerships in health and social care

Public sector Specific separate provision	Partnership/joint working	Private sector Specific separate provision
NHS health care provision Local authority community care provision	Private finance initiatives (PFI)[a] Public sector payments for private health care provision Public/private partnerships	Hospitals Dental care Osteopathy Physiotherapy Care homes

Note:
a PFI: A private sector consortium pays for a new hospital. The local NHS trust pays the consortium a regular fee for hospital use, which covers construction costs, the rent of the building, the cost of support services and the risks transferred to the private sector.

The next model concerns a review of mental health services for adults in which the Audit Commission (1994b) has acknowledged that a range of service provision is necessary to meet individual needs.

The interest in this field of work is, as Figure 27.3 displays, the wide range of different services involved that cut across the boundaries of social services, health care, social security and housing. Further, poverty and inadequate housing are high priorities for users but which are often overlooked by professionals who tend to focus on treatment and therapy (Audit Commission 1994b: 17). Therefore, one critique of the model is that the services tend to appear to be of an equal level of involvement and access to users, which is not necessarily the case. However, many people with mental health problems live in the community so mental health teams have a demanding role in seeking to coordinate the various services across different sectors to meet user needs.

A model for carers and services

Seen from the angle of carers, a wide range of services can be of benefit, either directly or indirectly. However, the way agencies and professions have structured themselves, services are often separately organised and packaged in an array of different arenas, as illustrated by Powell and Kocher (1996: 15).

The model (Figure 27.4) reflects a basic problem in that the support and provision for carers' needs do not fit neatly into the way services are organised and delivered. Unlike the field of mental health, no central team is necessarily available to coordinate the services. While the carer usually wants to be able to assemble a flexible package of care and support, a further issue is that needs are likely to change over time, both for the cared for and the carer. As Powell and Kocher (1996) contend, the key challenge for community care is the requisite to alter the system to become more responsive to the needs of service users and carers. By the twenty-first century, a further factor would

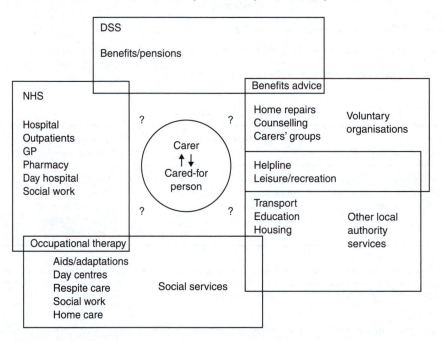

Figure 27.4 Carers and services.

Source: Powell and Kocher (1996: 15). Reproduced by kind permission of the King's Fund (www.kingsfund.org.uk).

be for interprofessional and interagency collaboration to play a lead part in this complex arena.

The jigsaw model

A rather different approach is to consider the purpose and outcome of working together. Drawing on the field of the mental health services, the Audit Commission (1994b: 55) has argued that the requirements for a comprehensive service must all be drawn together at a strategic level. In other words, strategic planning should determine the level and balance of resources, the priorities for the resources available and, importantly, the means of coordination and collaboration between them. Figure 27.5 shows how, starting with guidelines and information on needs, the steps towards strategy can interlock across the services, the authorities and user consultation, towards a strategic goal.

In the field of mental health, the potential sources of information on needs cover a range of arenas from directors of public health, contract managers, general practitioners, mental health teams, local authority social services and housing, voluntary organisations, users and carers, as well as the criminal justice system. By the mid-1990s, the Audit Commission (1994b: 54) still found that individuals and groups often worked in isolation nor was information shared, thus effort was often duplicated. The 2002 development of care trusts, based on integrated provision, should be in a better position to address a collaborative strategy.

Models for users

How far users have gained from interprofessional collaboration remains somewhat unclear but the first of two models show the potential. In Figure 27.6, Hornby and Atkins (2000) present a resource pool that represents the sum total of help to a particular individual or family living in a locality. From a user-centred and community-oriented perspective, rather than profession-central and agency-oriented viewpoint, the resource pool takes on a different look.

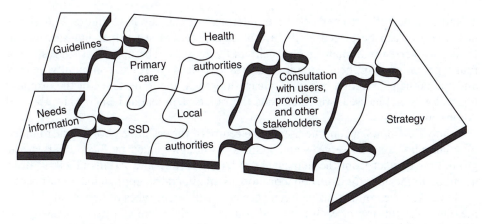

Figure 27.5 The jigsaw model: developing a strategy for mental health. (SSD = Social Services
          Department.)

Source: Audit Commission (1994b: 55), Exhibit 26. Reproduced by kind permission of the Audit
Commission.

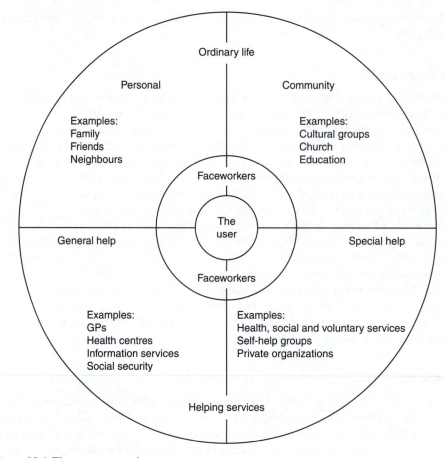

Figure 27.6 The resource pool.

Source: Hornby and Atkins (2000: 84) Reproduced by kind permission of Blackwell Science.

Rather differently from most other interprofessional models, Figure 27.6 shows how the user can be placed at the centre as a potential self-helper but surrounded by faceworkers: the human face of help and provision. The approach suggests that four types of help can then be applied according to need: personal, community, general and special help. Within a community care approach, the importance of the ordinary life sector is emphasised, which extends the range of potential helpers (Hornby and Atkins 2000: 83–4).

Figure 27.7 shows, again, the user at the centre of the resource pool but surrounded by a complex arena of services and settings. Although guided by faceworkers at the ground (as distinct from the management) level, Hornby and Atkins (2000: 9) draw attention to the need for close collaboration, as an integrative approach does not necessarily weaken the boundaries between agencies or different types of helper. In order to maximise the full use of each potential source of help, there is a need to clarify the differences of input and the areas of overlap.

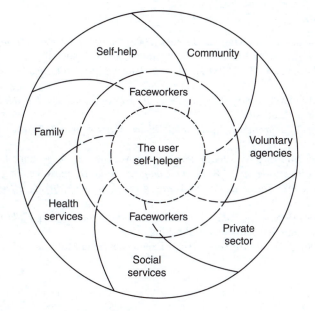

Figure 27.7 The user-centred model of help.

Source: Hornby and Atkins (2000: 9). Reproduced by kind permission of Blackwell Science.

References

Armitage, P. (1983) 'Joint working in primary health care' (Occasional Paper), *Nursing Times*, 79: 75–8.

Audit Commission (1994a) *Seen but Not Heard: Co-ordinating Community Child Health and Social Services for Children in Need*, London: HMSO.

Audit Commission (1994b) *Finding a Place: A Review of Mental Health Services for Adults*, London: HMSO.

Gregson, B., Cartlidge, A. and Bond, J. (1991) *Interprofessional Collaboration in Primary Health Care Organizations* (Occasional Paper 52), London: Royal College of General Practitioners.

—— (1992) 'Development of a measure of professional collaboration in primary health care', *Journal of Epidemiology and Community Health*, 46: 48–53.

Hornby, S. and Atkins, J. (2000) *Collaborative Care: Interprofessional, Interagency and Inter-personal*, 2nd edition, Oxford: Blackwell Science.

Hudson, B. (1998) 'Prospects of partnership', *Health Service Journal*, 108 (5600): 26–7.

Powell, M. and Kocher, P. (1996) *Strategies for Change: A Carers Impact Resource Book*, London: King's Fund Publishing.

Rawson, D. (1994) 'Models of inter-professional work: Likely theories and possibilities', in A. Leathard (ed.) *Going Inter-professional: Working Together for Health and Welfare*, London: Routledge.

Secretary of State for Health (1997) *The New NHS: Modern, Dependable*, CM. 3807, London: The Stationery Office.

Steinberg, D. (1989) *Interprofessional Consultation: Invitation and Imagination in Working Relationships*, Oxford: Blackwell Scientific Publications.

Further reading

Barrett, G., Sellman, D. and Thomas, J. (eds) (2005) *Interprofessional Working in Health and Social Care: Professional Perspectives*, Basingstoke: Palgrave Macmillan.

Glasby, J. and Dickinson, H. (2008) *Partnership Working in Health and Social Care*, Bristol: Policy Press.

Leathard, A. (ed.) (1994) *Going Inter-professional: Working Together for Health and Welfare*, London: Brunner-Routledge.

Loxley, A. (1997) *Collaboration in Health and Welfare: Working with Difference*, London: Jessica Kingsley.

Lymbery, M. and Millward, A. (2009) 'Partnership working', in R. Adams, L. Dominelli and M. Payne (eds) *Practising Social Work in a Complex World*, Basingstoke: Palgrave Macmillan.

Morris. K. (ed.) (2008) *Social Work and Multi-agency Working: Making a Difference*, Bristol: Policy Press.

Murphy, M. (2004) *Developing Collaborative Relationships in Interagency Child Protection Work*, 2nd edition, London: Russell House Publishing.

Quinney, A. (2006) *Collaborative Social Work*, Exeter: Learning Matters.

28 Theorising feminist social work practice

Lena Dominelli

This chapter marks the beginnings of a shift in orientation, from practice perspectives which focus on individuals (albeit in the context of their families and communities) to approaches which locate problems and issues not in the individual, but in society; the popular slogan, 'the personal is political', sums this up well. Feminism has had a major impact over the last 30 years or so, on public policy, on academic scholarship, on social work theory and practice, and on our personal lives and intimate relationships. Sometimes it has done so in an overt, unapologetically political way, for example, by drawing attention to men's violence against women. At other times, it has almost imperceptibly changed the way we think about ourselves and society, leading to a much more finely tuned appreciation of power, resistance and change. Feminist ideas have been particularly influential in social work, because social work has always been a profession which is largely performed by women, with women (see Walton 1975; Perry and Cree 2003). The selected extract is by Lena Dominelli, a Canadian social work academic (based in the UK) who has written extensively on feminism, anti-oppressive practice and community work. Here she provides an overview of feminism's contribution to theory and practice in social work.

From *Feminist Social Work Theory and Practice*, Basingstoke: Palgrave (2002): 17–40.

Introduction

Women have been at the centre of the struggle to define the appropriate role for social work in rapidly changing societies. Although crucial policies and legislation are formulated by men, women undertake the bulk of the caring tasks carried out within the home, and dominate the basic grades of paid professionals doing such work. Thus, arguments about the purpose of social work are intricately wound up with disputes over women's position in the social order.

Feminist social work has shed important insights on this issue because it takes women's well-being as the starting point, though not necessarily the end of its analyses and has made creating egalitarian social relations an integral part of practice. Feminist debates have provided conceptual frameworks with a fluidity and capacity to respond to criticisms and theorise the changing nature of women's lives. Key in feminists' rethinking of social work has been the questioning of positivist epistemological and ontological paradigms (Harding, 1990). These have included:

1   challenging men's experiences as the yardstick for measuring women's;
2   unpacking universalist standards and exposing their failure to describe, understand or value women's diverse lifestyles and contributions to society;
3   critiquing dualist thinking and the concepts that formulate knowledge as binary categories operating in opposition to each other;
4   recognising identity politics as a central dynamic in how social relations are organised and reproduced;
5   respecting women's multiple and fluid identities;
6   acknowledging the significance of gendered power relations in shaping the opportunities available for men and women to build their lives in accordance with their views of their needs; and
7   recognising the capacity of women to take action on their own behalf and to demonstrate solidarity across a range of social divisions.

These points become themes I explore throughout this book for these have given rise to what I consider crucial features that differentiate feminist social work from other forms of social work. Although I examine these in greater detail in subsequent chapters, I would summarise them here as the following:

1   assessing and working with the impact of patriarchal gender relations on men, women and children;
2   examining the impact of public and private patriarchy on women, men and children;
3   reconceptualising dependency;
4   avoiding false equality traps when building egalitarian relationships;
5   celebrating differences;
6   celebrating women's strengths and abilities;
7   valuing caring work and reforming the conditions under which it is carried out;
8   deconstructing community;
9   unpacking motherhood;
10   challenging monolithic descriptions of 'the family' and expanding the definition;
11   considering the social construction of gender;
12   separating the needs of women, children and men;
13   working as an insider/outsider;
14   mediating the power of the state; and
15   understanding agency and the capacity of the powerless to resist oppression.

Creating new understandings of women's lives

Feminist social work theory and practice is a fairly new theoretical construct, appearing formally on the academic social work scene in a significant way during the late 1970s and early 1980s. It originally sought to highlight the differing nature of women's experience in social work – the invisibility of it on the theoretical front where the 'universal' male personae held sway (Wilson, 1977); and identify the inadequacy of a practice that operated within the confines of a view of women as predominantly carers of others – their husbands, children and dependent older relatives (Dominelli and McLeod, 1989). Traditional social work practice has reflected the dominant social order which assumes women's dependency within the family (Segal, 1983) and fails to recognise women's struggles to be themselves through their daily work regardless of setting. Defining women as dependent has devalued their ability to act as agents who shape their lives in different directions by interacting with others (Dominelli, 1986).

Feminist practitioners and scholars have drawn on feminist theories and practice to place gender on the social work map by drawing upon and validating women's experiences as women. Early feminist analyses identified the gendered nature of social work profession where frontline work was undertaken predominantly by women working with other women (Wilson, 1977). The theorisation of social work as 'women's work' with a segregated division of labour characterised by women working with 'clients' and men in management making decisions about policies that impact on practice and allocate resources, came later (Hallet, 1991). Moves towards professionalisation and the centrally controlled reorganisation of social work within the British welfare state shifted it from being primarily a voluntary activity run on a shoestring to a large bureaucratic empire that has attracted men to its ranks, particularly at the top echelons (Walton, 1975).

Central to women's redefinition as a group different from men has been a re-examination of the division between public and private life (Gamarnikov *et al.*, 1983). Feminists have exposed women's exclusion from the former and demonstrated the close connection between the two. Caring work whether paid or not, has bridged the divide between them. White middle-class feminists have revealed how married women's (private) domestic labour enables their husbands to devote themselves to their careers (Gavron, 1966) and rise within the (public) hierarchical structures of the workplace. The price women have paid for undertaking this invisible private work has been incalculable (see Friedan, 1963).

In the West, the costs have been reflected in higher levels of depression (Rowe, 1988), lack of fulfilment, stymied aspirations (Brown and Harris, 1978), and rising levels of physical (Mama, 1989; Newburn and Stanko, 1995) and sexual (Wilson, 1993) violence sustained by women. In low income countries, women have paid with their lives when running away to escape confined existences within particular arrangements in the private domain (Kassinjda, 1998), committing suicide (Croll, 1978), or being killed by upholders of patriarchal norms (Basu, 1997). At the same time, substantial numbers of women have enjoyed their nurturing roles and gained satisfaction from successfully meeting these demands. They have been proud of their children's achievements and delighted to see their husbands' progress in a competitive world. For although visible as reflected glory, the accomplishments of the people that women have supported represent thousands of hours of hard work, love and devotion that have been energetically and willingly poured into sustaining the activities of loved ones.

In social work, feminist understandings of the public–private divide have been central to redefining social problems so as to: encourage women to see private troubles as public issues; involve women in collective action that improves their position; assist women in overcoming isolation and 'learned helplessness'; and create alternative forms of practice that respond to women's needs (Dominelli and McLeod, 1989). To achieve these goals, feminists have argued for the: integration of theory and practice; promotion of egalitarian social relations amongst women; valuing of women's responsibilities in the home and recognising their impact on women's capacity to engage in waged labour; awareness of gendered power relations in disadvantaging women; and acknowledgment of women's capacity to take action themselves (Wendall, 1996). Social workers' relationships with 'clients', colleagues in the workplace and employers have come under scrutiny and been accompanied by demands for changes (Benn and Sedgley, 1984). These seek to meet women's needs for respect; value their contributions to other people's lives; provide services women need; and promote their careers in paid employment. By openly discussing the links between public and private behaviours, feminists have highlighted the interdependent nature of the public and private domains. Their demands for change have impacted upon every aspect of women's lives and undermined a neat division between domestic and (waged) working lives.

Reconceptualising feminist social work theory and practice

Social work occupies an interesting position within the nation-state as the collective expression of its desire to care for others in difficult circumstances, and as a professional activity whose practitioners work in the interstices between the national and local levels, and between the personal and political planes. Social workers as public officials who represent the public's wish to intervene in the private lives of fellow citizens, if necessary without their consent in cases of mental illness or child protection, engage with the contradictions encapsulated by this divide. Consequently, the division between the public and private sphere is crossed at a number of different points in practice.

Feminist insights about the nature of the public–private divide can contribute to reconceptualising it. Identity formation and the politics of everyday life (Smith, 1987) are other analytical concepts relevant in enriching and subsequently transforming social workers' understandings. In social workers' encounters with women, the division of women's lives into public and private domains is important. Here, the private sphere is articulated and regulated through public social policies that control access to welfare resources by defining eligibility, and impact on women's relationships with each other and the state. The public realm also affects women's private family life for it is also the object of social policies enacted by the state (Showstack Sassoon, 1987).

Many ugly secrets about the horrific abuse of women and children within the privacy of family settings become routinised knowledges within the social work domain. Ironically, this knowledge becomes privately appropriated by remaining 'confidential' information between practitioners and 'clients', rarely being shared beyond the realm of supervisory relationships and case files. However, by drawing on detailed knowledge of their lives and experiential telling, women have recounted their suffering to astonished audiences, and people have begun to listen. Feminist social workers and researchers have documented their stories. These accounts have converted women's private troubles to public issues through feminist social action that has gained the support of a wide range of women including social workers (Dominelli and McLeod, 1989). Feminists have pressed for government action in subverting the public–private divide by passing laws against domestic violence and child abuse in the home (Dworkin, 1981; MacKinnon, 1993); proposing laws against rape in marriage (Jaggar, 1983); building women's shelters (Dobash and Dobash, 1992); and providing resources to help men desist from abusive behaviours (Cavanagh and Cree, 1996). These efforts have also unpacked the historically specific nature of the citizenship the nation-state provides women (Lister, 1997). Linked to women's identity as subordinate beings, it is a marginalised status that feminists reject.

Though extremely contentious, the concepts of language, discourse, difference, positionality, and deconstruction are central to a social work practice that aims to rectify matters that impede the realisation of individual well-being and social justice. By helping individuals in their social situation, such practice addresses the essentials of an individual's psychological growth within a social context. Deconstructing the category 'woman' enables social workers to focus on women's complex and fluid identities within and across a range of social divisions and variations across time and space. The process of deconstruction involves interrogating taken-forgranted assumptions about women and facilitates identifying their strengths and weaknesses in many dimensions of their lives.

Valuing women's capacities across the entire spectrum of abilities encourages a reconceptualisation of difference. By emphasising difference as a strength within an egalitarian framework, feminist social workers celebrate rather than disparage women's diverse and multiple identities or use these to pathologise the caring work women do simply because these differ from white middle-class male norms for (paid) work. Rather than proceeding to validate preconceived misconceptions and stereotypes, a strengths-based perspective fosters a critical stance that allows practitioners to make judgments based on a careful and thorough assessment of the specific realities of a given situation.

Other feminist concepts relevant to social work practice are: interconnectedness, reciprocity, mutuality, ambiguity, power and citizenship. These can be found in every aspect of women's lives, but are particularly evident in caring work. Interconnectedness signals the interdependence that exists between people – the ties that bind them together in mutuality and reciprocity. The notion of interconnectedness is useful in facilitating growth within egalitarian relationships and can be realised in social work relationships with 'clients', employers, employees, family, friends or strangers. Mutuality and reciprocity are the building blocks of egalitarian relationships for they permit each person involved in an exchange to contribute from her/his specific strengths to the interaction. Acting together, interdependency, mutuality and reciprocity give birth to social solidarity.

Women's relationship to change is not straightforward. Ambiguity underpins many struggles that aim to become more sensitive to the needs of others, particularly when women are uncertain about what to do, but desire to move away from previous patterns of interaction because their inadequacies have become so apparent. Social workers' attempts to address issues of oppression are replete with instances of ambiguity. Ambiguity is illustrated in women's roles as carers when women feel the double bind of being responsible for others and wanting to help, but also wishing to be free of the responsibility and focus on themselves. Feminist principles of solidarity assist in negotiating through the uncertainties of ambiguity to create an inclusive citizenship that celebrates difference. Citizenship in this framework is about obligations within reciprocal relationships. In it, ambiguity is not obviated, but provides the basis for reciprocity.

Citizenship draws upon interconnectedness, mutuality and reciprocity to build social solidarities through which individuals accept responsibility for each other and commit themselves to a jointly defined common good to ensure that the well-being of one is a concern of all. Both give and take are involved in reciprocated social interactions. Taking action consistent with the empowerment of self in creating egalitarian relationships with others is the basis of a non-exclusionary citizenship not limited to implementation within specific national borders (Dominelli, 1997; Lister, 1997). Feminist social workers aim to promote the capacities of women workers and 'clients' to become full citizens capable of taking control of their lives within empowering social contexts.

Empowerment relies on reconceptualising power as a 'transformative capacity' that is negotiated through social relations with others (Giddens, 1990). It sets the contours of a person's position in a specific social order (French, 1985). Understanding power relations – their creation and re-creation within social relationships, is essential to feminist theorising of oppression and developing alternative ways of organising daily life, and is crucial in identifying an individual's own 'standpoint' as socially constructed (Hartsock, 1987). Analysing the distribution of power and its impact on social relations assists in formulating plans of action that eliminate the privileging of one group over others.

Process issues are central to focusing on how to conduct empowering relationships (Humphries, 1996). Feminists' concern with process has been reflected in social work practice in the relationship between the worker and the 'client', between employees and their employers, and amongst employees. Feminist social workers engage in processual matters when establishing egalitarian relations between workers and 'clients', whether this is in a therapeutic relationship undertaken by a counsellor (Chaplin, 1988), a group involving a community worker (Jaggar, 1983), or a budgetary exercise executed by a case manager (Orme, 2000). Feminist social workers have questioned simplistic divisions between 'clients' and workers in contrasting professional expertise to experiential wisdoms, to also validate the latter. Recognising and valuing what has conventionally been depicted as lesser knowledges – those held by the person being helped, fosters egalitarian relations between professionals and service users (Belenky *et al.*, 1997). This has led feminists to re-examine the relationship between women and the state and expose its centrality in mediating and reproducing patriarchal relations between women and men and paternalistic relationships between workers and 'clients' (Showstack Sassoon, 1987).

Following through on these analyses, feminist social workers have begun building new parameters for a profession that has oppressed 'clients'. They have redefined the profession's loyalties more towards the people that they are committed to serve – the women whose chances in life have been shaped by unequal opportunities and the carrying of inordinate amounts of domestic responsibilities. As woman-centered practitioners seeking to establish equality, feminist social workers have sought to empower women rather than oppress them by listening to their stories, validating their analyses of situations and engaging them in decisions about their lives (Hanmer and Statham, 1988; Dominelli and McLeod, 1989). They have supported women through traumatic moments and rejoiced in their triumphs over adversity. In feminist social work, women are the starting point of any analysis. However, supporting women in gaining control of their lives involves challenging patriarchal arrangements and evaluating state interventions and men's activities in light of their impact on the oppression of women.

References

Basu, M. (1997) *The Challenge of Local Feminisms: Women's Movements in Global Perspective*, Boulder, CO: Westview Press.

Belenky, M.F., Clinchy, M.B., Goldberger, M.R. and Tarule, M.J. (1997) *Women's Ways of Knowing: The Development of Self, Voice and Mind*, New York: Basic Books.

Benn, M. and Sedgley, A. (1984) *Sexual Harassment*, London: Tavistock.

Brown, G. and Harris, T. (1978) *The Social Origins of Depression*, London: Tavistock.

Cavanagh, K. and Cree, V.E. (eds) (1996) *Working with Men: Feminism and Social Work*, London: Routledge.

Chaplin, J. (1988) *Feminist Counselling in Action*, London: Sage.

Croll, E. (1978) *Feminism and Socialism in China*, London: Routledge & Kegan Paul.

Dobash, R.E. and Dobash, R.P. (1992) *Women, Violence and Social Change*, London: Routledge.

Dominelli, L. (1986) *Love and Wages: The Impact of Imperialism, State Intervention and Women's Domestic Labour on Workers' Control in Algeria, 1962–1972*, Norwich: Novata Press.

—— (1997) 'Feminist theory', in M. Davies (ed.) *The Blackwell Companion to Social Work*, Oxford: Blackwell.

Dominelli, L. and McLeod, E. (1989) *Feminist Social Work*, Basingstoke: Macmillan.

Dworkin, A. (1981) *Pornography: Men Possessing Women*, New York: Perigree.

French, B. (1985) *The Power of Women*, Harmondsworth: Penguin.

Friedan, B. (1963) *The Feminine Mystique*, New York: Bell.

Gamarnikov, E., Morgan, D., Purvis, J. and Taylorson D. (eds) (1983) *The Public and the Private*, London: Heinemann.

Gavron, H. (1966) *The Captive Housewife*, London: Routledge & Kegan Paul.

Giddens, A. (1990) *The Consequences of Modernity*, Cambridge: Polity Press.

Hallett, C. (1991) *Women and Social Services*, London: Sage.

Hanmer, J. and Statham, D. (1988) *Women and Social Work: Towards a Woman Centred Practice*, London: Macmillan.

Harding, S. (1990) 'Feminism, science and the anti-Enlightenment critiques', in L. Nicolson (ed.) *Feminism/Postmodernism*, London: Routledge, 83–106.

Hartsock, N. (1987) 'The feminist standpoint: Developing the ground for a specifically feminist historical materialism', in S. Harding (ed.) *Feminism and Methodology*, Bloomington, IN: Indiana University Press, 157–80.

Humphries, B. (ed.) (1996) *Critical Perspectives on Empowerment*, Birmingham: Venture Press.

Jaggar, A. (1983) *Feminist Politics and Human Nature*, Totowa, NJ: Rowman & Allanheld.

Kassindja, K. (1998) *Do They Hear You When You Cry?*, New York: Delta Books.

Lister, R. (1997) *Citizenship: Feminist Perspectives*: London: Macmillan.

MacKinnon, C. (1993) *Only Words*, Cambridge: Harvard University Press.

Mama, A. (1989) *Hidden Struggle: Statutory and Voluntary Responses to Violence against Black Women in the Home*, London: Race and Housing Unit.

Newburn, T. and Stanko, E.A. (eds) (1995) *Just Boys Doing Business: Men, Masculinities and Crime*, London: Routledge.

Orme, J. (2000) *Gender and Community Care, Social Work and Social Care Perspectives*, Basingstoke: Palgrave.

Perry, R. and Cree, V.E. (2003) 'The changing gender profile of applicants to qualifying social work training in the UK', *Social Work Education*, 22 (4): 375–84.

Rowe, D. (1988) *Depression: The Way Out of Your Prison*, London: Routledge.

Segal, L. (1983) *What's To Be Done about the Family?*, Harmondsworth: Penguin.

Showstack Sassoon, A. (ed.) (1987) *Women and the State: The Shifting Boundaries of the Private and Public*, London: Hutchinson.

Smith, D.E. (1987) *The Everyday World as Problematic: A Feminist Sociology*, Toronto: University of Toronto Press.

Walton, R.G. (1975) *Women in Social Work*, London: Routledge & Kegan Paul.

Wendall, S. (1999) 'The loss of control', Community Care, 21–7 January: 22–3.

Wilson, E. (1977) *Women and the Welfare State*, London: Tavistock.

Wilson, M. (1993) *Crossing the Boundary: Black Women Survive Incest*, London: Virago.

Further reading

Brook, E. and Davis, A. (eds) (1985) *Women: The Family and Social Work*, London: Tavistock.

Cree, V.E. (1997) 'Surviving on the inside: Reflections on being a woman and a feminist in a male academic institution', *Social Work Education*, 16 (3): 37–60.

David, M.E. (2003) *Personal and Political: Feminisms, Sociology and Family Lives*, Stoke-on-Trent: Trentham Books.

Dominelli, L. (2008) 'Feminist theory', in M. Davies (ed.) *The Blackwell Companion to Social Work*, 3rd edition, Oxford: Blackwell.

Lloyd, M. (2005) *Beyond Identity Politics: Feminism, Power and Politics*, London: Sage.

McRobbie, A. (2009) *The Aftermath of Feminism: Gender, Culture and Social Change*, London: Sage.

Orme, J. (2002) 'Feminist social work', in R. Adams, L. Dominelli and M. Payne (eds) *Social Work: Themes, Issues and Critical Debates*, 2nd edition, Basingstoke: Palgrave.

—— (2002) 'Social work: Gender, care and justice', *British Journal of Social Work*, 32 (6): 799–814.

—— (2003) 'It's feminist because I say so!: Feminism, social work and critical practice in the UK', *Qualitative Social Work*, 2 (2): 131–54.

Phillips, R. (2006) 'Undoing an activist response: Feminism and the Australian government's domestic violence policy', *Critical Social Policy*, 26 (1): 192–219.

Ramazanoglu, C. (1989) *Feminism and the Contradictions of Oppression*, London: Routledge.

Stanley, L. and Wise, S. (1993) *Breaking Out Again: Feminist Ontology and Epistemology*, London: Routledge.

White, V. (2006) *The State of Feminist Social Work*, London: Routledge.

Wise, S. (1990) 'Becoming a feminist social worker', in L. Stanley and S. Wise (eds) *Feminist Praxis*, London: Routledge.

29 Contributions to a radical practice in social work

Roy Bailey and Mike Brake

Radical approaches, like feminist approaches, are concerned with changing society, not fitting individuals into society, or, as Bailey and Brake write in their classic text, 'our task is not to understand the world but to change it' (1980: 13). When I was a social worker, this meant bringing together the single parents with whom I was working to form a group, and, later, working with them to create a community-based resource for women and children. The women got far more from each other, individually and collectively, than I could ever have given them as 'my clients'. A great deal has been written from a radical perspective (sometimes called 'critical' or 'structural'), as illustrated from the many recommendations for further reading. I have chosen one of the seminal texts which, when it first appeared in 1975, was in the vanguard of a new way of thinking about, and practising, social work.

From *Radical Social Work and Practice,* London: Edward Arnold (1980): 7–24.

The question is often asked, somewhat sceptically, 'What is radical social work?' More often than not the questioner is not really expecting an answer. The question is posed as a sure way of changing the subject. Clearly, it is difficult and it certainly does not lend itself to an easy answer. However, before we get too worried that maybe there is no such thing as radical social work and that maybe we are all chasing shadows, we should remember that just about the same nervousness and anxiety is created by the question, 'What is social work?' Most of the people we know who are either engaged in the process of teaching social work students, or employed as professional social workers, steer clear of the question. The hesitation is often with good reason: after all, anyone who confronts it and attempts an answer leaves themselves open to attack and criticism.

In the brief introduction to our first volume (Bailey and Brake 1975) we made it clear there were no easy answers. This remains our position. However, it is no longer possible to dismiss critical questions from students about the general purposes of social work or about a particular practice. Social workers, *like other workers*, are trapped in a social structure which severely delimits their power and hence their ability to initiate significant change. Social workers, *unlike other workers*, confront daily, as their job, the victims of an economic and political structure that creates poverty and humiliation. Social workers and clients alike are bemused by forces beyond their control but to which we are all subject. The very weight of the institutional arrangements that bind us results in our hesitancy to make any grand-sounding claims for radical social work as a framework for practice that might resolve anything. Nevertheless, this is the task that radical social workers set themselves.

The issues of social work remain ideological. Theories and practices in social work are not detached propositions and techniques. The criticisms are not of case-work or working with individuals, not of group work or working with the family, not of youth work or working with and within a community: the criticisms are directed at the purposes to which these theories and methods are put. At the same time social workers are not above criticism by claiming that the consequences of their action were not intended by them. Most if not all our actions result in consequences either in addition to our intentions or in spite of them. We cannot abdicate responsibility for the consequences of our actions even if we did not initially desire or anticipate the results. No matter how well meaning a social worker, a criticism is justified if, as a result of dealing with a client, that client remains unaware of the public dimension of his or her problems. The problems and difficulties that are associated with a person becoming a client should be identified and located within some structural and political process. This is not to enable anyone, client or social worker, to avoid or deny responsibility for their personal decisions and choices, but rather to make it clear that their decisions and choices were made in circumstances not of their own choosing.

This criticism remains even if a client ceases to be a client. For example, a person about to have the gas or electricity cut off after failure to pay the necessary bills goes to a social worker, who with the best will in the world understands the problem and how it arose, can use his or her influence and persuade the appropriate authority not to take the action. This, coupled with social security payments, may 'resolve' the client's problem. The 'client' becomes a person again, albeit not quite the same person that he or she was before. The social worker can feel pleased with a job well done. For the client, however, the problem was experienced as personal and remains so. Other people, however, were and are facing the same problem. Circumstances out of their control, and common to many individuals and families, are rendered private and personal. (For discussion of this issue, see for example Mills 1959, Pearson 1973.) The very commonality and public nature of the conditions that create the poverty leading to a denial of fuel are not exposed. The social worker knows about it, of course, but so should the client. Introducing the client to others in like circumstances, or at least offering the introduction, assists in no small way in sustaining the individual's self respect and potentially makes him or her aware of wider problems associated with the production, distribution and consumption of fuel. It may further contribute to the arguments concerning the Right to Fuel as a social service. Social work as an institutional process can simultaneously assist people and render them less able to help themselves. Social workers cannot avoid criticisms of their practice by pleading that a consequence of their action was not their intention, indeed was nobody's intention. The focus on the public and collective nature of private and personal difficulties is left to the social worker. Each particular case has to be handled within the context of the sensitivities of both client and social worker. For radical practice, however, such connections should be taken for granted as dimensions of daily practice.

Radical practice is more than dealing with clients. The possibilities of doing much in the way of creating the conditions for real structural change are severely limited in the day-to-day working with clients, whether conceived of as individuals, groups, families or communities. Assisting in a positive fashion, trying to sustain mutual respect and self-respect, and trying to locate a client's position and problems within wider social groups and political processes are all important moments in a radical social worker's task. So too is the awareness of the social worker's own position within the structure, and the recognition of the many things they have in common with clients themselves. For example, government policy decisions may freeze local authority employment, which potentially throws newly-qualified social workers onto the unemployment queues where they find themselves alongside others who might well have been, in different circumstances, their clients. The crisis facing capitalism is translated into the conscious-ness of professionals and the middle classes in ways that have long been commonplace for significant proportions of the working class. Indeed, it is likely that one talks of the crisis of capitalism only when the uncertainties and insecurities that are normal experiences for social work clients are experienced by middle-class professionals. Only then do we read of the 'current crisis of capitalism'. For many the 'current crisis' has been with them for as as long as they can remember.

Arguably, a radical practice of social work and an overt admission by social workers of the political processes in which they are inextricably involved is not, in our terms, merely desirable, but in their terms urgently necessary. If 'It's alright for you to talk' was the expression that possibly enabled social workers to avoid some difficult ques-tions in the seventies, then 'Whose side are you on?' is the question that must re-emerge and be confronted in the eighties. The need to obtain some security from the trade union movement was never more important. Social workers committed to a radical stance must involve themselves in their union branches and work on behalf of their union in those places where they have access, in trades councils and in social services committees of the local authorities.

They should not, however, lose sight of their day-to-day work as social workers with clients. A radical social work can be practised with clients and considerable help can be given to people who, at that moment, arguably need it most. To practise radically is to present oneself with considerable difficulties. It is not enough to have 'in one's head' a theoretically-refined view of the class structure of our society and possibly, as a consequence, sympathy for and sensitivity towards clients and their problems. From different or indeed incompatible world views, similar sentiments may be expressed.

The difficult questions are concerned with practice as socialists. These we suggest are the critical issues. What if anything are the *distinctive* modes of social work practice from a marxist and a socialist perspective? The task for those engaged in the issues from a position of sympathy is to raise and hopefully to answer such questions.

Social workers, like the rest of us, are entering a period where profound changes in the occupation structure of our society are likely to occur, coupled with cultural and political change. Problems and severe hardships will persist and intensify. New problems will confront us. We haven't yet learned how to deal with existing ones. We have to translate our theories of society into a practice that at once helps and assists the victims of our system, and simultaneously, contributes to the creation of conditions which will transform that society into a socialist democracy. The idea that our task is not to understand the world but to change it is crucial to social work practice and, at the same time, a central dilemma for that practice.

One difficulty that arises for social workers who wish to develop a radical form of practice is that they need to develop their political and social analysis of the role of their profession and its historical development. Having understood that the problems which their clients experience are fundamentally related to the political economy, and faced with difficulties like structured unemployment, what can they do for individuals to relieve their exploitation and pain?

Implications for the practice of a radical social work

It is not possible to give a recipe for individual cases, but what is important is not so much the techniques used, but the analytical framework in which they are practised. There is a place for social work techniques traditionally used, such as casework, group work or community work, but these need to be used by a social worker who has analysed his/her relation to the State and has developed some form of political understanding of his/her role. The practice of social work needs to be divided into two forms of activism – collective action and individual practice.

1 Collective action

Ideally collective work involves the consumers in policy decisions. The common-sense view is that most social work consumers are too damaged or 'inadequate' to be involved. One method of practice is to organize the team so that a few regular meetings are arranged to discuss policy (and also frank interpersonal team dynamics), and that – separately at first – meetings are held with client groups and teams to assess what the former feel their needs are individually and in the community. The community has got considerable resources, as any community worker or voluntary worker finds out. There is no reason why consumers and workers should not work towards the breaking down of the professional hierarchy as community projects do.

The second area of collective action is that of welfare state trade union politics. The social worker not only needs to build up trade union consciousness within his/her own section, but also needs to develop links with other welfare state trade unions. This trade union base can be used to develop an informed opinion concerning the needs that welfare services consumers feel they need.

The third area is involvement in community issues, particularly community politics. It is certainly important, as Statham (1978) suggests, to develop involvement in radical alternatives which are occurring *outside* social work practice, as they will have relevance for that practice. They offer alternative views of reality, and emotional and ideological support. An obvious example is in the area of sexual politics, either in feminism or gay liberation. There are other groups involved in class politics, fighting racism, or sexual politics.

The fourth area of collective action is involved in the decentralizing and democratiz-ing of team work. It is important to develop a mode of operation which counteracts hierarchical structures in the team. One important element is to set aside weekly an allotted time to discuss what the goals of the team are, and to what extent these have been prevented by intra-group dynamics and by organizational problems. This is essen-tial if the team is to be developed in any collective sense. It also saves time in the end, because it can be used to delegate work, and to prevent the endless meetings that often bedevil social work. The actual work of the team needs to be community-based as far as possible, and obviously this raises problems for a team with statutory duties. This latter point is an important area for collective decisions. In attempting to gain a community-based social work, the social worker needs to know the area, rather in the way of the old 'patch system'.

An important area of collective work is welfare rights and advocacy, although this should not be seen as the only area of work for radicals. It is important that consumers understand their position, and this means assisting them to get all the benefits they are entitled to, and helping them agitate in the community for more.

2 *Working with consumers in individual practice*

No matter how collective team work is, the social worker is always faced with the one-to-one situation. A radical political perspective and a radical concept of psychology need to be used as an analytical base to build from, and not used to manipulate the powerless in a confrontation in which they lose considerably, and which leaves the social worker unscathed. This means that traditional techniques such as casework, group work and family work, and such traditional humanistic concepts as the aut-onomy of the client, are given a new meaning and a new dimension when affiliated to a radical socialist perspective. It is important to retain the client's perspective, including how the client sees the worker, and one important lesson is, to see their relation to the wider social structure, and not to romanticize them, which helps neither client nor the worker. It is important to make a distinction between radical work and the radicalization of consumers. The consumers of social services are not the vanguard of the revolution, and they mostly hold a mixture of reactionary and progressive views. They are the least likely group to be involved in progressive action, but at the same time they must not be written off. They often have a very realistic appraisal of their situation and what they feel the social services should provide. Radical social work is not an evangelical campaign, and many people who seek help are at a moment in their lives when they are too brutalized or desperate to be reached. The danger is that this may provoke a cynicism in the worker, which has its basis in despair over the difficulty of the situation, and eventually a contempt for the consumer. It is essential that this is resisted, which is why involvement in an alternative movement in the wider society is important. It is essential to work through people's feelings of depression, aggression or despair with the aims of helping them at both an individual and a collec-tive level. This means starting with their definition of the situation and their values, and then trying to extend these into a wider understanding of self and of society. It means trying to understand and work through the roots of depression or hostility and using this to prepare the person to become whole enough so that they can engage in struggle against their situation individually and then, perhaps, collectively. Society has developed a competitive ethos for scarce resources which accepts that there must by definition be casualties. Consequently failure is personalized by the most dispossessed and powerless groups. Consumers need to be helped to understand their position, and their feelings, and given insight into their motivation. Care must be taken that this does not become a form of social control, or used as a substitute to meeting material deprivation.

Social workers are caught up in a contradictory role, as implementers of state aid which they are powerless to change as individuals, and a mediators against the extreme forms of injustice of this aid. Social workers need to use their training courses to develop analysis and to work out strategies which will genuinely enable them to be activists on their consumers side.

References

Bailey, R. and Brake, M. (eds) (1975) *Radical Social Work,* London: Edward Arnold.
Mills, C.W. (1959) *The Sociological Imagination*, Oxford: Oxford University Press.
Pearson, G. (1973) 'Social work as the privatized solution to public ills', *British Journal of Social Work*, 3 (2): 209–27.
Statham, D. (1978) *Radicals in Social Work*, London: Routledge & Kegan Paul.

Further reading

Adams, R., Dominelli, L. and Payne, M. (eds) (2002) *Critical Practice in Social Work*, Basingstoke: Palgrave.
Barclay Report (1982) *Social Workers: Their Role and Tasks, Report of a Working Party (Chairman Peter Barclay)*, London: Bedford Square Press.
Corrigan, P. and Leonard, P. (1978) *Social Work Practice under Capitalism: A Marxist Approach,* London: Macmillan.
Davis, A. (2007) 'Structural approaches to social work', in J. Lishman (ed.) *Handbook for Practice Learning in Social Work and Social Care: Knowledge and Theory*, 2nd edition, London: Jessica Kingsley, 27–38.
Davis, A. and Garrett, P.M. (2004) 'Progressive practice for tough times: Social work, poverty and division in the twenty-first century', in M. Lymbery and S. Butler (eds) *Social Work Ideals and Practice Realities*, Basingstoke: Macmillan.
Ferguson, I. and Woodward, R. (2009) *Radical Social Work in Practice: Making a Difference*, Bristol: Policy Press.
Ferguson, I., Lavalette, M. and Mooney, G. (2002) *Rethinking Welfare: A Critical Perspective,* London: Sage.
Galper, J. (1975) *The Politics of Social Services*, Englewood Cliffs, NJ: Prentice-Hall.
Gray, M. and Webb, S.A. (2009) 'The return of the political in social work', *International Journal of Social Welfare*, 18: 111–15.
Healy, K. (2005) *Social Work Theories in Context: Creating Frameworks for Practice,* Basingstoke: Palgrave Macmillan.
Hick, S.F. and Murray, K. (2009) 'Structural social work', M. Gray and S.A. Webb (eds) *Social Work Theories and Methods*, London: Sage, 86–97.
Jones, K., Cooper, B. and Ferguson, H. (eds) (2008) *Best Practice in Social Work. Critical Perspectives*, Basingstoke: Palgrave Macmillan.
Jordan, B. and Parton, N. (eds) (1983) *The Political Dimension of Social Work*: Oxford: Blackwell.
Langan, M. (2002) 'The legacy of radical social work', in R. Adams, L. Dominelli and M. Payne (eds) *Social Work: Themes, Issues and Critical Debates*, 2nd edition, London: Palgrave Macmillan.
Langan, M. and Lee, P. (eds) (1989) *Radical Social Work Today*, London: Unwin Hyman.
Ledwith, M. (2005) *Community Development: A Critical Approach,* Bristol: Policy Press.
McLaughlin, K. (2008) *Social Work, Politics and Society: From Radicalism to Orthodoxy*, Bristol: Policy Press.
Mullaly, B. (1997) *Structural Social Work: Ideology, Theory and Practice*, 2nd edition, Oxford: Oxford University Press.
Stepney, P. (2006) 'Mission impossible? Critical practice in social work', *British Journal of Social Work*, 36: 1289–307.
White, S., Fook, J. and Gardner, F. (eds) (2006) *Critical Reflection in Health and Social Care*, Maidenhead: Open University Press.

30 Post-modernism in social work

Barbara Fawcett

It seems fitting to end the reader with a chapter on post-modern approaches, because 'post-modern' probably sums up best the condition in which we find ourselves, in society and in social work. As outlined in Part I, social work today takes place in a fragmented, risky and changing policy and practice context. Some of the certainties which encouraged us to make claims on behalf of social work theory and knowledge look decidedly shaky, and social work practice is pulled simultaneously in a number of competing directions; its future, as ever, uncertain. But post-modernism is not just a counsel of despair. If everything is changing, then, as I have argued previously (Cree 1995, 2008), we can do something about it. We, as practitioners, service users, students and academics can come together to make social work the positive, enabling, strengths-based, community-focused resource it can be. The extract is taken from Barbara Fawcett's chapter in an edited collection. Fawcett has written extensively on post-modernism and social work. She is Professor of Social Work who is originally from the UK and is now based in Australia.

From M. Gray and S. Webb (eds) *Social Work Theories and Methods*, Sage: London (2009): 119–28.

Introducing postimodernism

Postmodernism, postmodernity and 'the postmodern' are all terms that have been used in a variety of ways. A common thread that runs throughout is the distinction made and the associated distancing from concepts relating to modernism, modernity and 'the modern'.

This chapter explores the terminology and the many ways in which the associated conceptual orientations have been developed. Given the size of the topic, three main areas are explored. These relate to the operation of knowledge and power, understandings of the 'self' and the different interpretitions given to, inter alia, unity, fragmentation and contradiction. As a means of making links between modernism and postmodernism, a form of critical postmodernism is developed throughout this chapter and the implications for social work are explored.

The theory of postmodernism

Terminology

Fiona Williams in 1992 memorably referred to *postmodernity* as a way of referring to the postmodern condition and to *postmodernism* as a means of understanding the condition. This establishes a helpful distinction between postmodernity (and a postmodern era) and postmodernism, which can be seen to encompass a wide range of theoretical perspectives that both influence and inform the era or condition. In a similar way, 'modernity' can be regarded as a useful means of referring to the modern condition, with modernism being used to denote a range of theoretical orientations that characterize the modern period.

In relation to the timeframe we can currently be seen to occupy, there is wide-ranging variation and dispute, with arguments and associated terminology veering from modernity to late modernity to postmodernity with the imposition of the 'small certainties' of modernism (Bauman, 1992; Callincos, 1989; Fawcett and Featherstone, 1998; Giddens, 1990; Lyotard, 1994).

The relationship between postmodernism and poststructuralism is also contested, with some writers making a clear distinction between the concepts and others arguing that there are so many similarities that a conceptual blurring has taken place. Madan Sarup (1993), for example, maintains that it is difficult to maintain a distinction between poststructural theories and postmodern practices. However, others, such as Andreas Huyssen (1990), insist on a clear distinction being made between the concepts. It can also be argued that to concentrate on definitional issues and associations is to miss the point of the postmodernist project. However, in order to apply concepts as slippery as postmodernism to social work practice, there is a need to forge links and associations, however impermanent these may turn out to be.

Conceptual frameworks

In order to apply theoretical concepts to practice contexts, it is necessary, to some extent, to both simplify and generalize. In this, the importance of layering the analysis has to be recognized. Accordingly, there are the outer layers, which, in some instances, may be all that is required. However, there are also further layers that can be uncovered when further interrogation is called for. In this chapter, emphasis is placed on the outer layers, although certain areas are explored in greater depth. As highlighted above, these focus on the operation of knowledge and power, understandings of 'self' and the interpretation of concepts such as unity, fragmentation and contradiction.

Modernism

It is useful, although not a prerequisite, to start an exploration of postmodernism by looking at what *modernism* is broadly seen to represent.

Modernism is generally regarded as being characterized by the key ideas and values of the Enlightenment. These rested on strong notions of order and the belief in unity and included an acceptance of the importance and the inevitability of progress, the belief that rational scientific objective facts will continue to be revealed and that incontrovertible and essential truths relating to not only science but also social and psychological phenomena will continue to be discovered.

Drawing from the work of Zygmunt Bauman (1992) and Sarup (1993), modernism can be seen as being dominated by the operation of grand narratives or 'big stories' that are viewed as having a universal application and a universal set of principles. Examples of these grand narratives or 'big stories' include liberalism, Marxism, psychoanalysis, economic rationalism, biosocial determinism and structurally orientated analyses. These 'big stories', at various points, have claimed infallibility and have provided all-embracing explanations that have lended to ignore the possibility of large gaps or omissions or criteria that simply do not fit. These metanarratives have provided pervasive ways of seeing the world at particular points in time. Although Westernized concepts have dominated, there has also been a tendency to assume a global applicability or relevance. Said (2003), for example, presents the discourse of orientalism as a systematic way of demonstrating how European culture has been able to manage and produce the 'orient' politically, sociologically, militarily, ideologically, scientifically and imaginatively during the post-Enlightenment period.

Modernism, as writers such as Michel Foucault (1972, 1979, 1980) have highlighted, can be associated with a tendency to associate knowledge and power with expert knowledge. The intertwining of knowledge and power can then be used to draw a dividing line between the knowledge of the expert and that of the service user, client or consumer. As a result, experiential knowledge is downgraded and this can be seen in the ways in which, for example, various government documents, such as *The National Service Framework for Mental Health* (UK Department of Health, 1999) published in England and Wales, equates 'gold standard' research with the carrying out of randomized controlled trials and relegates research that focuses on the experiences of service users to fifth position. In relation to social work, the doctor, social worker or professional assumes the mantle of the expert and the accompanying power of position and influence is used to determine what constitutes acceptable and unacceptable knowledge. Psychiatric or clinical knowledge of schizophrenia, for example, is prioritized over other forms of knowledge relating to belief systems or experiential criteria. Since the onset of the Enlightenment in the eighteenth century, medicalized knowledge obtained by going to university has been ascribed a much higher status than that of the folk healer, even though, for a while at least, the levels of success were probably similar.

With regard to 'self', modernist understandings tend to refer to individuals as having a unified or essentialist core self. This 'self' remains the same in all situations and types of 'self' can be identified and categorized. This also allows personal experience to be referred to in a straightforward, factual and uncomplicated way. The feminist phrase 'the personal is political' has clear modernist overtones, in that it is accepted that personal experiences have a unique validity that can straightforwardly lead to the adoption of political positions.

In a similar manner, language is regarded as comprising fixed meanings, referring to objects and events that are tangible and factual (Sarup, 1993). However, Ferdinand de Saussure (1974, 1916), who is seen as the founder of modern structural linguistics, moved away from this interpretation when he developed an analysis that presented language as structuring meaning rather than referring to something real and tangible. Saussure regarded meaning as socially generated and viewed language as an abstract system comprising signs, made up of a signifier (sound or written image) and signified (meaning). Prior to being combined in language, he maintained that signifiers and signified had no natural connection. However, once a signifier and a signified had been combined, a fixed meaning or a 'positive fact' (de Saussure, 1974, 1916: 120) was produced.

With regard to concepts such as 'unity', 'fragmentation' and 'contradiction', modernism focuses on *unity* and there is a marked tendency to make facts fit the perspective being presented, rather than emphasis being placed on exploring fragmentation, diversity and contradiction. Gendered binaries are perhaps one of the most significant examples. Here, the unity category 'man' is set against the unitary category 'woman' and there is a focus on homogeneity rather than heterogeneity within the gender categories. However, the establishment of these binaries has presented an opportunity to challenge clevalued binary positionings and proponents of 'second wave feminism', to give an example, concentrated on re-examining, repositioning and revaluing the unitary category 'woman' in relation to the unitary category 'man'. This proved to be a very significant project and served to place women's rights firmly on the political agenda. However, like any rights-based movement, these constitute social movements embedded within the modernist conceptual frame of reference.

Postmodernism

Judith Butler (1995: 35) asked: 'The question of postmodernism is surely a question, for is there, after all, something called postmodernism?' This is a pertinent quote for there are those who reject postmodernism for its relativism, fluidity and the difficulties involved in weighting criteria to separate 'the acceptable' from 'the unacceptable'. Stevi Jackson (1992: 31), for example, fiercely opposed poststructuralist critiques of radical feminism, stating that 'Women are being deconstructed out of existence'. Similarly, Christine Di Stefano (1990) raised concerns as to whether or not feminism without an essentialist subject and some kind of standpoint could survive. She drew attention to becoming 'an other amongst others' (1990: 77) in a pluralist world. However, there are feminists who have embraced forms of postmodern feminism and their work will be considered later in a discussion of 'critical postmodernism'. These matters aside, a key question to address at this point echoes the one posed by Butler above. What is postmodernism?

A range of authors (for example, Best and Kellner, 1991; Dickens and Fontana, 1994; Howe, 1994; Parton, 1994; Featherstone and Fawcett, 1995; Fawcett, 2000, 2007) have looked at the ways in which postmodernism has placed emphasis on areas such as deconstruction, plurality, relativity and anti-foundationalist methodology generally. Although, as highlighted, attempts at definition can be regarded as a modernist enterprise, postmodernism can be broadly characterized by an emphasis on deconstruction, or the questioning and taking apart of taken-for-granted assumptions and accepted theoretical frameworks. This lends itself to dominant understandings – clinical psychiatric criteria, for example – being deconstructed and interrogated. Accordingly, questions are asked about how, at a particular point in time, psychiatry became the dominant discourse, with 'discourse', drawing from Foucault, understood to mean the way in which, at specific historical junctures, power, language and institutional practices come together to produce taken-for-granted or accepted social practices.

Postmodern critique emphasizes that all knowledge claims – no matter how powerfully they are embedded in social, political and individual ways of viewing the world – have to be opened up for critical questioning. It also means that, to continue with the example given, opening up dominant discourse to critical scrutiny is not simply a question of mental health survivor perspectives replacing clinical psychiatric understandings. Postmodern perspectives place emphasis on the necessity for the operation of a wide range of understandings. However, a key point to restate is that, as a result of everything being viewed in plural terms, postmodern orientations render it impossible to give one perspective greater weight than another as all have claims to validity and all are relative. A consequence is that it becomes difficult to take a political, moral or ethical position and separate out what might be regarded as the unjust from the just. Similarly, in relation to modernist notions of 'expert knowledge', post-modern orientations draw attention to the way in which such forms of knowledge operate and dismantle the corresponding power relationships. As all knowledge is regarded as relative, it is no longer possible for one individual or group to claim particular expertise or justify their dominance.

It is, however, also important to note that postmodern orientations cannot claim a monopoly on deconstructive forms of analysis. Critical theory, for example, focuses on deconstructing accepted or taken-for-granted tenets, such as the claims made by economic rationalists or proponents of neoliberal managerialist frameworks. The difference is that Critical theory aims to uncover the truth of a situation or what is really going on (Harvey, 1992), while, as far as postmodern orientations are concerned, there is an absence of a central core, only an endless series of layers.

With regard to understandings of the 'self', postmodern perspectives replace a modernist 'core ' unitary self that remains the same in all situations, with a fluid and fragmented 'self', which is continually constructed and reconstructed by social practices and the interplay of dominant discourses. This tends to result in a view of 'self' that is continually being constructed and where individual agency or will is limited. This conceptualization has been subject to considerable modernist critique. From a feminist perspective, for example, Seyla Benhabib (1995) notably said that postmodern concepts of subjectivity were not compatible with feminist politics. She differentiated between strong and weak postmodern analyses, equating strong positions with 'the death of the autonomous, self-reflective subject, capable of acting on principle' (Benhabib, 1995: 29). She regarded weak analyses as those that deconstruct to reconstruct and are amenable to being utilized as a form of feminist critique.

Language, similarly – drawing from Jacques Derrida's pivotal (1978) work on deconstructionism – is never fixed, not even when signifier and signified are combined. Rather, by means of what he called the concept of *différance*, meaning can only be produced by the never-ending juxtaposition of signified and signifier in discursive contexts. Accordingly, meaning and meanings continually change and are always in process, with the person producing the sound or written image playing no part in the creation of meaning. To give an example, the combination of 'hallucination' and 'psychiatric' temporarily produces one set of meanings, while the juxtaposition of 'hallucination' and 'spirituality' temporarily produces another. In short, there are no essentialist or immutable connections between language and meaning and both are in a constant state of flux.

Critical postmodernism

What critical postmodern perspectives do is to draw from both modern and postmodern orientations to produce forms of critical analysis that critique, interrogate, deconstruct and reject foundational underpinnings for particular conceptual frames, yet facilitate the identification of inequalities and the mounting of effective challenges in particular contexts.

Modernism and postmodernism are not opposite sides of the same coin. Postmodernism cannot be explained by simply looking at modernism and formulating antithetical positions. Critical postmodernism is about drawing from *both* orientations to produce a form of analysis that makes links and explores tensions (Fawcett, 2000). Accordingly, with regard to modernism, the universal 'big stories' based on rationalist foundations are rejected and claims related to the operation of expert knowledge are dismissed. With regard to postmodernism, the emphasis on relativism, pluralism and anti-foundationalism is challenged, as it becomes impossible to ground ideas or make distinctions between what is acceptable and what is not. As has been highlighted, within postmodernism all ideas and actions are plural and relative and, as a result, none can carry more weight than another, leaving power imbalances and oppressive forces, such as sexism, racism and 'disablism', to be dismissed as irrelevant.

When looking at the ways in which *critical postmodernism* differs from *postmodernism* in relation to the operation of knowledge and power, emphasis can be placed on posing a series of questions at macro and micro levels – that is, at the level of society and the level of the individual. Drawing from Fook (2002), these questions include the following.

- What constitutes 'acceptable knowledge'?
- Why are some forms of knowledge valued over other forms at particular points in time?
- How do we know what we know?
- What has informed what we know?
- How has the perspective of the knower influenced what is known and how it is known?

Interrogation of these aspects serves to deconstruct and dismantle accepted tenets and knowledge/power configurations. In terms of weighting criteria and addressing structural inequalities and social divisions, critical postmodern perspectives ensure that this is still possible, but only in specific contexts or particular situations (Fawcett, 2000; Fraser and Nicholson, 1993; Williams, 1996). This is important and is where critical postmodern perspectives differ most markedly from postmodern orientations. Accordingly, a social worker using a critical postmodern perspective – and addressing the questions outlined above – would acknowledge the operation of competing power and knowledge frameworks. He or she would do this by drawing attention to information that, it would appear, was being privileged and responded to and information that was being downgraded and ignored in a particular context or situation. The multiplicity of meanings an event can have for a particular person at a particular time and the way in which understandings can vary is another area to attend to as social workers and service users may not be making similar connections or sharing meanings. Similarly, in any interaction, both the social worker and the service user draw from a variety of underpinning conceptual frames – for example, from medicalized or social models of disability, child protection understandings, welfare orientations, rights-based underpinnings, 'commonsense' viewpoints and so on – and this also has to be acknowledged.

Significance for social work practice

With regard to social work practice, postmodern orientations have been criticized for promoting fragmented rather than unified and coherent analyses. They have shifted the focus away from the big canvas of modernism and concerns with global poverty and Inequality and have instead concentrated on relative and competing claims about small and, some would argue, insignificant and disconnected facets. However, the continuing Importance of postmodernism – particularly critical postmodernism – can be seen to lie in the emphasis placed on context and process.

In modernist analyses, there is an element of the 'taken-for-granted' with regard to unquestioned underlying tenets or 'truths', expert opinion or the power and authority of established institutions. Postmodern perspectives question and deconstruct all prevailing power/knowledge frameworks, so that none can claim a privileged position or contend that there is a 'right' way forward or an enduring and incontrovertible fact. As a result, nothing can be regarded as fixed and 'everything' has to be regarded as fluid and transitory, with a temporary stasis only being achievable in specific contexts. This can be seen to constitute a challenging and what can be described as a liberatory aspect of postmodernism. Indeed, it is in this irreverent and unremitting examination and exploration of everything that postmodernism's more enduring and significant contribution to social work practice can be seen to lie.

In conclusion postmodern perspectives have been explored using modernist and critical postmodernist orientations as a form of critique and a way of applying theory to practice. Critical postmodern perspectives have been presented as having the capacity to provide the conceptual tools to interrogate, deconstruct, construct and negotiate ways that are responsive to context, knowledge and power dynamics, and to the varying ways in which the 'self' is presented in different situations. Critical postmodern orientations draw attention to all aspects of a situation and focus on inclusion and negotiation the weighting of criteria in context and the making of intercontextual links. These attributes, it is contended, can be seen to have an ongoing relevance for social work and its commitment to constructive critique, theoretically nuanced practice and the need for social workers to continually differentiate between acceptable and unacceptable social practices in a variety of complex contextual situations.

References

Bauman, Z. (1992) *Intimations of Postmodernity*, London: Routledge.

Benhabib, S. (1995) 'Feminism and Postmodernism', in L. Nicholson (ed.) *Feminist Contentions: A Philosophical Exchange*, London: Routledge.

Best, S. and Kellner, D. (1991) *Postmodern Theory: Critical Interrogations*, Basingstoke: Macmillan.

Butler, J. (1995) 'Contingent foundations', in L. Nicholson (ed.) *Feminist Contentions: A Philosophical Exchange*, London: Routledge.

Callincos, A. (1989) *Against Postmodernism: A Marxist Critique*, Cambridge: Polity Press.

Cree, V.E. (1995) *From Public Streets to Private Lives: The Changing Task of Social Work*, Aldershot: Avebury.

—— (2008) 'Social work and society', in M. Davies (ed.) *Blackwell Companion to Social Work*, 3rd edition, Oxford: Blackwell, 289–302.

Derrida, J. (1978) *Writing and Difference*, Chicago: University of Chicago Press (trans) A. Bass.

Dickens, D.R. and Fontana, A. (1994) *Postmodernism and Social Enquiry*, London: UCL Press.

Di Stefano, C. (1990) 'Dilemmas of Difference', in L. Nicholson (ed.) *Feminism/Postmodernism*, London: Routledge, 63–82.

Fawcett, B. (2000) *Feminist Perspectives on Disability*, Harlow: Prentice Hall/Thompson.

—— (2007) 'Women and violence', in B. Fawcett and F. Waugh (eds) *Addressing Violence, Abuse and Oppression: Debates and Challenges*, London: Routledge.

Fawcett, B. and Featherstone, B. (1998) 'Quality assurance and evaluation in social work in a postmodern era', in J. Carter (ed.) *Postmodernity and the Fragmentation of Welfare*, London: Routledge, 67–84.

Featherstone, B. and Fawcett, B. (1995) 'Oh no! Not more isms: Feminism, postmodernism, poststructuralism and social work education', *Social Work Education*, 14 (3): 25–43.

Fook, J. (2002) *Social Work: Critical Theory and Practice*, London: Sage.

Foucault, M. (1972) *The Archaeology of Knowledge*, London: Tavistock.

—— (1979) *Discipline and Punishment*, Harmondsworth: Penguin.

—— (1980) *Michel Foucault: Power/Knowledge; Selected Interviews and other Writings 1972–1977*, in C. Gordon (ed.) Hemel Hempstead: Harvester Wheatsheaf.

Fraser, N. and Nicholson, L. (1993) 'Social criticism without philosophy: an encounter between feminism and postmodernism', in M. Docherty (ed.) *Postmodernism: A Reader*, Hemel Hempstead: Harvester Wheatsheaf.

Giddens. A. (1990) *The Consequences of Modernity*, Cambridge: Polity Press.

Harvey, L. (1992) *Critical Social Research*, London: Unwin Hyman.

Howe, D. (1994) 'Modernity, postmodernity and social work', *British Journal of Social Work*, 24: 513–32.

Huyssen, A. (1990) 'Mapping the postmodern', in L. Nicholson (ed.) *Feminism/Postmodernism*, London: Routledege, 234–80.

Jackson, S. (1992) 'The amazing deconstructing woman', *Trouble and Strife*, 25: 25–31.

Lyotard, J.F. (1994) *The Postmodern Condition: A Report on Knowledge*, Manchester: Manchester University Press (Original 1984).

Parton, N. (1994) ' "Problematics of government", (post)modernity and social work', *British Journal of Social Work*, 24: 9–32.

Said, E.W. (2003) *Orientalism*, London: Penguin.

Sarup, M. (1993) *Poststructuralism and Postmodernism*, Hemel Hempstead: Harvester Wheatsheaf.

de Saussure, F. (1974 [1916]) *Course in General Linguistics*, London: Fontana.

UK Department of Health (1999) *The National Service Framework for Mental Health*, London: Stationery Office.

Williams, F. (1992) 'Somewhere over the rainbow: Universality and diversity in social policy' in N. Manning and R. Page (eds) *Social Policy Review 4*, London: Social Policy Association, 200–18.

—— (1996) 'Postmodernism, feminism and the question of difference', in N. Parton (ed.) *Social Theory, Social Change and Social Work*, London: Routledge, 61–76.

Further reading

Agger, B. (1991) 'Critical theory, poststructuralism, postmodernism: Their sociological relevance', *Annual Review of Sociology*, 17: 105–31.

Bauman, Z. (2007) *Liquid Times: Living in an Age of Uncertainty*, Cambridge: Polity Press.

Bracken, P. and Thomas, P. (2005) *'Postpsychiatry' Mental Health in a Postmodern World*, Oxford: Oxford University Press

Cahoone, L. (1996) (ed.) *From Modernism to Postmodernism: An Anthology*, Oxford, Blackwell.

Cree, V.E. (2009) 'The changing nature of social work', in R. Adams, L. Dominelli and M. Payne (eds) *Social Work: Themes Issues and Critical Debates*, 3rd edition, Basingstoke: Palgrave Macmillan, 26–36.

—— (2010) *Sociology for Social Workers and Probation Officers*, 2nd edition, London: Routledge.

Dominelli, L. (2009) 'The postmodern "turn" in social work: The challenges of identity and equality, *Social Work & Society*, 7 (1), available at www.socwork.net/2007/festschrift/arsw/dominelli/ (accessed on 16 June 2010).

Healy, K. (2000) *Social Work Practices: Contemporary Perspectives on Change*, London: Sage.

—— (2005) *Social Work Theories in Context: Creating Frameworks for Practice*, Basingstoke: Palgrave Macmillan.

Leonard, P. (1997) *Postmodern Welfare: Reconstructing an Emancipatory Project*, London: Sage.

Lewis, G. (2000) *'Race', Gender, Social Welfare: Encounters in a Postcolonial Society*, Cambridge: Polity Press.

Napier, L. and Fook, J. (eds) (2000) *Breakthroughs in Practice: Theorising Critical Moments in Social Work*, London: Whiting & Birch.

Parton, N. (2000) 'Some thoughts on the relationship between theory and practice in and for social work', *British Journal of Social Work*, 30: 449–63.

Parton, N. and O'Byrne, P. (2000) *Constructive Social Work: Towards a New Practice*, Basingstoke: Macmillan.

Pease, B. and Fook, J. (eds) (1999) *Transforming Social Work Practice: Critical Postmodern Perspectives*, Sydney: Allen & Unwin.

Said, E. (1993) *Culture and Imperialism*. London: Chatto & Windus.

Sawicki, J. (1991) *Disciplining Foucault: Feminism, Power and the Body*, London: Routledge.

Seidman, S. (ed.) (1994) *The Postmodern Turn*, Cambridge: Cambridge University Press.

Taylor, C. and White, S. (2000) *Practising Reflexivity in Health and Welfare: Making Knowledge*, Buckingham: Open University Press.

White, M. and Epston, D. (1990) *Narrative Means to Therapeutic Ends*, New York: W.W. Norton.

White, S., Fook, J. and Gardner, F. (2006) *Critical Reflection in Health and Social Care*, Maidenhead: Open University Press.

Index

Page numbers in *Italics* represent tables.
Page numbers in **Bold** represent figures.